GLORIA JEAN SESSLER is a noted medical writer and studied cardiology with Dr. Paul Dudley White. She is the author of a previous book entitled **Orchids and How to Grow Them**.

STROKE

How to prevent it/ How to survive it

GLORIA JEAN SESSLER

A SPECTRUM BOOK

PRENTICE-HALL, INC. / Englewood Cliffs, N.J. 07632

Library of Congress Cataloging in Publication Data

Sessler, Gloria Jean.
Stroke: how to prevent it/how to survive it.

(A Spectrum Book)
Includes index.
1. Cerebrovascular disease. I. Title. [DNLM:
1. Cerebrovasular disorders--Popular works. WL 355
S492s]
RC388.5.S46 616.8′1 80-26867
ISBN 0-13-852913-2
ISBN 0-13-852905-1 (pbk.)

To my husband
with love and gratitude

A SPECTRUM BOOK

Printed in the United States of America

10 9 8 7 6 5 4 3 2 1

Prentice-Hall International, Inc., London
Prentice-Hall of Australia Pty. Limited, Sydney
Prentice-Hall of Canada, Ltd., Toronto
Prentice-Hall of India Private Limited, New Delhi
Prentice-Hall of Japan, Inc., Tokyo
Prentice-Hall of Southeast Asia Pte. Ltd., Singapore
Whitehall Books Limited, Wellington, New Zealand

CONTENTS

FOREWORDS, vii

ACKNOWLEDGMENTS, ix

CHAPTER ONE
THE INCIDENCE OF STROKES, 1

CHAPTER TWO
EARLY WARNING SIGNS OF AN IMPENDING STROKE, 28

CHAPTER THREE
RISK FACTORS YOU CAN CONTROL, 45

CHAPTER FOUR
ATHEROSCLEROSIS, 88

CHAPTER FIVE
CHOLESTEROL AND TRIGLYCERIDES, 99

CHAPTER SIX
DIABETES, 122

CHAPTER SEVEN
SMOKING, 143

CHAPTER EIGHT
ORAL CONTRACEPTIVES, 164

CHAPTER NINE
STRESS, 176

CHAPTER TEN
LABORATORY TESTS AND DIAGNOSTIC PROCEDURES, 189

CHAPTER ELEVEN
THE COMPLETED STROKE, 206

CHAPTER TWELVE
MEDICAL AND SURGICAL TREATMENT OF A STROKE, 226

CHAPTER THIRTEEN
REHABILITATION, 245

CHAPTER FOURTEEN
SOME SELF HELP AIDS, 266

CHAPTER FIFTEEN
FAMOUS PERSONS WHO HAVE HAD STROKES, 269

INDEX, 274

FOREWORDS

Five hundred thousand persons are victims of strokes each year in the United States. Not only are they, their families, and their friends profoundly affected; stroke lurks as a hidden threat for all. Hence, this is a book for you and for everyone. It is not a medical text full of dry statistics, although the author has collected an immense amount of information about the cause, prevention, and treatment of the disease. In this volume she speaks to you personally as a wise, compassionate friend comparable to the influence exerted on her by that great teacher, Dr. Paul Dudley White. She introduces a pervading air of optimism and of vitality that effectively dispels the despair that accompanied this disease only a decade ago. And she proves that after a stroke one need not feel that fate has singled out the victim; the book closes with short biographies of famous men who had the same disease. This meld of medicine, philosophy, and history has produced a volume that not only is authentic but is totally absorbing for the reader.

Claude E. Welch, M.D.

Senior Surgeon, Massachusetts General Hospital
Clinical Professor of Surgery Emeritus, Harvard Medical School
President, Massachusetts Political Society (ret.)
President, American College of Surgery (ret.), U.S. Chapter

As a physician particularly interested in cardiovascular disease, I am pleased with this comprehensive book on strokes and all its ramifications. Strokes represent one of the most common serious ailments in this country, and it is obviously very important that the public understand what strokes are, what the risk factors are that cause strokes, and how to avoid them, what the early warning signs of stroke are so that the patient may receive early appropriate medical help, what the diagnostic and treatment procedures are, and, very importantly, what stroke rehabilitation is.

This book is consistent with the modern day wish of patients to understand as much as possible about their bodies and potential health problems. Because stroke is so clearly affected by a number of factors that can be controlled—such as smoking, high blood pressure, diet, stress, and contraceptives—it is particularly important that potential victims are fully knowledgeable about these factors. Because rehabilitation is so important and helpful in this problem, it is crucial that the patients be aware of this important endeavor and in the same context, that they should be aware of the marvelous results from rehabilitation as described in this manuscript. All these important points and a number of others are beautifully described in this manuscript. Perhaps the most important point is the fact that this book is written in a way that is understandable to the potential patient.

W. Gerald Austen, M.D.

Chief of Surgical Services, Mass. General Hospital
Edward D. Churchill Prof. of Surgery, Harvard Medical School
American Heart Association Past President

ACKNOWLEDGMENTS

A great teacher's influence knows no bounds, and I have been blessed with having had the greatest. As teacher, counselor, friend, and physician, the late Dr. Paul Dudley White opened wide the gates of medical knowledge and history for me. He made learning both an exciting and an enjoyable experience. So it is with great affection and an everlasting sense of gratitude that I salute his memory.

Without the devoted assistance of my husband who put up with an enormous amount of inconvenience while I was writing and who read every page of the manuscript, offering invaluable suggestions all along the way, this book could never have been written.

My great appreciation and very warmest thanks go to Theresa O'Brien who, despite an exremely busy schedule, spent many weeks deciphering my handwriting, and who with several of her friends typed the final manuscript. Without her perseverance and long hours of dedication it would have been impossible to complete this book on schedule.

I also wish to express my appreciation to the following:

To Phyllis von Herrlich of the Greater Boston Chapter of the American Heart Association for her many kindnesses, not the least of which was spending so much time locating material on strokes from the Heart Association files.

To the staff of the Putterham Branch of the Brookline Library—Deborah Abraham, Thelma M. Katz, Cynthia Ann Monahan, and the late Doris Fincher—for their never-failing graciousness and kindness in providing reference material.

To Dr. Jacob Lerman, esteemed endocrinologist and dearest friend who has so generously given of his time and expertise in guiding me along the pathways of medical knowledge.

To Marguerite O'Shea, who throughout the long year during which this book was being written never failed to extend both understanding and encouragement. To Grayce Carney Gavin, who was always there to offer support and reassurance when I needed them most. To Dr. Helen C. Atwood, who constantly shored up my spirits with an understanding born of her own literary efforts. To Regina A. O'Shea, R.D., whose expertise in the field of nutrition and experience in a rehabilitation hospital proved so very helpful in reviewing the manuscript. To Teresa O'Shea, who made me constantly aware of the importance of never losing sight of a patient as a person. And to all who in any way have made the writing of this book such an enjoyable and rewarding experience, my heartfelt and grateful thanks.

CHAPTER ONE

THE INCIDENCE OF STROKES

A stroke is no respecter of age or position in life. From the newborn infant to the oldest citizen bowed down with the weight of his years, from kings to peasants, from popes to paupers, no one is immune. Having a stroke is undoubtedly one of the most devastating experiences in anyone's life.

Because for so many years there really was not very much that could be done for the victims of a stroke, the idea that having a stroke literally meant the end of one's world became an accepted belief. Fortunately this is no longer so.

In these last years of the twentieth century, much progress has been made and is continuing to be made in controlling and even eliminating many of the risk factors that bring on a stroke. So many new surgical techniques have been developed that can not only aid the person who has had a stroke but can even prevent an impending stroke from occurring, and so many remarkable new concepts in the field of rehabilitation are taking place that can restore those who have had strokes so that they can lead useful, self-sustaining lives, that the prospect of having a stroke need no longer strike terror into the heart of anyone.

Yet until everyone is made aware of these advances, strokes will continue to constitute a modern-day plague.

Any disease that affects 500,000 people a year, kills 200,000, and leaves 300,000 others with some permanent form of disability must be considered a major health problem.

Two and a half times as many people survive a stroke as die from one, and complete recovery is always a possibility. Strokes rank as the third major cause of death and the leading cause of disability in the United States.

About 30 per cent of those who survive a stroke are able to return to normal activity and productive work. The majority of those who are left with a permanent disability or impairment are in most cases capable of tending to their daily requirements with little or no assistance. It has been estimated that nearly two million people in this country alone are living with some form of disability, either slight or severe, as the result of a stroke. Only 15 per cent of those who are stricken will require total nursing care for the rest of their lives, showing that a stroke is not the hopeless disease it was once thought to be nor does it have to have the tragic aftereffects so long associated with it.

There was a time not so many years ago when the person who was taken to a hospital emergency room and diagnosed as having had a stroke was either sent back home or to a nursing facility because it was felt that there was nothing very much that could be done. And to tell the truth, not many medical professionals wanted to be bothered with these so-called hopeless cases.

But all this has changed. The great advances that have been made in medicine and surgery during the past two decades have resulted in a steady decline in stroke-related deaths. This trend has been particularly noticeable since 1973.

Thanks to the pioneering efforts of Dr. Howard A. Rusk, it is now realized that much can be done through rehabilitation for those with stroke-related disabilities. As newer, more successful methods of treating hypertension (high blood pressure)—the number one cause of strokes—have become available and as other risk factors for a stroke have been recognized as such and methods for treating them successfully discovered, no longer does one have to wait around helplessly for a stroke to strike like a bolt out of the blue.

Now it has become possible to strike back when a stroke occurs and, even more important, to prevent one from occurring in the first place.

A whole new concept of stroke therapy has emerged as the result of a better understanding of the reasons that strokes occur, leading to intensive efforts on the part of all medical personnel to return those who have been stricken to useful, productive lives and to educate everyone everywhere to the fact that strokes can be prevented.

We fear only what we do not understand. As we learn more

about strokes, their causes, the risk factors, and the preventive measures that can be taken, we can at last take a positive stand against this killer and crippler. It is hoped that one day, as with so many other devastating diseases, medical science will make the stroke a relic of a bygone era.

Although strokes have felled men since the beginning of recorded history, it was not until the time of Hippocrates that the disease was given the name of *apoplexy.* The word *apoplexy* comes from the Greek word *apoplexia,* meaning to strike down. Although the term *apoplexy* is still occasionally used, over the years it has gradually given way to the word *stroke.* Another frequently used term is *cerebrovascular accident,* known as a CVA—cerebro because it is the brain that is affected, vascular because it occurs in the blood vessels, and accident because it is unexpected.

WHAT A STROKE IS

Stroke is the word that is used to describe a sudden attack of *ischemia* (i.e., an interruption of, a cutting off of, or an interference with the flow of blood to the brain), which results in signs and symptoms of neurological deficit. The nerve cells in that part of the brain deprived of blood cannot function, which sometimes results in total or partial loss of consciousness. The brain is dependent on having a steady supply of oxygen. Because there is no reserve supply of oxygen in the cerebral tissues, cerebral metabolism cannot be sustained during periods of reduced or total loss of cerebral blood flow.

When the brain is completely deprived of oxygen, changes within the brain that can result in extensive damage occur within 10 to 20 seconds. Irreversible damage can occur in the cerebral hemispheres after three to 10 minutes.

Ischemia, whether resulting in cerebral infarction (i.e., blockage) or resulting in an intracranial hemorrhage, is one of the most frequent precipitating causes of a stroke. There are many more. The Committee of the National Institute of Neurological Diseases and Stroke of the National Institutes of Health classifies more than 50 different diseases as potential causes of a stroke.

Both infarction and ischemia result from an interruption in the flow of blood to the brain and from tissue perfusion. A cerebral hemorrhage results from a ruptured vessel which, because of the spurting blood from the injured vessel, destroys some of the nerve cells. A blood clot can also form around the area of spurting blood.

CLASSIFICATION OF STROKES

Strokes are classified according to their severity, as follows:

MAXIMAL —a stroke that has resulted in the severest possible deficits.

SUBMAXIMAL —a stroke in which the deficit is less severe.

EVOLVING or PROGRESSING —a stroke causing damage that results in neurological deficits that have not stabilized but are still occurring, a situation that can continue for hours, days, or even weeks.

STABLE —a submaximal stroke in which there has been no further progression or evolution in neurological deficits for a period of about two weeks.

MAJOR —a stroke that results in severe neurological deficits.

MINOR —a stroke in which both the symptoms and deficits are slight.

PURE MOTOR HEMIPLEGIA —a condition in which the face, arm, and leg are weakened or paralyzed on one side of the body only, with no visual or speech deficits.

PURE SENSORY STROKE —a condition in which there is numbness of the face, arm, or leg without weakness or paralysis.

Those parts of the brain that control such body activities as walking, talking, moving, seeing, hearing, tasting, smelling, and so on and that have been damaged because of the loss of their blood supply are no longer able to control these functions. The result is paralysis of or a loss of some function in these affected areas. These effects can be slight or severe, temporary or permanent.

Although death may occur within hours or days after the onset of a stroke, most patients do survive for many years. Recovery depends on which brain cells have been affected, how widespread the damage is, how fast the body can repair itself, and whether other parts of the brain that have been less damaged can compensate by taking over the functions of the severely damaged brain cells.

A stroke never affects all areas of the brain equally. Fortunately, most strokes affect only a small area of the brain and result in the loss of only a few vital functions. It is only when a stroke is so massive or when many areas of the brain have been affected that the damage then becomes irreversible and there is widespread paralysis and loss of vital functions.

HOW TO RECOGNIZE A STROKE

The characteristic that differentiates a stroke from most other diseases is its sudden onset. A stroke usually results in collapse and unconsciousness, and at times in convulsions and coma.

A feeling of numbness is often experienced in a leg or arm. The numbness rapidly progresses to a state of paralysis, which usually occurs on only one side of the body.

The pupils of the eyes are often unequal in size, the larger pupil being in the eye on the paralyzed side of the body. Often the eye lids tend to droop. Seeing double, a condition known as *diplopia,* may occur. Blindness in one eye is also common.

A sudden headache that is rather severe in intensity or a dizzy spell that results in a sudden fall are signs that may indicate a stroke. Breathing may be difficult, slow, and labored, and the sounds may be stenorous and torturous.

The cheeks tend to puff out with each exhalation. The neck may be stiff and rigid. There may be a temporary loss of speech or difficulty in speaking, as well as difficulty in understanding what is spoken. If the person remains conscious, he or she may show signs of mental confusion, slurred speech, and a noticeable inability to concentrate.

Difficulty in swallowing is often experienced. The face and mouth tend to pull to one side. Although the face is usually warm and flushed, it may also be ashen gray.

Nausea and vomiting may occur.

THE BRAIN'S PARTS AND FUNCTIONS AND THE AREAS OF THE BODY THEY CONTROL

To better understand how and why a stroke affects the various parts of the body in the way it does, an understanding of the brain and its components and the functions of these components is necessary.

The brain, that most marvelous of organs, the seat of thought and the center of reason, contains the control centers of every idea, thought, and movement of which the body is capable. Although the brain is the most complex organ in the body, it weighs only three pounds yet is composed of over 10 billion cells. It is a mass of soft, spongy, gray nerve tissue that is so extremely intricate in detail that it completely fills the cranial cavity, which is formed by the bones of the skull.

The brain and the spinal cord are covered by three membranes. The outer membrane is a tough, fibrous covering that lies close to the skull itself. Next to this comes a web-like, much more delicate membrane. Finally, there is the inner membrane, which rests against the brain itself. There is a cavity between the middle weblike membrane and the inner membrane that contains the cerebrospinal fluid. This fluid, which is watery, clear, and colorless, acts as a water cushion to protect the brain and the spinal cord from shock. It also receives waste products from the nerve tissues. It is this fluid that is removed in a spinal tap, which is done either to relieve cranial pressure or to analyze the fluid to determine the presence of an infection in the brain.

The brain has several regions, each one of which controls a different function. Each region interacts closely with every other region. It is these regions that constitute the control centers of the brain.

CEREBRUM

The region of the brain known as the cerebrum (also called the forebrain) is the largest part of the brain and represents two thirds of the brain's total weight. It is divided into two sections. or hemispheres, one in which the sensory stimuli are received and a second in which the motor impulses originate.

The cerebrum is considered to be the center of the intellect and of the will and the seat of the emotions. Memory, thought, learning, and association are all controlled by the cerebrum, as are all voluntary acts.

On the outside the cerebrum is wrinkled and folded. Deep inside these folds are fissures that separate the cerebrum into rounded projections called *lobes*.

FOUR MAIN LOBES

The *frontal-lobes* are so called because of their location. Here are located the centers of coordination, voluntary muscle control, and memory association. These lobes also control respiration. Because this area is considered to be the seat of intelligence and the emotions, it is easy to see why a prefrontal lobotomy, the surgical procedure by which the nerve tracts from the front part of the brain connecting to other areas of the brain are severed, can alleviate excruciating pain and effectively change a person's personality.

The *parietal-lobes* are located at the sides of the cerebrum. This is the region governing such senses as temperature, pain, touch, and skin sensation.

The *temporal-lobes* are located near the temples. Hearing, taste, and smell are controlled here.

The *occipital-lobes* are located at the back of the cerebrum. It is here that the sensory areas that regulate sight are located. The visual speech area that enables you to memorize pictures and words is located here.

The insula or Island of Reil is also found in the cerebrum within the lateral fissures.

The cortex, whose name comes from the Latin word meaning rind, is made up of the gray matter formed by cell bodies. It covers the outside of the cerebrum. These cell bodies also form the white matter of the cerebrum. Fibers from these cells lead to all parts of the brain. In their journey through the brain these fibers cross over one another. Thus a fiber or an axon, which is the conducting part of a nerve cell, enters the brain on the left side of the body and crosses over to the right side of the brain. This is why the right side of the cerebrum controls the left side of the body and the left side of the cerebrum controls the right side of the body.

A reduction in or a slowing of the circulation of blood on the left side of the brain will cause weakness on the right side of the body, and vice versa. In the right-handed person it is the left hemisphere of the brain that is dominant. For a left-handed person, it is the right side that is dominant.

Studies have shown that in 97 per cent of the population the language center is located on the left side of the brain. Eighty-nine per cent of the population are right-handed. A small group of people are ambidextrous—that is, they can use both hands with equal ease. In only 3 per cent of the population is the language or speech center on the right side of the brain.

What this means is that if the left side of the brain is damaged in a person who is right-handed, a speech impairment known as *aphasia* (which is discussed in detail in a later chapter), as well as paralysis on the right side of the body, will result. If, in these same right-handed persons the nondominant right side of the brain is damaged, there will be no speech impairment. Right-handed persons are controlled by the left side of the brain, and left-handed persons are controlled by the right side. There are some persons, notably those who are left-handed, whose speech is controlled by the left side of the brain whereas the speech of others who are left-handed is controlled by the right side of the brain.

This fact may explain such speech difficulties as stuttering and stammering, which occur when one tries to forcibly change the pattern of left-handed writing to right-handed writing. Such a change involves not only the act of changing the hand that is doing the writing; it also entails changing or trying to change the dominant part of the brain from one side to another. And this is no small task.

The cerebrum controls all mental activities and all motor, sensory, and association activities such as memory and learning. For example, the sensory areas receive impulses from the sensory organs and translate these impulses into seeing, hearing, tasting, smelling, and into sensations appropriate to the skin and joints. If these areas are damaged, blindness, deafness, and a loss of smell and taste result.

The motor areas of the cerebrum control the muscles of the body. Any damage to these areas causes paralysis.

There are also speech areas of the cerebrum that bring together both seeing and hearing and the mechanisms of speaking and writing.

The association areas are considered to be the centers of emotions and intelligence. Because these are the areas concerned with moral sense and values, any damage to them can result in a loss of moral sense and social responsibility.

All these control centers are connected to one another by the fibers previously mentioned that transport nerve impulses in the brain. Thus these various centers never operate in an isolated manner or independently of one another. They always act in unison. Every part of the cerebrum influences everything you do. For example, writing is the result of the cooperation between the visual center and the motor area, with the motor area controlling the muscles used in writing.

CEREBELLUM

The cerebellum is the second largest area of the brain and is often referred to as the "little brain" or lower or back brain because of its location under the back part of the cerebrum. Like the cerebrum, it has two hemispheres. The cerebellum can easily be distinguished from the cerebrum because the grooves of the cerebellum are straighter and shallower.

The function of the cerebellum is to maintain balance and

muscle coordination. It receives impulses from the inner ear, which contains the balance mechanism, and also from the muscles and joints. It then coordinates these impulses to achieve both coordination and balance. Any damage to this part of the brain results in a loss of muscular control.

THE BRAIN STEM

Near the center of the brain are several small but important regions. Their function is to act as relay stations for the system of nerve fibers going from the brain to the spinal column. They are part of the brain stem.

The first of these regions is the *midbrain.* The midbrain is also called the *mesencephalon,* from the Greek words *mesos* (middle) and *enkephalos* (brain). Its location is just above the pons, between the cerebrum and cerebellum, and it is the lightest and shortest part of the brain stem. It contains many important nerve cells and fibers that go from the cerebral cortex to the reflex centers of the brain.

The second region near the center of the brain is the *pons.* The word *pons* comes from the Latin word meaning bridge and describes its function. It connects the two halves of the cerebellum and acts as a bridge from the cerebrum to the spinal cord. The pons is the area where nerve impulses can pass between the various other parts of the brain. Injury to this section of the brain can result in lack of muscle tone, the loss of reflexes, and deep coma.

The third part of the brain stem is the *medulla,* which is the lowest region of the brain and is located at the base of the skull. Its shape is that of a walnut. Its function is to regulate heart action and to dilate and constrict the blood vessels, thereby helping to retain normal blood pressure, breathing, and swallowing.

THE SPINAL CORD

The spinal cord, which is almost 18 inches long and half an inch wide and weighs about an ounce, resembles a cable or cylinder that has been formed by the bones of the spine. Like the brain itself, it too contains cerebrospinal fluid between the middle and inner membranes that cushions it from shocks. The sensory and motor nerves meet here in the spinal cord, which acts as a place for the simple reflex actions occurring in the trunk and the limbs of the body. Nerve fibers go all along the spinal cord and into the brain.

CIRCULATION—THE BLOOD SUPPLY TO THE BRAIN

The supply of blood to the brain is actually more vital than the supply of blood to any other region of the body. Blood flowing through the brain at the rate of one and a half pints a minute furnishes the brain with both oxygen and glucose, which are the brain's foods and without which it would die.

Interestingly, although the brain represents only 2 per cent of the weight of the entire body, it uses up to 25 per cent of the oxygen in the blood. It has very little capacity for storing reserves and thus must have a constant supply of both oxygen and glucose.

COLLATERAL CIRCULATION

Among the many wonders of the brain is a built-in mechanism called the *collateral circulation*. The word *collateral* comes from the Latin words *con* (together) and *lateralis* (to the side). The collateral circulation is a sort of backup system to assure that there will be a constant circulation of blood to the brain even if one of the major arteries should be partially, yet not completely, blocked. The collateral arteries may be able to carry the blood around the blocked area and in so doing keep the brain supplied with blood.

Under ordinary circumstances, the circulation of blood to and through the brain delivers an amount of oxygen and glucose in excess of the brain's requirements. This flow to the brain is carefully controlled by the body and is not subject to fluctuation as is the blood supply to the other organs of the body. This is important because the brain is unable to tolerate any reduction in its blood supply for more than a few minutes. Any decrease in the supply of oxygen to the brain from any cause whatsoever leads to a mentally confused state that can progress to unconsciousness. Irreparable damage to the brain results when there has been a lack of oxygen for a period of eight minutes.

A decrease in the amount of glucose available to the brain can also be disastrous. Glucose is a form of sugar that is circulated in the blood. Hypoglycemia, which comes from the Greek words *hypo* (less than), *glykos* (sugar), and *haima* (blood), is a condition in which there is a deficiency of sugar in the blood. It can lead to mental confusion, muscular uncoordination, sometimes convulsions, and if serious enough, unconsciousness.

Eating may affect the quality of blood to the brain by helping to provide the necessary glucose. However, neither eating nor intellectual activities themselves affect the flow of blood. Even exercise causes only a slight decrease in the flow of blood despite the fact that the muscles of the body when used in exercise will then demand more than their normal share. Conversely, during sleep, when the body is at rest, there is only a slight increase in the blood supply to the brain.

Collateral circulation is truly quite remarkable. When an artery or blood vessel has been damaged, other smaller arteries and blood vessels tend to increase in size (dilate), and they then take over part of the function of the damaged artery. This enables cells that temporarily lack a supply of blood to recover because the collateral circulation has rushed to the rescue before those cells have had a chance to die. The availability of collateral circulation may be decisive in determining the extent of the damage caused by a stroke because any cells that do not receive an adequate supply of blood die.

Remarkable, too, is the fact that the parts of the body affected by a stroke caused by the loss of the supply of blood to the cells in the various control centers of the brain may improve and even return to normal when and as the other brain cells take over the functions of the damaged cells. This is why there is always hope that a loss of speech, an impaired memory, or paralyzed muscles may improve and return to normal.

ARTERIES OF THE BRAIN

The supply of blood to the brain originates in the aortic arch, which is part of the aorta (the main artery of the trunk of the body). Two large pairs of arteries from the aortic arch to the brain: the internal carotid arteries and the vertebral arteries that are located at the back of the neck near the spine.

THE CAROTID ARTERY

The carotid artery is the principal artery of the neck. It is divided into a right and left branch just below the jaw. The majority of strokes occur in those areas of the brain whose blood supply is received through the branches of the carotid artery.

One of the branches is called the *external carotid artery,* and it supplies blood to the neck and the face.

Upon entering the skull, the *internal carotid artery* supplies blood to the eyes and the front part of the brain. Any decrease in the flow of blood through, or any obstruction in, the internal carotid artery brings about some impairment in the front part of the brain, which controls memory, muscular movements, and sensations of temperature, touch, and pain. This impairment may result in weakness, paralysis, or a tingling or numbness on the side of the body opposite to the side where the artery is obstructed. The name *carotid* comes from the Greek word *karos* (heavy with sleep). The artery was so called because the ancient Greeks believed that the carotid arteries caused sleep. Pressure on these two arteries can produce unconsciousness, which is what happens when a person is strangled.

THE VERTEBRAL ARTERIES

The vertebral arteries and their branches provide blood to the back half of the brain. An obstruction in the vertebral arteries can result in a difficulty with vision, which usually occurs in both eyes.

BASILAR ARTERY

One of the vertebral arteries is called the *basilar artery.* Damage to this artery can cause difficulty in both swallowing and talking, numbness of the face, weakness in the arms and legs, unsteadiness, and even collapse.

THE CIRCLE OF WILLIS

The two main pairs of arteries, the carotid and the vertebral, form a circle at the base of the brain known as the Circle of Willis. If one of the blood vessels of these arteries becomes blocked, the arteries that normally would be receiving blood from the blocked blood vessel can now receive it from one of the other blood vessels of the artery, thanks to the circle that these arteries form. Other arteries branch upward from the Circle of Willis. Their function is to carry blood, oxygen, and glucose into the remaining areas of the brain. Any damage that occurs in this area and interrupts the supply of blood can result in an inability to move a leg or an arm. It can also cause a loss of sensation in a leg.

THE POSTERIOR CEREBRAL ARTERY

Another branch of the vertebrobasilar artery is the posterior cerebral artery. As its name indicates, it is located at the back of the brain. Any blockage of this artery results in visual disturbance because this is the artery that supplies blood to the visual control center. Memory and reading disturbances may also result. Speech, however, remains normal. At the onset of a stroke in this area, it is not uncommon for a person to experience total blindness, which usually abates within several hours.

THE MIDDLE CEREBRAL ARTERY

Another artery, the middle cerebral artery, quite frequently is the site of a stroke. Any interruption of blood in this artery results in paralysis, either total or partial, or numbness of the face, arm, or leg on the nondominant side of the body (i.e., the left side of a right-handed person or the right side of a left-handed person). There may also be some speech and vision problems. The flow of blood to the brain is automatically regulated by the widening (dilating) or constricting (narrowing) of the blood vessels. If an area of the brain becomes extremely active and is thus using more oxygen and releasing more carbon dioxide into the blood stream than it normally would, the blood vessels automatically dilate (widen) so that more oxygen-filled blood can reach this area.

THE CAPILLARIES

The arteries in the brain further subdivide into even smaller branches, and then into capillaries, which are minute blood vessels and, hairlike, as is implied by the source of the term from the Latin *capillaris*. The capillaries connect the smallest arteries with the smallest veins and form a bridge between those arteries and veins. It is through them that the food and oxygen in the blood are exchanged for the waste matter from the tissues. The veins then carry this so-called "used" or exchanged blood back through the network of blood vessels to the heart. The capillaries further emerge into very small veins which, after ascending to the uppermost surface of the brain, drain into cavities, called venous sinuses, that empty into the internal jugular veins located on each side of the neck at the throat. These then join together with the other veins and arteries that go to the heart itself.

The blood is thus pumped from the heart to the brain through a vast network of arteries, ranging from the two main arteries, the carotid and vertebral, through the smaller arteries, and finally into the hairlike capillaries which enable the blood to reach into the millions of nerve cells that make up the brain tissues.

The underlying cause of all strokes is a lack of oxygenated blood to any part of the brain. It is this oxygenated blood that is necessary to maintain brain function.

THE DIFFERENCE BETWEEN A HEART ATTACK AND A STROKE

Although both a stroke and a heart attack, or coronary as a heart attack is sometimes called, may occur suddenly, this is where the similarity ends. A stroke is the result of an impairment of the circulation of the blood in the brain, whereas a heart attack is the result of an impairment of the circulation of blood to the heart itself.

KINDS OF STROKES

There are four kinds of strokes. Their names derive from the manner in which the blood supply to the brain is disturbed: cerebral thrombosis, cerebral embolism, cerebral hemorrhage, and cerebral infarction.

CEREBRAL THROMBOSIS

The word *thrombosis* comes from the Greek words *thrombos* (clot) and *osis* (condition). A cerebral thrombosis occurs when a clot forms in an artery that supplies blood to a particular part of the brain, preventing the free flow of blood in the brain. Any blockage of an artery leading to the brain or in the brain itself causes those brain cells supplied by that artery to die within eight minutes.

It is highly unusual and unlikely for a clot to form in a healthy artery. Rather, it forms in an artery that has been damaged by a buildup of plaque, which has caused the walls of that artery to become thickened and narrowed. This condition is called *atherosclerosis*. The word comes from the Greek words *sklērosis* (hardness) and *athērē* (porridge), and it aptly describes the fatty degeneration or thickening of the walls of an artery.

Arteriosclerosis is another word often used to describe this condition. It further refines the meaning to pertain more fully to arteries by using the prefix *arteria,* which in Greek means artery. Arteriosclerosis is discussed in greater depth in Chapter 5.

A thrombosis, which signifies a blockage, most often occurs when yellow fatty plaques accumulate and harden inside the wall of an artery. As plaque accumulates and hardens, it causes the space inside the artery where the blood flows to become narrow, much as rust and dirt clog up and narrow a water pipe. The place where the artery has become narrowed is the place where a thrombosis may form. This thrombosis further plugs up the artery and then prevents the blood from flowing through.

When thrombosis happens, the tissues in the brain that cannot receive the blood they need to survive die, resulting in a stroke. The term *cerebrovascular occlusion,* meaning to close up or to obstruct a cerebral artery, is still another term used to describe this condition.

A cerebral thrombosis is a type of stroke in which a disturbance to the brain's blood supply because of the formation of clots has tended to accelerate, usually while the patient is sleeping. It is then upon awakening that the damage becomes apparent. A cerebral thrombosis is unrelated to activity. In fact, when a person awakens from sleep with a neruological deficit, it usually means that he or she has experienced a cerebral thrombosis.

Cerebral thrombosis tends to occur where there is a history not only of atherosclerosis but also of hypertension (high blood pressure), of cardiovascular diseases and diabetes mellitus, of hyperlipidemia, and in acute and chronic meningitis. The word *meningitis* comes from the Greek word *mēnigx* (membrane) and is an inflammation of the membranes of the spinal cord or of the brain. *Encephalitis,* which comes from the Greek word *egkephalos* (brain) and *itis* (inflammation), refers to an inflammation of the brain and can also contribute to a cerebral thrombosis. Inflammation around the blood vessels in the brain can also cause a cerebral thrombosis.

Polycythemia, which derives from the Greek words *poly* (much, or many), *lytos* (cell), and *haima* (blood), refers to an excess of red blood cells and can, because of the increased viscosity or thickness of the blood, also lead to the formation of blood clots in the brain.

If tumors are present in the brain and if they begin to grow, they tend to constrict or compress the blood vessels, and this too can result in the formation of blood clots.

The complete blockage of a major blood vessel such as the carotid artery may cause a major infarction. The word *infarction* comes from the Latin word *infarctus* (to stuff). Infarctions can cause death. In a heart attack, an infarction leaves a dead area in the heart's tissues that is later scarred over. An infarction in the brain results in the same type of dead area that is later filled in with scar tissue, but this scarred area cannot in any way contribute to the flow of blood in the brain. Fortunately, for most persons, their collateral or secondary circulation is sufficiently adequate so that death does not occur. Conversely, a cerebral thrombosis can occur when the collateral circulation is so well developed that an occlusion of an artery will be asymptomatic (i.e., without symptoms).

If the obstruction to an artery in the brain causes a complete blockage, it is called a *cerebral arterial thrombosis,* whereas if the blockage is only partial, it is called a *cerebral arterial stenosis.* The word *stenosis* denotes a narrowing rather than a blockage of an artery.

If the carotid artery on only one side of the body is blocked by a thrombosis, a stroke results, with paralysis on the opposite side of the body. Or there may be a lesser degree of loss of function involving the arms and legs on the same side of the body.

A physician using a stethoscope listens to the sounds in the carotid arteries on both sides of the neck to determine if there are any bruits, or noise. If one of the carotid arteries is completely blocked, the bruit, or noise, may be absent in that artery but heard instead over the carotid artery on the other side of the neck because of the increased flow of blood through the artery,

A thrombosis in a blood vessel may occur in minutes or take hours or even years to develop. Many signs warn that a thrombosis is developing. One of the most important warnings is a transient ischemic attack (transient meaning fleeting, ischemic from the Greek *ischein* (to hold back, in this case the blood supply), and attack referring to its sudden onset. This symptom is discussed in greater detail in Chapter 2, which deals with the early warning signs of an impending stroke.

A thrombosis is most likely to occur during periods of inactivity, such as sleeping and, surprisingly, when the blood pressure is normally lower. The amount of damage that occurs tends to reach its maximum extent within one to three days. Then the patient's condition stabilizes and can even improve.

The effects of a stroke caused by a thrombosis depend on just which brain tissues have been impaired and where the interruption in the flow of blood took place. In other words, the affected control centers of the brain determine the damage.

A large blood vessel can take longer to become clogged than a smaller one, and it is much more apt to be accompanied by a headache than is a clot in a smaller blood vessel.

If the blockage is transitory, lasting less than 10 to 15 minutes, there are usually no neurological deficits. But if the blockage lasts longer, certainly more than 24 hours, the neural damage that results can bring on neurological dysfunction, disability, and even death.

CEREBRAL EMBOLISM

The word *embolus* comes from the Greek and means plug, or clot, as does thrombosis. Therefore, an embolism like a thrombosis, denotes that a blood vessel has become plugged or obstructed. But the term *embolism* is reserved for those clots that form in one area, break off, and move along with the blood flow to another area that is usually some distance away.

Most emboli originate in the left side of the head, in the aorta, or in the large blood vessels in the neck.

An embolism occurs suddenly and without warning. The maximum amount of damage that results from an embolus is apparent within minutes of its onset.

Although a blood vessel of any size in the brain may become plugged by an embolus, the middle and posterior cerebral arteries, because of their location as pathways or routes for the flow of blood from the carotid and basilar arteries, are most frequently the areas involved. Cerebral embolism also usually occurs in more than one blood vessel.

We have seen that a cerebral thrombosis is often noticed just after a person has awakened from a night's rest, and we can assume the thrombosis occurred during sleep. A cerebral embolism, on the other hand, occurs while the person is awake and active.

Whereas a thrombosis forms along an arterial wall that has already been plugged with fatty plaque, an embolism often develops as the plaque travels through the blood vessels. In this case embolism denotes a wandering clot, usually from the area of the heart, which in some way has been damaged. Emboli frequently occur after a recent myocardial infarction or a coronary. In some instances fragments of atherosclerotic lesions or plaque may break apart and be carried as an embolus through the blood vessels until such time as either the blood vessel through which it is traveling becomes too narrow for the embolus to get through, or it joins up with another piece of plaque or a clot and forms an obstruction that is called an *occlusion*.

The small clots, or emboli, from the heart itself can travel or wander in the blood stream until they become wedged in one of the arteries of the brain and block the flow of blood in the brain. This type of stroke may also occur with rheumatic heart disease, as well as with an infection or inflammation of the heart valves.

An ophthalmologist, a physician whose specialty is diseases of the eye, can tell in his routine examination with an ophthalmoscope (an instrument used for seeing into the interior of the eye) if there are any small embolic fragments in the retina of the eye. This would be a clear indication that immediate treatment and evaluation of the person's cerebrovascular and cardiovascular systems is imperative.

CEREBRAL HEMORRHAGE

Originally the term *apoplexy* was used to describe the group of symptoms that indicate a hemorrhaging in the brain. Today the word *apoplexy* has given way to the word *stroke* to describe a whole range of conditions causing interference with the blood supply of the brain. The term *cerebral hemorrhage* describes what occurs when a diseased or fragile artery in the brain bursts and floods the surrounding tissues with blood.

A diseased artery is one that has been narrowed by the formation of plaque or fatty deposits on the walls of the artery. A fragile artery is one that has been weakened over a long period of time, usually as the result of hypertension. An *aneurysm,* which comes from the Greek word *aneurysma* (widening), is a blood-filled pouch that balloons out from a weak spot in the wall of an artery that often has resulted from hypertension. When an aneurysm bursts in the brain, it causes a cerebral hemorrhage. Not all aneurysms burst, but enough of them do to give cause for concern.

As with a water pipe, to which an artery is often compared, a leak in the wall of an artery is much more likely to occur under high pressure than under low pressure. This is what happens in an artery when an aneurysm is ballooning out.

When the artery bursts, it can no longer act as a conduit to supply blood to other parts of the brain. Because the brain cells deprived of blood fail to get the necessary glucose and oxygen, they cannot function. As the blood leaking from the artery begins to accumulate, it soon forms a solid clot, which then displaces brain tissue. Thus, along with the hemorrhage, there is also a thrombosis.

Ten per cent of all strokes are caused by cerebral hemorrhages, which occur most often in a person who has both atherosclerosis (i.e., hardening of the arteries) and hypertension (i.e., high blood pressure).

There are also indications, though as yet not conclusively proven, that a hemorrhage may result from the softening of the brain tissue surrounding a blood vessel. Exertion or emotional excitement can cause changes in the blood vessels, which can also contribute to their rupture and hemorrhage.

A cerebral hemorrhage may occur as the result of a head injury (trauma), as the result of an acute infection that causes damage to the blood vessels in the brain, and in acute leukemia.

Leukemia is a disease characterized by an excess of white blood corpuscles, indicating the presence of an anemic condition caused by a decrease in hemoglobin or red blood corpuscles. Leukemia can occur in conjunction with periarteritis nodosa, which is an inflammation of the external covering of an artery that results in the formation of nodules or small protuberances along the artery. It can also occur in conjunction with polycythemia, a condition in which there is an excess of red blood cells.

Sixty per cent of all cerebral hemorrhages occur in the deep parts of the cerebrum, the putamen; 10 per cent occur in the thalamus; 10 per cent in the cerebellum; and 10 per cent in the brain stem.

Actually, however, a hemorrhage can occur anywhere in the brain with the bleeding being continuous until a clot has formed. The clot that forms in this instance usually does so deep inside the brain, most often in the motor area. Because the clot causes pressure on the nerves located in this area, there is paralysis of the muscles these nerves control.

Recovery from a cerebral hemorrhage may occur with no damaging effects if, and it is a big if, the bleeding stops before it has a chance to destroy vital areas of the brain. Any clots that do form absorb very slowly, but they can be absorbed in the blood stream. The extent of the damage to the brain depends in large measure on the speed with which the blood flows from the site of the hemorrhage to the other areas of the brain.

One marked difference between a cerebral hemorrhage and a cerebral thrombosis is that there is a sudden loss of consciousness when a hemorrhage occurs, whereas there is a gradual loss of consciousness with a thrombosis.

TYPES OF CEREBRAL HEMORRHAGES

INTRACEREBRAL HEMORRHAGE There are several kinds of cerebral hemorrhages. One is an intracerebral (within the brain) hemorrhage, which leads to a condition known as hemiparesis. The word *hemiparesis* comes from the Greek prefix *hemi* (half) and the

Greek word *paresis* (weakness). It refers to a slight weakness on one side of the body only. The other condition is known as *hemiplegia,* from the Greek words *hemi* (half) and *plēgē* (paralysis). It refers to paralysis of only one half of the body.

An intracerebral hemorrhage occurs most often when there is severe hypertension and/or an aneurysm. It accounts for nearly 25 per cent of all cerebral hemorrhages. Even a small hemorrhage can cause major neurological deficits.

With a cerebral hemorrhage there are no warning signs, such as there are with a cerebral thrombosis or embolism. When the hemorrhage occurs, the person is usually awake and active.

A massive cerebral hemorrhage results in decreasing consciousness, severe headache, and vomiting, along with paralysis. The outlook for survival is not good. From 75 to 90 per cent of those persons afflicted die within one to two weeks. As the bleeding progresses, unconsciousness may deepen into coma, the pupils of the eyes become fixed and dilated, and death usually follows within 48 hours.

In 10 per cent of the incidents of intracerebral hemorrhage, seizures may occur soon after the hemorrhaging begins. These seizures, from the Middle English word *seizen* (to take possession of), resemble an attack of epilepsy. The word *epilepsy* comes from the Greek word *epilēpsia* (seizure). Epilepsy is a disturbance of consciousness accompanied by convulsions. There are two types of seizures. One is called *grand mal,* from the French word for great evil, and is marked by violent clonic movements. The word *clonic* comes from the Greek word *klonos* (turmoil), and this aptly describes this type of seizure. The face becomes cyanosed (i.e., a dark blue in color), and there is frothing at the mouth.

The second type of seizure is known as *petit mal,* which in French means little illness. It consists of a period of momentary unconsciousness with no convulsions.

Those who do manage to survive a cerebral hemorrhage make a remarkable recovery, and a recurrence is rare.

PARENCHYMATOUS HEMORRHAGE Another type of intracerebral hemorrhage is the parenchymatous hemorrhage. The word *parenchyma* comes from the Greek words *para* (beside), *en* (in), and *chein* (to pour). It refers to the escaping of blood into the substance of the brain and is considered to be a grave condition. It most frequently occurs as a result of hypertension of long duration and is suspected when there has been an acute headache of sudden onset followed by some impairments of consciousness ending in a coma. The mortality for this type of a hemorrhage is extremely high.

SUBARACHNOID HEMORRHAGE Yet another type of intracerebral hemorrhage is the subarachnoid hemorrhage. The word *subarachoid* derives from the Latin word *sub* (under) and the Greek words *arachnē* (spider) and *eidos* (form). This type of hemorrhage is so called because the bleeding occurs in the space between the two layers of membrane that cover the brain. It is most often associated with aneurysms and is considered to be extremely serious. It occurs most often in middle age, with hypertension usually not being a factor.

For the most part there are no warning signs. The onset is sudden, occurring when the person is awake and often after physical exercise and stress. The neck becomes stiff, and there may also be back pain and a severe headache. There is either drowsiness or unconsciousness and a lateral Babinski sign on both sides of the body. The Babinski sign, also called Babinski's toe sign, refers to the manner in which the big toe bends backward when the sole of the foot is stimulated with a sharp instrument. The Babinski sign indicates that there is organic rather than hysterical hemiplegia (i.e., hemiplegia occurring as a symptom of hysteria).

About 5 per cent of all strokes are caused by a subarachnoid hemorrhage. The prognosis is poor. At least 50 per cent of those persons stricken die as a result of the first episode of bleeding. Of those who do survive this phase, 25 per cent have a recurrence of bleeding within a few weeks. With each episode of bleeding there is a higher risk of dying. In fact, this is the only type of stroke that causes death within minutes in those persons who have been considered to be otherwise healthy.

INFARCTIONS

Infarction, which comes from the Latin word *infarcere* (to stuff into), refers to the stoppage or blockage of a blood vessel occurring as a result of foreign matter, such as clots of blood, plaque, and so on, in the blood. An infarction reduces or completely stops the flow of blood through the blood vessel, resulting in the death of the brain tissues thus deprived of blood.

The size of the infarct depends on the availability of the collateral circulation to take over the supply of blood to those tissues surrounding the area of the infarct as well as to other areas of the brain. Persons with atherosclerosis are prone to having small infarcts called *lacunas,* which are less than a centimeter in diameter. Lacunas are most often found in the pons and in the deeper areas of the brain and in the thalamus.

Infarcts caused by thromboses in the large blood vessels may be either large or small in size, depending again on the amount of collateral circulation available. Hypertension is also a factor in causing infarcts, as is diabetes.

Lacunar infarcts give rise to symptoms such as the clumsy-hand syndrome along with the more serious hemiplegia or paralysis of one half of the body.

Cerebral edema, from the Greek word *oidēma* (swelling), and which in this case refers to an abnormally large amount of fluid in the tissues of the brain, may last up to two weeks when the infarct is large. It usually lasts only three to five days. Most of the deaths that take place within a week of a massive cerebral infarction are caused by cerebral edema. When death occurs after a week, it is usually because of complications of a nonneurological nature, such as a pulmonary embolism. The word *pulmonary* comes from the Latin word *pulmonarius* (lung). A pulmonary embolism is a blood clot in the lung. Another complication can be a myocardial infarction. The word *myocardial* derives from the Greek word for muscle (myo) and the word for heart (kardio). A myocardial infarction is a blockage in the muscle tissue of the heart. A urinary tract infection that spreads throughout the body can also cause cerebral infarction.

An infarct of recent origin shows up on a scan as a small, soft area of the brain. A scan maps the distribution of radioactive material in the brain and provides pictures of cross sections of the brain. After a week or two the infarct undergoes changes until there is a final shrinking and scarring over of the affected area.

Pure motor stroke (i.e., paralysis on one side of the body without any sensory deficits), pure sensory stroke involving only one side of the body, the clumsy-hand syndrome, central facial weakness, and ataxia (i.e., failure of muscle coordination and weakness involving the legs more than the arms) are all characteristic signs of lacunar infarcts.

Lacunar infarcts produce a set of symptoms similar to those produced in pseudo bulbar palsy. These symptoms consist of bilateral motor difficulties and loss of emotional control. Some of the symptoms resemble those characteristic of Parkinson's disease.

Not all lacunar infarcts have these recognizable symptoms. Some have no discernible symptoms at all.

OTHER CAUSES OF A STROKE

LESIONS AND INFLAMMATION

Although most strokes are vascular (i.e., pertaining to the blood vessels) in origin, some are caused by lesions in the brain or an inflammatory or degenerative condition in the body itself.

COMPRESSION

Strokes can also be caused by pressure on the brain tissues or arteries when a hemorrhage occurs because the blood flowing out of a blood vessel that has been compressed at one section causes another section to swell. A blood clot may then develop, and this in turn presses against an artery resulting in a closing or blocking off of that artery. This is known as compression. A brain tumor is a good example of what is meant by compression. As the tumor enlarges, it may either compress an artery or cause pressure on the tissues that surround the artery.

SUBDURAL HEMATOMA

The word *subdural* comes from the Latin words *sub* (beneath) and *duros* (hard). In this case the word refers to the area of the outer membrane covering of the brain. The word *hematoma* comes from the Greek words *haima* (blood) and *oma* (tumor) and refers to a tumor enfused with blood and located between the surface of the brain and the dura. A subdural hematoma can be a precipitating factor in a stroke. Many times this type of tumor results from a trauma, a wound, or an accident. Subdural hematomas develop in one and a half to 10 per cent of all head injuries.

MULTIPLE SCLEROSIS

Multiple sclerosis, a disease marked by sclerosis (the Greek word for hardness) is characterized by hardening of patches in the brain and the spinal column, can also be a factor in causing a stroke.

ENCEPHALITIS, SEPTICEMIA, AND HYPOGLYCEMIA

Encephalitis is an inflammation of the brain caused by abscesses filled with pus that result from mastoiditis. Septicemia, the name of which comes from the Greek word *septikos* (putrid) and *haima* (blood) is exactly what the name implies—putrid blood. Hypoglycemia, or low blood sugar, is a condition in which the amount of glucose or sugar in the blood is not sufficient to keep the brain nourished. All three of these conditions can cause a stroke.

AGES AT WHICH STROKES OCCUR

Although 60 per cent of the victims of a stroke are over 65 years of age, no age is immune from them. Strokes can occur in infancy through childhood, in adolescence, in young adulthood, in middle and old age. Perhaps most incredible of all is the fact that newborn babies can also have strokes.

STROKES IN CHILDREN AND ADOLESCENTS

Although hypertension and atherosclerosis can and do occur in children, there is no definite cause-and-effect association between these diseases and a stroke, as there is in the older age groups. The precipitating cause can be congenital heart disease. "Congenital" does not mean "hereditary." *Congenital* refers to heart disease that begins during the life of the fetus. Such heart disease can be caused by a venous thrombosis—that is, a blockage occurring in the veins. It can result from the trauma of a wound or injury to the head. It can result from sickle cell anemia, which is a hereditary form of anemia more prevalent among Blacks but also occurring in whites. It can be caused by an intercranial hemorrhage (i.e., bleeding within the skull) or by an aneurysm. Aneurysms are rare in infants but are more common in adolescents.

Strokes that occur in children are often quite severe. The collateral circulation in this age group has not developed to the point of usefulness, and this gives rise to paralysis and convulsions that may prove fatal.

Loss of sight, of speech, of intellectual function, and of initiative all leave a child severely handicapped with both emotional and physical needs that must be met. When you consider that this is a lifetime problem, you will realize that the expenditure of resources needed to help the child is enormous.

STROKES IN YOUNG ADULTS

In young adults the underlying cause of strokes is usually hypertension, no doubt caused in part by an early development of atherosclerosis. Under the age of 30 females seem to outnumber males in the incidence of stroke. This is believed to be caused by the use of oral contraceptives. The rate of strokes is four times greater in those who use oral contraceptives than it is in those who do not. A woman who is both taking the pill and is also a heavy smoker has a 16 per cent greater risk of having a stroke than a woman who does neither.

The recovery rate in this age group is good. Many young adults who have had strokes become functionally independent.

STROKES IN MIDDLE AGE

About 15 per cent of all strokes occur in persons under age 50; 45 per cent occur in those under age 59. As you can see, middle age is a particularly threatening age for strokes. These are the persons who are in their most productive years, and it is in this age group that the greatest economic impact is felt. Great hardships occur when a stroke hits the provider of the family.

STROKES IN THE ELDERLY

As might be expected, the greatest incidence of strokes occurs in the elderly—that is, in those persons over 65 years of age. Primarily this is because the older you get, the more likely you are to have atherosclerosis and some degenerative changes in the blood vessels. Therefore, the risk of having a stroke does increase with age. Because most stroke victims in this age group have already retired from the work force, the loss of bodily function is not as crucial to them as it would have been during their wage-earning years.

As a result of therapy and the ways that are devised by the individual person to compensate for any residual weakness or paralysis, persons in this age group seems to function better than might otherwise have been expected. Because of their age, their collateral circulation has had a chance to become more fully developed and is able to take over the function of the damaged arteries before severe and extensive damage can be done to the brain itself.

PERSONALITY CHARACTERISTICS OF STROKE VICTIMS

It is in the young adult and the middle-aged groups that a stroke profile begins to emerge. In these age groups a stroke often occurs after a severe emotional upset that has intensified just before the onset of the stroke.

In the middle-aged group, those who are in their years of highest achievement, there is a pattern of pressure in their daily lives resulting from their determination to meet previously set goals within a short period of time. The image they have of themselves is that of active, hard-working people with high standards and a great sense of responsibility. They feel they must at all costs live up to this image. They always have a sense of urgency, of there never being quite enough time to accomplish all they want and to meet those never-ending deadlines. The stroke-prone persons in this group have been shown to have a tremendous sense of determination and a strong will. They also find it difficult to control their anger.

It is in this group in particular that a feeling of anger, of hopelessness, and even at times of shame, of a feeling of not performing up to their own high standards, that quite often set the stage for a stroke.

PREVENTION OF STROKES

One of the wisest observations ever made was that an ounce of prevention is worth a pound of cure. Nowhere in medicine is this more true than in dealing with the risk factors that lead to a stroke. The regular physical checkup assumes the greatest importance in the prevention of a stroke, for it is during these checkups that any of the risk factors that have been shown to cause strokes can be detected and treated.

Even if you have already had a stroke, any further strokes may be prevented. The chances are that what caused the first stroke will eventually contribute to subsequent ones unless the cause is treated and controlled.

Through years of observation and particularly through the efforts of the Framingham Heart Study Group, there has emerged evidence of what have come to be known as *risk factors*. The presence of these risk factors enables the stroke-prone individual to be identified. The more risk factors there are, the greater the risk of having a stroke. The modification or elimination of these factors is of paramount importance because brain cells that have been damaged as the result of a stroke cannot rejuvenate themselves.

Not to be overlooked is the fact that treating and controlling the risk factors costs a whole lot less than does a stroke, both economically and in terms of suffering. There are only a few risk factors—heredity, sex, race, and age—that can neither be modified nor controlled.

A history of strokes in one or more branches of a family, along with a history of any of those diseases that have come to be recognized as definite risk factors (such as hypertension, atherosclerosis, diabetes, and hyperlipidemia, i.e., an excess amount of fat in the blood) suggest that there is an inherited tendency toward, but not an absolute certainty of, developing a stroke.

Men tend to have more strokes than do women and at a younger age.

Nonwhites have strokes more often than do whites. As you grow older, the risk of having a stroke increases because the normal progressive degenerative changes in the blood vessels that occur after years of pumping blood through the body cannot be completely prevented.

But because we do know the risk factors leading to a stroke, we can, in the case of those factors we can control, make a change in our lifestyle that will either prevent them from developing at all or, if they do develop, will lessen their severity.

In the case of those risk factors that cannot be controlled, we can be aware that although they do tend to increase the risk of our some day having a stroke, with good medical care and a healthy lifestyle, a stroke is not inevitable.

CHAPTER TWO

EARLY WARNING SIGNS OF AN IMPENDING STROKE

It is small consolation after a stroke has occurred to recall that yes, the patient had indeed experienced moments of loss of memory, or had lost the use of an arm or a leg for a few moments, or had problems with vision. How much better it would be to become familiar with the warning signs of a stroke and, more important, to act promptly when they do occur. Fortunately most strokes do give warning signs that, if heeded, can prevent those strokes from ever occurring. The most important of these signs is a transient ischemic attack.

TRANSIENT ISCHEMIC ATTACK (TIA)

WHAT A TIA IS

By definition, a transient ischemic attack is an episode of transient, focal neurological abnormality or deficit that lasts from a matter of minutes to a few hours, but never more than 24 hours. In most instances, the entire episode is over within minutes. The characteristic sign of a TIA is a rapid overall improvement. Generally, there are no aftereffects. The only exception might be when several

TIAs have occurred in rapid succession or when a TIA has lasted longer than 24 hours, yet did not progress to a completed stroke.

Another type of attack similar to the TIA in nature is a reversible ischemic neurological deficit (RIND) or a prolonged reversible ischemic neurological deficit (PRIND). The difference between the TIA and the RIND or PRIND is that in the latter the neurological deficit does not clear up within a 24-hour period. It does, however, completely disappear within one to two weeks. Were the deficit, usually in the form of paralysis, not to disappear, a completed stroke would have occurred.

A TIA is often called a "little stroke". It is caused by ischemia—that is, a blockage in one of the carotid arteries, the vertobasilar arteries, and cerebrum, or the cerebellum. A TIA occurs when the blood supply to a localized area of the brain is temporarily inadequate.

THE SIGNIFICANCE OF A TIA

A TIA is the principal warning sign of an impending stroke—a harbinger, as it were. Although figures vary as to the number of people who, having had a TIA, go on to having a full-blown stroke within the next five years, the average rate is from 35 to 75 per cent, a statistic that emphasizes the importance of a TIA as a warning sign.

The risk of a stroke occurring after a TIA is highest during the first year after the occurrence of the TIA. Risk decreases with each succeeding year that is free from further attacks.

The significance of a TIA as a warning sign was first understood in the early 1900s. However, little was done about it until 1951 when Dr. Derek E. Deney-Brown, a professor of neurology at Harvard Medical School, and Sir George W. Pickering, a neurologist from England, began emphasizing the importance of these attacks and submitting their findings to the medical journals.

A TIA indicates that there is underlying vascular (blood vessel) disease. Thus, its early recognition and treatment unquestionably helps to prevent the development of a stroke.

THE FREQUENCY OF TIAs

The number of TIAs experienced by an individual can vary widely from as few as only one or two a year to as many as 50 such episodes in a single day. Once a TIA has occurred, it tends to recur unless the underlying cause is eliminated.

THE INCIDENCE OF TIAs

As might be expected, a TIA occurs most frequently in the elderly. This does not mean, however, that it cannot and does not occur at much younger ages. In the 55-to-65 age group, a TIA is more likely to precede an incapacitating stroke than it is the 65 or older group.

The incidence of TIAs increases with age, going from the rate of 31 in every 100,000 persons in the general under-65 population, to about two in every 1,000 in the over-65 age group. A TIA can even occur in children, particularly when the children have atherosclerosis. And women as well as men are at risk.

A TIA is serious at any age because it indicates that at the time it occurred there was an insufficient blood supply to some part of the brain. It is symptomatic of a vascular problem that, if left untreated, can and many times does lead to a stroke.

THE CAUSE OF TIAs

An embolism resulting from a buildup of plaque due to atherosclerosis in the walls of a blood vessel is the most common cause of a TIA. Small emboli, pieces of plaque that have formed on the walls of an artery, break off and, in attempting to flow through the blood stream, sometimes get lodged temporarily in an artery or blood vessel that controls a vital function. It is then that a TIA occurs. When these emboli pass on through the blood vessel and past a vital control center, the transient ischemic episode ends and there is a return to normal function.

These emboli limit the flow of blood to and through the arteries, particularly to those small branches of arteries located in the various control centers of the brain. The progressive narrowing of an artery because of the buildup of plaque can also limit the flow of blood in an artery.

In a TIA the blockage from these emboli is not as complete as it would be in the case of a stroke. The constant breaking off of small pieces of plaque, particularly in the arteries of the neck, can contribute to repeated TIAs when they begin to go through the blood stream.

When larger pieces of plaque break off, the TIA may be more severe, more areas of the body may be affected, and the episode may last longer. Yet this still is called a TIA, not a stroke, provided that the resulting neurological deficit does not last any longer than 24 hours. Recovery occurs either because the plaque breaks up and allows the blood to flow through normally, or the collateral circulation is sufficient to maintain a flow of blood to all the vital areas of the brain.

Both a decrease in cardiac output and hypotension (low blood pressure)—that is, a transitory drop in blood pressure from its normal level—can also cause a TIA. A TIA can occur as the result of a momentary cardiac arrhythmia (irregular heart beat)—in other words, during a period when the heart is temporarily out of rhythm.

The heart normally beats at about 72 beats per minute. This is known as the heart rate. When the rate goes below 60 beats per minute, it is called *bradycardia*, from the Greek words *brady* (slow) and *kardia* (heart). When the heart rate accelerates to over 100 beats per minute, it is known as tachycardia, from the Greek words *tachys* (swift) and *kardia* (heart). The rate of the heart and its rhythm are two different things. Rhythm refers to the steadiness of the heart beat. If the heart beat is unsteady or irregular, such as occurs when there is skipping, fluttering, or fibrillating (i.e., quivering), or if the heart beats are irregularly spaced (such as when there is a premature beat or a long pause between beats), the heart is then said to have arrhythmia, an abnormal rhythm.

It should, however, be strongly emphasized that chronic cardiac arrhythmias do not of themselves cause TIAs. The TIA caused by an arrhythmia is the result of an isolated episode of abnormal rhythm that is serious enough to cause a disruption in the blood supply.

A TIA can be caused by an artery that has become kinked. It can be caused by polycythemia, a condition in which there are too many red cells in the blood. A decrease in the oxygen-carrying capacity of the blood can also cause a TIA.

When TIAs occur in the carotid artery, they produce transient hemiparesis—that is, a slight paralysis on one side of the body. They also result in aphasia, which denotes difficulty in speaking and communicating, and in transient difficulties with vision.

The TIAs that occur in the vertebrobasilar system produce dizziness, drop attacks (see page 33), sudden fainting known as syncope, difficulty in identifying people and objectives, and blindness in half of the field of vision in the eye, along with numbness on only one side of the body.

SYMPTOMS OF A TIA

A TIA may manifest itself as a sudden, fleeting, or blurring of the vision in one eye or as the complete loss of vision in one eye. There may be signs of diplopia (double vision), vertigo (a sensation of whirling, either of oneself or of the objects around oneself), a weakness or numbness on one side of the body, difficulty in speaking, motor uncoordination (ataxia), or headaches. These symptoms may come singly, or there may be several of them simultaneously. But again, the characteristic that differentiates a stroke from a TIA is that the deficits in a TIA disappear suddenly with no residual aftereffects, whereas the deficits from a stroke become fixed.

Generalized feelings of dizziness, fainting, or a loss of consciousness are not always indicative of a TIA, although they can be. Most of the time their causes are associated with other diseases. A TIA is a focal deficit—that is, a disturbance of blood circulation in a specific blood vessel in the brain that controls a specific function.

When a person who has had a TIA is examined by a physician, a history of the onset and symptoms of the episode is taken so that a determination can be made as to which blood vessels are involved. If it is the carotid artery that is involved in the episode, the treatment may necessitate surgery, but if it is the vertebrobasilar artery, medical management, usually with drugs, is indicated. The TIAs associated with a vertebrobasilar artery have a lower incidence of ending in a completed stroke than those associated with the carotid artery.

It is true that many of the deficits associated with a TIA are also present during a full-blown stroke, but these deficits when associated with a stroke last longer and indeed may become permanent disabilities. These permanent disabilities are discussed more fully in Chapter 12, which deals with the completed stroke.

Should any of the symptoms mentioned occur, they should be immediately brought to the attention of a physician for prompt treatment. They all indicate that there has been a decrease in the blood supply to some area of the brain. Because these symptoms are truly warning signals, they should be heeded.

The art of language is indeed strange. Not everyone's idea of the meaning of a word or a phrase is the same. A clarification, therefore, of just what is meant by each of the symptoms associated with a TIA might prove helpful. As we have said, many of these symptoms also occur in a completed stroke, but here they are discussed only as they pertain to the early warning signs in the TIA before a stroke has a chance to occur.

WEAKNESS AND NUMBNESS

When speaking of weakness and numbness in an arm or leg, it is important to determine whether that numbness or weakness is constant or whether it started in one area of the arm or leg, such as in a finger or in a toe, and then proceeded to march on to include the entire limb.

With a TIA the weakness does not march. It appears all at one time and remains where it started. Most people describe the sensation of weakness or numbness that is experienced in a TIA as sort of "just being there, of being all over the arm or leg."

Numbness denotes a loss of sensation, making it impossible to use the affected leg, arm, or hand in a normal manner. Some people describe the feeling as one of heaviness. There is an inability to pick up something from the floor or to walk in a normal manner. Weakness denotes a lack of strength—for example, difficulty in forming a fist with the weakened hand.

TEMPORARY DIZZINESS AND UNSTEADINESS

What is known as *drop attack*—that is, falling suddenly with no warning that it was about to happen and with only a brief period of unconsciousness—is another symptom of a TIA. Sometimes there is a period of unsteadiness or of losing one's balance. Not all episodes of dizziness and unsteadiness are indicative of a TIA. Unless they are accompanied by a short period of unconsciousness, they are not considered to be manifestations of a TIA.

Vertigo, the Latin word for turning around, is a sensation of whirling motion in which either you have a feeling of whilring around or the objects around you seem to be whirling around. Although it is a form of dizziness, more often vertigo is a symptom of an inner ear disturbance. Although it is sometimes quite frightening, it is not by itself evidence of either a TIA or a stroke.

Attacks of lightheadedness, even though they occur fairly frequently, are not by themselves an indication of either a TIA or a stroke.

TEMPORARY LOSS OF SPEECH AND DIFFICULTY IN UNDERSTANDING SPEECH

Difficulty in speaking, in writing, in understanding language, and in reading indicate that the TIA is localized in the speech-control center of the brain.

Aphasia, from the Greek words *a* (not) and *phasis* (to speak), which means an inability to speak or to express oneself in words, is yet another symptom of a TIA (see Chapter 12). Aphasia lasts but a very short time, and there is complete recovery with the restoration of the ability to speak and to understand words. When aphasia occurs in a TIA, it is usually caused by a disturbance located in the dominant hemisphere of the brain that controls the language center and that affects both speech and reading. As the result of a temporarily diminished supply of blood to this part of the brain, the language center is unable to function normally.

SUDDEN LOSS OF VISION OR A TEMPORARY DIMNESS IN VISION

Disturbances in vision can include seeing many of the colors, weird shapes, and flashes or sparks of light that are often seen by those persons experiencing a migraine attack. These visual disturbances can occur in both eyes, although usually only one eye is affected. If these symptoms were caused by a migraine headache, they would not disappear within the short period of time that a TIA lasts, but rather could last for as long as three or four days. In some instances of TIAs, vision can be lost completely, resulting in blindness for the short period of time during which the TIA is in progress. Whenever a TIA occurs in a branch of the internal carotid artery that leads to the eye, there are visual difficulties.

HEADACHES OR CHANGE IN PREVIOUS PATTERNS OF HEADACHES

Although a migraine is the most familiar form of a headache, it is not the only kind. There is the cluster type of headache which, although severe and paroxysmal (sharp, sudden, and periodic), lasts a much shorter length of time than does a migraine.

Then there is the depressive headache, which accompanies an episode of depression.

Any change in the normal pattern of a headache resulting from tension or a head cold should be evaluated by a physician because headaches can be a first indication of a more serious problem, not only of a potential stroke but also of many abnormalities of the brain itself, such as a tumor.

DIPLOPIA (DOUBLE VISION)

The word *diplopia* comes from two Greek words, *diplo* (double) and *opsis* (sight)—hence the term double vision. Diplopia is a very important warning sign demanding prompt attention.

CHANGE IN PERSONALITY AND EMOTIONS

Some distinct changes of personality do at times develop in the elderly. Elderly persons often tend to become irritable, quick-tempered, suspicious, and demanding—in short, hard to get along with.

Their emotions are easily aroused, ranging from spells of crying to outbursts of rage and anger. This behavior is particularly hard to understand in a person who has always heretofore been cheerful, considerate, kind, helpful, and optimistic in his or her outlook on life. These changes may be the result of atherosclerosis, a normal aging process, but one that is accelerated. In some people, atherosclerosis is so advanced that these symptoms develop while they are in their sixties, whereas in others these changes do not begin to show up until they are well into their seventies or eighties.

Atherosclerosis is a prime risk factor in the cause of both TIAs and strokes. However, just because an elderly person experiences these symptoms, it does not necessarily mean the person is having either a TIA or a stroke. Perhaps both will eventually develop, but if these personality traits are the only symptoms shown, no focal neurological deficit is present, and no unconsciousness ensues, then the traits are more apt to be the marks of senility rather than of a TIA or a stroke.

RISK FACTORS LEADING TO A TIA

Cigarette smoking, hypertension, atherosclerosis, diabetes mellitus, hypercholesterolemia (i.e., excessive amount of cholesterol in the blood), hyperlipidemia (i.e., too many fat droplets in the blood), the use of oral contraceptives, a family history of stroke, and any cardiovascular disease that is left untreated are all considered to be risk factors in bringing about those conditions that can result in a TIA. Each of these risk factors is discussed in detail along with their treatment in the following chapters.

TREATMENT OF TRANSIENT ISCHEMIC ATTACKS

MEDICAL TREATMENT

Because episodes of TIA are the precursors of a stroke, it is of paramount importance that they be prevented. This can best be done by a careful and thorough physical examination at least once a year. If a TIA does occur, steps can be taken to prevent its recurrence by treating the underlying causes—the risk factors.

The choice of treatment is determined by a person's overall physical condition, age, type of work, the frequency of the attacks, and so on. And not all physicians agree on what is the best mode of treatment. The treatments most often used include anticoagulants, antiplatelet drugs, aspirin, anturane, and vasodilators.

ANTICOAGULANTS

The word *anticoagulant* comes from the Latin words *anti* (against) and *coagulans* (congealing). Anticoagulants are substances such as dicoumarol, coumarin, and heparin, which prevent the blood from clotting.

Heparin has a direct anticoagulant effect. It primarily activates a plasma protein called antithrombin III, which inactivates the thrombus or blood clot. The extracts of many organs of the body produce heparin. The lungs and intestinal mucosa of domestic animals are especially important sources for clinical usage.

Heparin has a direct effect on the coagulation of blood, but coumarin has an indirect effect. Heparin is also a far more potent anticoagulant than is coumarin. In a patient taking heparin, bleeding occurs much more frequently than in a patient taking coumarin. It takes time for a dose of coumarin, which is an oral drug, to become effective, whereas heparin, which is given as an intravenous injection, works almost immediately.

Coumarin is similar to warfarin, the rat poison, and operates in the same manner. Oral anticoagulants such as coumarin do not directly inhibit coagulation. Rather, they inhibit the synthesis of the Vitamin K factors in the liver, thereby decreasing the production of those clotting factors in the liver that afford protection against development of a clot. Because anticoagulants decrease the ability of the blood to clot, they help to prevent thrombi or clots from forming in the blood vessels. They do not, however, dissolve clots that have already formed.

The history of anticoagulants goes back to the 1920s when an anticoagulant substance was found in the sweet clover that was being fed to some cattle and which was causing them to bleed to death. The improperly cured or spoiled sweet clover hay contained a toxic element that interfered with normal blood clotting. The cattle were cured when the ranchers stopped feeding them the spoiled sweet clover.

In 1934 Link and Campbell of the University of Wisconsin successfully isolated the active bleeding agent in crystalline form, and it became known as dicoumarol. Anticoagulants have a tendency to thin the blood out. This decreases its viscosity—that is, its stickiness—decreasing the chance for the blood to clot. The purpose of anticoagulants is to prevent a clot from forming or to prevent an extension of an existing clot. They are not intended to dissolve the clot itself.

Anticoagulants are not recommended as a form of treatment when there is severe hypertension and a tendency to bleed. Whether they are used or not is entirely up to the physician treating the patient. There is no blanket rule for their use, nor is there agreement as to their benefits. Complications can result from their use, and the benefits must be carefully weighed against these complications.

Whenever an anticoagulant is being used, the patient has a great responsibility in following all the instructions received from the prescribing physician. There is an imperative need for weekly prothrombin time tests, familiarly known as pro time, which determine the length of time it takes the blood to clot. The test is simple to perform. A calcium-binding anticoagulant is added to a sample of blood along with an extract of crude lipid and emulsified rabbit brain, which is used as a source of tissue factor. The time between the addition of calcium to the plasma and the appearance of a visible clot is called the *prothrombin time* (pro time). The normal time is less than a two-second deviation from the control. The clotting time of normal plasma is about 12 seconds. The length of time recorded as the prothrombin time indicates the degree of clotability of the blood. The longer the time, the less apt the blood is to clot too readily. If a laboratory uses a different method for determining the pro time, the normal values determined by that laboratory are the ones that apply.

Another prothrombin test is called the partial thromboplastin time test (PTT). This test also determines the length of time it takes the blood to clot.

During anticoagulant therapy, it is essential to make certain that the length of time it takes the blood to clot is no longer than normal. A longer time would indicate that the blood had been thinned out so much that bleeding could too easily occur. Then there would be concern about the possibility of cerebral bleeding that could develop into a hemorrhage. On the other hand, if the blood clots in less than the normal period of time, it is an indication that in all probability the blood is clot-prone, and this could result in a thrombosis.

Anticoagulant therapy for a period of six months to a year does reduce the risk of recurrent TIAs, provided all precautions are taken. But no firm determination has been made as to whether it can prevent a stroke.

Anticoagulant therapy cannot prevent emboli already thickened with plaque from breaking off the arterial walls. Blood that is thin might help prevent small clots from causing an obstruction by enabling them to flow along through the blood stream with greater ease, but so long as pieces of plaque are dislodged from the arterial walls, there will be emboli.

ANTIPLATELET DRUGS

Whenever a break occurs in the endothelial lining of an artery, platelets tend to adhere to this spot and form a thrombus, or clot. Diabetes, hyperlipoproteinemia, atherosclerosis, and heavy smoking all contribute to the tendency of platelets to form emboli. Aspirin and anturane are two of the most promising of the antiplatelet drugs.

ASPIRIN Aspirin has recently come into use as a treatment in TIAs as well as in the treatment of strokes, mostly as the result of a study made by the Canadian Cooperative Study Group in which it was found that aspirin significantly lowered the risk of repeated TIAs in males by 48 per cent. No such effect was found in women.

It was also shown that aspirin could prevent a TIA because of its action as an anticoagulant. The recommended dose is one 300 mg tablet twice a day, although in the Canadian study the dose was four 100 mg tablets a day. The group who benefited most from aspirin therapy were those who were having many TIAs in a short period of time.

The effect of aspirin on the blood appears to be to make the blood less viscous. Aspirin can prevent the blood platelets from aggregating or clumping together for as long as eight days, which is their entire life span. Aspirin is the only antiplatelet drug whose effect is so long-lasting that it need be taken only once a day.

Not everyone benefits from aspirin's anticoagulant effect, however. And as do the anticoagulants Dicumoral and Coumadin, aspirin also has some risks. It can trigger bleeding in those persons who have an ulcer or who are ulcer prone.

Sulfenpyrazone inhibits blood platelets from aggregating (i.e., clustering together and perhaps forming a clot), as does dipyridanole. However, neither of these drugs has the prolonged effect of aspirin and therefore must be taken more than once a day in order for their effect to remain in the body.

ANTURANE Anturane, which is the trade name for sulfenpryazone, was also used by the Canadian Cooperative Study Group in its research. The principal use of Anturane had been in gout therapy because of its action in lowering uric acid. It is this property that is proving effective in both TIA and stroke-prevention therapy.

It is thought that there is a relationship between hyperuricemia (i.e., an abnormal amount of uric acid in the blood) and atherosclerosis. The action of Anturane is thus twofold: It lowers the level of uric acid, and it has an inhibiting effect on the tendency of blood platelets to cluster together.

These two drugs, aspirin and Anturane, interfere with the agglutination or the clustering together of the platelets in the blood. Masses of these platelets, plus fibrin, cause the blood to clot. The use of these two drugs helps to alleviate a buildup of clots, which have a tendency to break off into emboli.

VASODILATORS

Vasodilators, of which Persantine is an example, are drugs that relax the blood vessels and thereby help to widen them. Many physicians are still not convinced that these drugs prevent either TIAs or strokes. Their use, therefore, is on a highly individualized basis.

ALCOHOL

Many people believe that alcohol has the power to dilate the arteries; this sometimes becomes the excuse for having a drink. Before long, this leads to the second, the third, and eventually, perhaps, alcoholism. There is no available data to prove that alcohol does widen the arteries in the brain. It does, however, tend to cause a rise in blood pressure (hypertension), which has been proven to be a risk factor in both TIAs and strokes. This does not mean that everyone must or should abstain from alcohol, but as in all things, drinking should be done in moderation. If your physician tells you that you have any of the risk factors associated with a stroke, if you must drink, ask his opinion as to whether you should continue to do so and above all, follow his instructions.

DRIVING A CAR AFTER A TIA

The physician must use extremely good judgment in advising a patient who has had a TIA about driving. No one can possibly predict when another TIA will occur if multiple TIAs are occurring every week or so. Many of these attacks cause periods of blindness lasting several minutes. Because the time of the next TIA cannot be predicted, driving necessarily should be prohibited until it is felt that the underlying conditions causing the TIAs have been satisfactorily corrected and/or controlled.

If the incidences of TIAs continue and become even more frequent, hospitalization is then necessary for further testing and evaluation, and driving is then, of course, not an issue.

SURGERY

The second method of treating a TIA is surgery. Surgery may seem like a drastic measure for dealing with a TIA, but it may alleviate the cause when multiple episodes are originating in the carotid artery. Indeed, surgery may be mandatory when all medical measures fail to provide relief.

Not everyone is a candidate for surgical intervention. Surgery at an advanced age in a person in a weakened condition and with widespread atherosclerosis is not practical and is of no benefit.

Surgery should be considered only when one of the blood vessels is almost occluded and, because of this, is causing multiple TIAs. Surgery can be considered only when the occluded area is easily accessible to the surgeon and the occlusion can be removed by surgical procedures currently in use.

CAROTID ENDARTERECTOMY

The surgical procedure used in transient ischemic attacks is known as a *carotid endarterectomy,* a procedure in which the inner lining of the blood vessel is removed and the lesions scraped out. The area heals extremely well. As in all surgical procedures, there is a risk that must be taken into consideration.

Before surgery is even considered, a brain scan and an angiograph must be done to actually map out the arterial walls and show where there is severe stenosis, or narrowing, of the carotid artery because of the buildup of plaque. If the patient is able to tolerate surgery, then an endarterectomy may be of significant help.

GRAFTS

In some instances, notably when the plaque on the walls of the arteries has calcified to such an extent that it goes right through the artery wall, it may be necessary to use a graft to repair the artery. In grafting, a vein is permanently attached to an artery. Then the grafted vein takes over the function of that portion of the artery to which the vein was grafted. Usually the vein chosen for the graft is taken from the patient's leg. However, the surgeon sometimes uses a graft made from dacron instead.

ANASTOMOSIS

Anastomosis is the Greek word for opening, in this instance denoting a means of communication between two blood vessels. Anastomosis is a comparatively new approach used for connecting a superficial temporal artery (i.e., an artery in the area of the temples) to a branch of the middle cerebral artery. This type of surgery results in an increase in the rate of blood flow in those blood vessels now supplied through this graft connection.

SOME DISORDERS THAT MIMIC A STROKE

When there is a particular set of symptoms that could apply to more than one disease, the physician is called on to make what is known as a differential diagnosis. This is where experience and expertise come into play. A confirmed diagnosis is seldom, if ever, made without seeing the results of laboratory tests and other diagnostic tests such as X-rays and scans. These tests are discussed in Chapter 10.

Some of the disorders that can mimic a stroke, particularly those that occur during a TIA, are migraine, vertigo, epilepsy, heart irregularities (arrhythmia), and hypoglycemia. Others are intoxication from drugs or from alcohol, postural hypotension (that feeling of dizziness that occurs when one goes from a lying or sitting position to one of standing), and electrolytic unbalance, which often occurs while one is taking diuretics to reduce the amount of fluid in the body. Diuretics are often prescribed for reducing an elevated blood pressure (hypertension), and they can result in a depletion of one of the electrolytes, potassium. This condition is known as hypokolemia (low potassium). Its symptoms are leg cramps and dizziness. It can be alleviated with either a potassium supplement such as K–Lyte or K–Ciel, or by drinking or eating food rich in potassium—such as prune, orange, tomato, or grapefruit juice, or bananas, cantaloupe, oranges, raisins, watermelon, carrots, celery, lima beans, spinach, and tomatoes. Nearly all vegetables are rich in potassium when they are eaten raw. However, in cooking, much if not all the potassium is lost if the water used in cooking the vegetables is discarded (see Chapter 5).

HYPONATREMIA

Hyponatremia is a condition in which there is not enough sodium or salt in the blood. It, too, is another condition whose symptoms can mimic a stroke. Fortunately, this condition occurs only occasionally, and it does so when a patient has not followed the physician's advice to restrict water consumption when on a salt-free diet and taking diuretics at the same time.

Hyponatremia results from edema (excess fluid) that is brought about by drinking large amounts of water, the low sodium (salt) content of the blood because of the diet, plus the diuretic that tends to flush out such minerals as sodium and potassium.

Hyponatremia can also lead to so-called water intoxication, with its feelings of lethargy, confusion, and even coma. Treatment consists of restricting the intake of water and eliminating the diuretics.

HYPOTENSION

Hypotension, that is low blood pressure, can also mimic a stroke because when the blood pressure is lower than normal, the blood cannot flow through the blood vessels at the normal rate. This decrease in blood flow can result in cerebral insufficiency because the quantity of blood getting to the brain may not be enough for normal functioning. Slow, sometimes muddled, thinking and the feeling of not being one's usual self are some of the symptoms of hypotension. Once the reason for low blood pressure has been determined, it can be corrected.

HYPERVENTILATION

Emotional upsets and anxiety can cause what is known as the hyperventilation syndrome, which is simply overbreathing. Although this can be a frightening experience by itself, it is not an indication of either a TIA or a stroke.

In hyperventilation the carbon dioxide and carbon dioxide pressure fall rapidly and pH or acidity tends to rise, resulting in symptoms that resemble both a cardiovascular and a neurological problem.

In hyperventilation there can be a rapid drop in blood pressure, possibly a low blood sugar, some heart irregularities, and even chest pain. The mouth and throat are unusually dry. There may be some belching, bloating, and flatulence because of gas in the digestive tract. Dizziness, along with numbness and tingling, and sensations of being hot or cold may occur.

Treatment consists of getting the person to breathe quietly into a paper bag the opening of which has been placed securely over the nose and mouth. The bag will fill and empty with each breath. If any air seems to be escaping from the bag, the bag should be held tightly against the cheeks, the nose, and the chin. By having the person rebreathe his own carbon dioxide, an elevation in the pressure of carbon dioxide takes place in the body, and in less than a minute the attack of hyperventilation begins to subside.

Anyone experiencing an attack of hyperventilation is promptly evaluated for any underlying emotional problems that might have caused the overbreathing. Usually an understanding of what causes and what can be done to prevent these attacks—such as relief of emotional tension and anxiety, possibly with medication—brings an end to them.

BRAIN TUMORS AND HEMATOMAS

Brain tumors and subdural hematomas can cause vision disturbances as well as convulsions and periods of unconsciousness. These are all symptoms also present in TIAs and strokes.

ANEMIA

Some symptoms of anemia can mimic a stroke. Blood that is anemic (i.e., deficient in red blood corpuscles, hemoglobin, or both) cannot supply the amount of oxygen that the body and the brain need to function properly. Headache, fatigue, poor appetite, and often a tendency to faint are all associated with anemia. If there is severe anemia, the resulting symptoms can mimic the symptoms of a TIA or a stroke.

The tests for anemia are relatively simple. They consist of a CBC (complete blood count) with a differential [i.e., a determination of each of the many varieties of leukocytes (white blood corpuscles) that are in the blood], a hemoglobin test to determine the number of red blood cells, and an hematrocrit to indicate the values of the red cells per unit in the circulating blood. These tests are discussed in Chapter 10.

ADRENAL INSUFFICIENCY

Adrenal insufficiency is another disease whose symptoms can mimic the symptoms of a stroke. The adrenal glands are located near the kidneys. The hormone secreted by them is called *adrenalin.* During periods of intense excitement or of great fear, the amount of adrenalin that is secreted is increased. This in turn causes an elevation in blood pressure and an increase in the heart rate.

Here, however, we are concerned not so much with the overfunctioning of these glands but, rather, with a deficiency in their functioning.

A common form of adrenal insufficiency is known as Addison's disease. Its manifestations are many. Among them are muscle weakness, a lack of strength known as asthenia, some anemia, loss of weight, low blood pressure, faintness, dizziness, twitching, nervousness, pain, possible dehydration, and lack of proper kidney function.

President John F. Kennedy was believed to have had Addison's disease. This belief was so widespread that when he was taken into the Parkland Memorial Hospital in Dallas after his assassination, the first thing the emergency room physician did was to administer a massive dose of cortisone to compensate for the glands' deficiency.

Two hormones, ACTH and cortisone, are used as treatment of Addison's disease, and the correct level of both as determined by the physician must be maintained for the life of the patient.

CHAPTER THREE

RISK FACTORS YOU CAN CONTROL

HYPERTENSION

THE EFFECTS OF HYPERTENSION ON THE BODY

The number-one risk factor leading to a stroke is a silent one: hypertension, or high blood pressure. It is silent because for most people there are few, if any, symptoms. Unless their blood pressure is checked, they never know they have it. Waiting for symptoms to develop before having your blood pressure checked is like playing Russian roulette. Too often there are no symptoms before the heart attack, the stroke, or even death.

Once hypertension has reached the point where it is causing heart, brain, and kidney problems, there is an increased risk of death. In 38 per cent of untreated cases of moderate and severe hypertension, death occurs within five years.

One out of every 10 adult Americans, or about 23,000,000 people, have some degree of hypertension, be it moderate or severe. Another 20,000,000 have what is called *labile hypertension.* The term *labile* is used to describe the situation in which the blood pressure tends to fluctuate at higher-than-normal levels. The word comes from the Latin word *labi* (to glide). Thus, the labile hypertensive's pressure is normal one time and high the next.

Life insurance statistics indicate that the mortality rate from hypertension increases as the blood pressure rises, resulting in as much as a 35 percent reduction in life expectancy. Hypertension is fast becoming a major health problem worldwide. It is also a chronic illness requiring constant monitoring and treatment. But hypertension can be controlled. In most instances an elevated blood pressure can be returned to normal levels and kept that way with medication. Most sobering of all is the fact that the death rate from strokes could decline drastically if hypertension were diagnosed and treated soon enough.

Hypertension can cause many problems in the brain, in the heart, and in the kidneys. When blood pressure is excessively high, it can cause the blood vessels in the brain to burst. The resulting flow of blood damages the surrounding areas of the brain, terminating in a stroke. Hypertension can contribute to the development of a transient ischemic attach (TIA) (see Chapter 2).

Hypertension can cause heart disease, because when the blood pressure is elevated the heart has to work much harder to supply the body's tissues with blood. This results in an increased load being placed on the heart, which in turn causes heart strain. Because the heart has to pump against this high pressure, it eventually becomes enlarged. Carried to an extreme, the heart could go into failure because of its inability to pump the blood hard enough. This failure is called *congestive heart failure* because the heart becomes congested from all the extra effort and actually does fail.

Hypertension also speeds up the development of atherosclerosis. This means that the rate at which the fatty deposits or plaque plugs up the arteries and reduces the flow of blood through these arteries is accelerated.

Hypertension can both cause atherosclerosis and be the result of it. This effect is most often seen in the elderly. When the blood pressure is constantly elevated, the arteries are then always under stress. Blood pressure that is elevated for only a short period of time does not do irreparable damage, but over a long period of time it certainly does. The arteries tend to lose their elasticity because of the increased pressure on the arterial walls.

Hypertension also causes kidney disease because it damages the small blood vessels in the kidneys, making it much more difficult for them to filter out waste products and excess fluid from the blood. This can result in kidney failure.

When there is an increase in blood pressure in the veins and arteries of the brain over a long period of time, it can lead to either a hemorrhage in one or more of these arteries or in the formation of a clot or thrombosis. The Framingham Heart Study Group showed that in those persons with hypertension, strokes develop seven times more frequently than they do in those whose blood pressure is normal. The risk of having a stroke increases 30 per cent for each 10 mmHg increase in blood pressure. Those persons whose blood pressure is within normal limits seldom have a stroke.

Fortunately, hypertension ranks as the most treatable of the risk factors that contribute to bringing on a stroke. Early treatment of hypertension can afford great protection against the strokes caused by atherosclerosis or ruptured blood vessels in the brain.

The progress of hypertension is insidious. Even the headache and dizziness that only rarely accompany hypertension, and then usually only when the hypertension is severe, are often attributed to other causes. Of course, many times a headache is caused by simple tension, nervousness, or anxiety. If these headaches are left untreated, the increase in nervousness and anxiety they engender can lead to hypertension, but the underlying reason for their occurrence may be nervousness, and in this case this is the condition that must be treated. Headaches are not considered to be a common symptom of hypertension.

It is truly tragic that it should be only after a stroke or a myocardial infarction (heart attack) has occurred that many persons first become aware that they have hypertension. Often they have had it for a long period of time. It is doubly tragic because normal or near normal levels of blood pressure can be achieved in over 80 per cent of our population.

WHAT BLOOD PRESSURE IS

The term *blood pressure* refers to the force of the blood against the walls of the arteries. It is the force that is generated by the heart as it beats and pumps the blood throughout the body.

The walls of the arteries stretch and contract as the force or pressure of the blood goes up and down. Each time the heart contracts (i.e., each time it beats), which normally is about 72 to 75 times a minute, the blood pressure increases. This is called the systolic pressure, from the Greek word *systoli* (contraction). Systolic pressure is expressed as the first, or high, number in the blood pressure reading.

Each time the heart relaxes, which it does between beats, the blood pressure goes down. This is known as the diastolic pressure, from the Greek word *diastellein* (to expand). The diastolic pressure is expressed as the lower number in the blood pressure reading. For example, in a blood pressure reading of 120/80, the 120 denotes the systolic pressure and the 80, the diastolic pressure.

Blood pressure varies, not only from day to day but from minute to minute. During sleep the blood pressure goes down. Agitation and excitement cause it to rise. These are normal changes. Blood pressure also tends to be somewhat lower during periods of extremely hot weather. It is usually at its highest level in the morning and then tends to fall during the day. The lowest point is reached at about 3:00 A.M., during sleep, after which time it begins to rise.

In those persons whose blood pressure is normal, the pressure once again rises after that midsleep 3:00 A.M. low level. However, it does not continue to rise as much after awakening as it does in the case of those who are hypertensive. Blood pressure tends to reach a peak at about 10:00 A.M. At midafternoon the blood pressure again begins to fall until about 3:00 A.M. when it once again begins to rise. These facts are interesting because most, not all, but most strokes not caused by a thrombosis or an embolism but by a hemorrhage seem to occur between the hours of 6:00 A.M. and 2:00 P.M. when the blood pressure is highest.

Many cerebral hemorrhages seem to occur about 10:00 A.M. when the blood pressure in the person who is hypertensive is at its highest level. This points up the important part hypertension plays in bringing on a stroke.

It is only when the blood pressure is elevated and remains elevated and when the resting blood pressure is higher than normal that a person is considered to be hypertensive.

With age the arteries become less supple, less flexible so that when the same amount of blood tries to get through aged arteries, the result is an increase in blood pressure.

A diagnosis of hypertension is never made after only one reading. Several readings are taken, preferably at daily or biweekly intervals to give time for any transient, emotional upset that might have caused the elevation in the blood pressure to pass.

NORMAL VS. ABNORMAL BLOOD PRESSURE

Traditionally, physicians have considered that blood pressure consistently at or above 140/90 should be treated. Normal blood pressure is 120/80, allowing for slightly higher levels in both systolic and diastolic pressures in the elderly.

Any elevation in blood pressure, however, even in the elderly, should be carefully monitored by a physician. When the level of blood pressure reaches 140/90 or sometimes a bit higher, the physician will start treatment if it seems warranted. This fact assumes importance when it is realized that even mild hypertension results in a decrease in life expectancy. For example, the life span of a man aged 35 years whose blood pressure is 140/95 is decreased by nine years over that of a man whose blood pressure is normal. A man the same age, whose blood pressure is 150/100 has a life expectancy of 16 years less than he would have if his blood pressure were in the normal range.

The systolic pressure is not any less important than is the diastolic. Both are significant.

Hypertension is classified as mild when it is in the 140/90 to 160/95 range, moderate when it is between 160/95 and 180/95 and 180/115, and severe when it is at 180/115 and above. It is also considered severe if, in addition to an elevated blood pressure, there are convulsions and severe neurological changes that indicate a stroke is imminent. Quite often heart failure is experienced when the diastolic pressure goes above 140.

Each stage of hypertension from mild to severe is determined by the level of the blood pressure itself, the person's age, any change in the blood vessels or in the kidneys, and the length of time the blood pressure has been elevated.

ROLE OF STRESS IN BLOOD PRESSURE

Emotions and stress play a vital role in hypertension. Anger and fear cause a rise in blood pressure, and this is normal. It dates back to the beginnings of civilization to the so-called fight-or-flight pattern of response to pressure. If, instead of overtly fighting or fleeing from an upsetting situation, a person remains in the stressful situation, his blood pressure rises. This signifies a frustrated inward reaction.

What is not normal is an overreaction to even mild forms of stress. Those who overreact are known as hyperreactors. They respond to every little upset in daily life as if it were a life-threatening emergency. This abnormal reaction within the sympathetic nervous system, which regulates body functions that are not voluntarily controlled, causes an excess of activity within the system. Because the nervous system controls blood pressure, an increase in pressure results. At one time this reaction was believed to be of such great significance that a surgical procedure was devised to correct it. The operation was first performed in Boston by Dr. Reginald Smithwick. It was called a sympathectomy, and its results were so promising that it was held in high regard for some time. This surgical procedure succeeded in bringing about an interruption in the function of parts of the sympathetic nervous system, which controls the glands, the heart, and the smooth muscles. The sympathetic nerves in the thorax and lower part of the back were cut so to dilate or widen the arteries in both the pelvis and the legs. The result was a continuous reduction in blood pressure.

After a few years, though, sympathectomy was replaced by the antihypertensive drugs that were just coming into existence. Technically, the use of drugs in controlling hypertension could be called a clinical sympathectomy because the results achieved are the same as those obtained by surgical sympathectomy.

The person who experiences excessive reactions to stress and strain is usually tense and highstrung. Many times, although failing to show his reactions outwardly, inwardly he is constantly overreacting. The result is that his blood pressure is constantly elevated. As this elevated blood pressure becomes a permanent part of his everyday reaction to stress and strain, his system becomes either used to it or learns to tolerate this elevation in blood pressure. The mechanism that controls this blood pressure gets stuck at this higher level and then does not allow the pressure to decrease as it normally would at the end of the period of stress and strain. The blood pressure then tends to remain elevated.

The mechanisms that control the rise and fall of the blood pressure are known as *baroceptors*, a group of specialized, pressure-sensitive nerve cells that detect any unusual rise or fall in blood pressure. They act through the automatic nervous system to stabilize the blood pressure within normal limits.

Baroceptors have a narrow range. If the blood pressure rises above or falls below this range, they try to regulate the pressure by bringing about changes in the way the heart and the blood vessels react. It is when the baroceptors are constantly forced to act on the heart and blood vessels in an effort to keep the blood pressure within normal limits and cannot do so that trouble begins.

With proper treatment, blood pressure can be reduced and can be maintained at normal or near normal levels. The baroceptors are then not called on constantly to react in an emergency manner on the heart and blood vessels.

ROLE OF ENVIRONMENT IN BLOOD PRESSURE

Environmental factors—ranging from an excessive intake of salt, to cigarette smoking, to a lack of exercise, and to noise—may also influence the development of hypertension.

The Federal Health Agency in West Berlin monitored workers with hypertension in a bottling plant where the noise level was around 95 decibels. When the workers wore ear covers, their blood pressure went down, but when their ears were uncovered, their blood pressure rose.

It is not absolutely certain whether environmental factors are of themselves the cause of hypertension or whether they are only a part of the total hypertension picture.

KINDS OF HYPERTENSION

Hypertension may be divided into two main types. One type is gradual, progressing quite slowly over a 10-to-20-year period with little if any kidney failure. This type is known as *essential hypertension*. In this group, death will usually result from a heart attack or a stroke if the hypertension is not controlled.

Then there is *accelerated* or *malignant* hypertension, which can have a rapid onset. It develops at a younger age and is quite predictable (see p. 52). If it is not treated, the survival time is short, usually less than a year. The mortality rate for untreated malignant hypertension is close to 100 per cent within a two-year period.

ESSENTIAL HYPERTENSION

Essential hypertension, also known as primary hypertension, is the most common disease in the United States today. Many researchers firmly believe that hypertension is largely hereditary, that it does tend to run in families. If a person's parents are or were hypertensive, the chances of that person's having hypertension are thereby doubled.

Along with heredity, there is also a race factor. Hypertension is much more common in blacks than in whites. It has been estimated that 20 per cent of the general population is hypertensive whereas 50 per cent of the black population is hypertensive. The word *essential* used in this sense does not mean necessary but rather is used as is the original Latin word from which it is derived—*essentialis* (essence). It is so used to indicate a type of hypertension that has no underlying disease as its cause.

Although the exact cause of essential hypertension is not known, extensive research has shown that those persons who have this form of hypertension seem to have certain characteristics in common. Certain personality factors seem to predominate (see page 62).

MALIGNANT HYPERTENSION

Malignant hypertension, often called secondary hypertension, is an accelerated form of the disease that has as its main characteristic acute changes in the blood vessels themselves, usually in the arterioles, which are the smallest arteries, which in turn lead to the tiny capillaries.

Malignant hypertension causes both vascular disease and kidney damage. Even though the term malignant is used to describe this particular form of hypertension, it is well to remember that there is no such thing as benign or good hypertension. The word *malignant* comes from the Latin word *malignus* (bad) and is used to describe this form of hypertension because it indicates that the disease is worsening. This type of hypertension often leads to the life-threatening hypertensive emergency or crisis in which the dangerously elevated blood pressure must be lowered as fast as is safely possible.

For hypertension to be considered malignant the diastolic pressure must be in excess of 120 mm Hg. There is also usually some evidence of retinopathy—that is, a hemorrhage or an accumulation of fluid in the eye's retina, which receives images and is the instrument of vision.

Papilledema (i.e., edema or swelling of the optic nerve as it enters the eyeball) indicates that there is a blurring of the margin of the optic disc. This is a characteristic sign of malignant hypertension.

Some persons have many of these symptoms with lower levels of blood pressure than that normally considered to be severe hypertension. There are others whose diastolic pressure is extremely high and yet who never do develop malignant hypertension. Actually less than 1 per cent of those persons considered to be hypertensive ever develop the malignant form. The greastest incidence of malignant hypertension is found in the 45-to-55 age group. Beyond this age it rapidly decreases.

In those persons who have malignant hypertension the disease usually develops within two to seven years, following the first indication of hypertension. It can, however, develop in a month's time or take as long as 25 years. It can also develop as a complication of essential hypertension. In other words, hypertension that started out as essential can reach a point at which other organs of the body, notably the kidneys, become affected.

Two situations can lead to malignant hypertension. The first is when a case of so-called renal (kidney) disease grows worse over a period of years and finally reaches the stage at which it can be classified as malignant. This is the course the disease usually takes in Whites. In Blacks, however, the malignant type of hypertension comes on suddenly with no previous years of buildup and progresses rapidly, sometimes resulting in death within a month of its onset. It is also the form of hypertension that most often affects Blacks.

RENOVASCULAR HYPERTENSION

When the underlying cause of hypertension is caused by kidney disease, the kidney that is damaged tends to secrete a larger-than-normal amount of the hormone renin. This excessive secretion of renin, combined with a narrowing of the main renal artery (perhaps caused by atherosclerosis), causes what is known as *renovascular hypertension*—that is, hypertension caused by an abnormality in the blood vessels of the kidneys.

Renin catalyzes or speeds up the formation of antiotensin, which is the most powerful known agent for raising blood pressure. Studies have shown that low plasma renin levels appear to afford protection against both heart attacks and strokes. A high level of renin thus emerges as a potential risk factor.

It has also been shown that those persons who have essential hypertension that is accompanied by below-normal levels of renin do not experience either strokes or heart attacks. On the other hand, those who have essential hypertension and also a high level of renin, do have strokes and heart attacks. Although the reasons for these findings are still being investigated, they do explain why some people with known hypertension that has never been treated still live to a ripe old age, and it also points up why the laboratory tests discussed in Chapter 10 are so important. If a high level of renin is discovered during testing, proper and prompt treatment can be life-saving.

Aldosterone is another of the hormones secreted by the kidneys;

it causes the kidneys to retain both salt and water. Excessive amounts of aldosterone cause the blood pressure to rise.

In recent years greater emphasis has been placed on the role of a pheochromocytoma (tumor) in the development of hypertension. Pheochromocytoma comes from the Greek words *phaios* (dark), *chroma* (color), *kytos* (cell), and *oma* (tumor). Such tumors are found in the adrenal glands, and although usually benign and not given to spreading to other areas of the body, they produce and secrete large quantities of norepinephrine and epinephrine, two hormones that elevate blood pressure by acting as heart stimulants.

HYPERTENSION IN CHILDREN AND ADOLESCENTS

Until quite recently adult hypertension was of the greatest concern to the physician. Now, however, evidence is piling up to suggest that hypertension begins in childhood—the so-called juvenile hypertension. Hypertension has even been found in newborn babies. If it were diagnosed and treated at an early age, the strokes and heart attacks that occur later on in life could be substantially reduced.

It has been estimated that among the general population, 1.2 per cent of children ranging in age from 6 to 9 years will have a blood pressure higher than that considered to be in the normal range. From ages 14 to 18 years, the rate rises to as high as 12.2 per cent.

CAUSES OF JUVENILE HYPERTENSION

Hypertension in children is seldom of the essential or primary type, that is, without a known cause. In the majority of cases it can be directly traced to problems in the heart and kidneys, with kidney disease being the more common cause. Hypertension also accompanies many childhood diseases.

Usually there has been a history of recurring urinary tract infections, a gain in weight above the normal levels for the child's size and age, some episodes of excessive perspiration, and perhaps even some weakness. Yet, as many as half of all the children who are found to be hypertensive have had no such symptoms.

To detect hypertension in children, the physician must check their blood pressure at least once a year. Treatment should be begun promptly, if necessary. Dr. Paul Dudley White felt strongly that the prevention of hypertension should start with the young before the disease could become established.

TREATMENT OF JUVENILE HYPERTENSION

Before initiating an active program of drug therapy, the usual procedure is to check the blood pressure at frequent intervals to achieve a reduction in weight if the child is overweight. It is also suggested that the child be more active physically and on a moderately restricted salt diet (which, by the way, would rule out most of the "junk" foods that youngsters love). Five gm of salt a day for adolescents and somewhat less for children is considered to be sufficient to fulfill the requirements of moderate salt restriction.

Children's blood pressure is very labile, that is, it tends to fluctuate. This is a normal pattern that is taken into consideration by the physician before arriving at a diagnosis.

An interesting fact has emerged from studies of blood pressure in children and adolescents in that at age 14 the normal blood pressure is at the children's level, whereas two years later at age 16 it begins to shift to an adult level, and at age 18 the blood pressure is at the level of the more mature young adult.

The Georgia Heart Association has developed a superb program for detecting hypertension in children while at the same time making it interesting and fun. It is done in school as part of the health education curriculum. The basics of blood pressure are explained to the students, as well as how and why it fluctuates. The students are taught how to take blood pressure readings, and then they are loaned a sphygmomanometer (blood pressure cuff and gauge) and a stethoscope so that they can go home and take their parents' blood pressure. This has a twofold purpose. Not only is the blood pressure of the children taken but also that of their parents. When blood pressure is elevated, the family physician can be seen and treatment instituted at once.

The National Heart, Lung and Blood Institute has urgently recommended that a blood pressure check be made on every child over the age of three years as part of the annual physical checkup. Many adults who have hypertension also had hypertension as children.

This recommendation is in line with Dr. Paul Dudley White's idea of the Children's Crusade by which he strove in his later years to educate the public to the concept that strokes and heart attacks are the ultimate results of risk factors, such as hypertension, which in many cases begin not immediately before the stroke or heart attack but years previously in the presumably carefree days of childhood.

HYPERTENSION IN YOUNG ADULTS

For a young adult a diastolic pressure over 90 mm Hg is considered to be abnormal; over 95 mm Hg requires treatment. A systolic pressure above 120 mm Hg in a young adult should be monitored regularly for any sign of a further rise. Most young adults have labile blood pressure so that the blood pressure may have to be taken on quite a few occasions before an average reading can be determined.

Anxiety seems to be the underlying cause of hypertension in young adults. Once this anxiety has been controlled, the blood pressure invariably becomes stabilized at normal levels and remains at normal levels with no need of further medication. Anxiety is controlled in many ways. By tranquilizers–reassurance, periods of meditation, and the chance to talk out problems with an understanding adult.

A systolic reading of 130 mm Hg in this age group has been found to be a significant sign of a death rate in later life that is 60 per cent above the norm.

The same levels of blood pressure considered to be normal in middle-aged persons apply to young adults. The World Health Organization has suggested the following classification of blood pressure at both the young adult and older adult level:

Blood pressure under 140/90	Normal
Blood pressure between 140/90 to 160/95	Borderline hypertension that should be carefully and regularly monitored by a physician.
Blood pressure over 160/95	Definite hypertension; treatment is essential.

Many physicians have found through experience that any blood pressure level above 140/90 should be subjected to some form of treatment—be it drugs, diet, exercise, or meditation to prevent a further elevation in the pressure. Such treatment, it is hoped, can go a long way toward the prevention of a future stroke or heart attack.

HYPERTENSION IN MIDDLE AGE

In middle-aged persons, a systolic blood pressure reading over 140 mm Hg should be carefully watched. A pressure over 150 mm Hg should be treated, particularly so if the diastolic pressure is also elevated. In those persons near 60 years of age, a systolic pressure of 165 mm Hg must be treated even if the diastolic pressure is not much above the 90 mm Hg cut-off mark. This is the age when strokes and heart attacks are most frequent and most lethal. Hypertension must be treated and brought under control before it is too late.

HYPERTENSION IN THE ELDERLY

What would be considered as hypertension in a young adult cannot necessarily be considered as such in the elderly. Because hypertension is the number one risk factor in a stroke, every effort must be made to maintain blood pressure within normal limits. "Normal limits" needs to be further defined as it pertains to older persons.

Blood pressure does tend to increase with age owing, in great measure, to a loss of elasticity in the arteries as a result of atherosclerosis. Therefore, in the elderly it is to be expected that blood pressure levels tend to be somewhat higher than those in the young adult and the middle age groups.

Indeed, having a somewhat higher level of blood pressure may be necessary in the elderly in order for an adequate flow of blood to be maintained in an aging body with its aging arteries. This allowable elevation in blood pressure, however, should not exceed 180/105 mm Hg. Whenever the level of blood pressure is reduced in the elderly, it must be done gradually and over an extended period of time.

Continued observation by the physician to see that the blood pressure does not rise any further may be all that is necessary, particularly if the pressure remains stable at this somewhat elevated level. If, however, the blood pressure begins to rise to a new high, treatment is necessary to lower it.

The elderly are especially sensitive to most of the antihypertension drugs. The drugs side effects, such as dizziness when going from a lying or sitting position to a standing one, can be extremely annoying and can result in falls. The dizziness is caused by orthostatic or postural hypotension. The word *orthostatic* comes from the Greek words *orthos* (straight) and *statikos* (causing to stand). The dizziness is caused by a momentary drop in blood pressure that occurs when the person first stands up, but it quickly adjusts itself within a minute or two.

When orthostatic or postural hypotension occurs, both the systolic and diastolic pressures can drop as much as 20 mm Hg. The reasons for this drop vary from the presence of cerebrovascular diseases to kidney and neurological diseases. Postural hypotension can bring about a momentary insufficiency in the circulation of blood in the areas of the brain or in the heart (see Chapter 1). The symptoms of postural hypotension occur mostly in the morning when the person gets out of bed. They can also occur when the person exercises strenuously and perspires excessively.

Often the elevated blood pressure of an elderly patient can be lowered by complete bed rest for several days, either at home or in a hospital. These measures apply only to those elderly persons whose sole problem is hypertension. Any additional symptoms, such as an abnormal electrocardiagram, any changes in the eye grounds, and any signs of kidney disease, would all necessitate much more vigorous forms of treatment.

HYPERTENSION IN WOMEN

Women are by no means immune to hypertension. Death from strokes and heart attacks is substantially higher in the hypertensive woman than in the woman whose blood pressure is normal. And women enjoy no advantage over men in the incidence of stroke, particularly after menopause.

Since the advent of oral contraceptives, an elevation in blood pressure has occurred in many women who take these pills, particularly when they also smoke. About 5 per cent of the women who take oral contraceptives for a period of five years become hypertensive. The reason for this development is not clear. Weight gain may be one factor because the estrogen in the pill tends to cause an increase in weight and a retention of fluid. This is particularly true in the woman who has mild kidney disease along with a family history of hypertension.

Recognizing that there is a relationship between the use of oral contraceptives and hypertension, particularly when the woman smokes, and because of the high incidence of strokes in women taking oral contraceptives, physicians have been taking a long, hard look as to the advisability of the use of this medication.

Pregnancy is another period of a woman's life when hypertension may occur. Even in those women whose blood pressure has always been normal, hypertension tends to develop quite rapidly toward the end of pregnancy, returning to normal after the birth of the child.

The toxemia (i.e., blood poisoning) of pregnancy is also associated with hypertension. One of the more serious aspects of toxemia is preeclampsia, which is characterized by hypertension, edema, and proteinuria (albumin or protein) in the urine. The severity of this condition is comparable to the extent in the rise of the blood pressure.

Eclampsia is another major toxemia in pregnancy that is associated with hypertension. Convulsions and clonic movements are its features. Obstetricians are extremely conscious of the importance of hypertension in their patients, and they do an outstanding job in its treatment and control

Menopause is yet another phase in a woman's life when hypertension may become a problem. In this instance, hypertension is caused by the body's forced adjustment to a decreased supply of estrogen. Menopause is a time in life of lessened physical activity and of a resultant increase in weight, both of which contribute to an elevation in blood pressure. A rise in blood pressure may first occur during the menopause, reinforcing the need for an annual checkup.

In women as well as men, middle and old age are the times when strokes most often occur. Hypertension is one risk factor that is easily and satisfactorily controlled.

MEASURING BLOOD PRESSURE

Blood pressure readings are expressed as millimeters of mercury. The higher number, called the systolic pressure, records the pumping action of the heart or the heart at work. The lower number, the diastolic pressure, records the pressure when the heart is at rest and is refilling with blood. It is quite generally agreed that the diastolic pressure is more indicative of the severity of hypertension than is the systolic pressure. Systolic pressure, however, is an excellent predictor of cardiovascular problems in the making.

In recent years more and more emphasis has been placed on the elevation of the systolic pressure than was the case in the past. An elevation in systolic pressure has been shown to be a risk factor for both strokes and heart attacks in men who are over 45 years of age and in women of any age. This is so even when the diastolic pressure is not greatly elevated.

To have some means of comparison, the blood pressure should be taken under the same conditions each time—that is, either sitting comfortably in a chair or lying down. Whatever the position when the blood pressure is first taken, it should be continued during subsequent checks.

HOW BLOOD PRESSURE IS MEASURED

Two pieces of equipment are all that are needed to measure blood pressure: a sphygmotonometer and a stethoscope. Although none of those persons who were involved in the development of the sphygmotonometer ever received a medical award for their efforts, they probably should have. This instrument, along with the stethoscope, is undoubtedly the most used piece of equipment any physician has. The word *sphygmotonometer* comes from the Greek words *sphygmos* (pulse), *manos* (thin), and *metron* (measure).

Although blood pressure was first measured in 1711 in one of his mares by the Reverend Stephen Hales by a rather cumbersome means, it was not until 1880 that the first practical device for recording blood pressure in a human being was developed. The developer was a Viennese physician, Dr. Samuel S. K. von Bosch.

After the process for the vulcanization of rubber had been invented, an Italian physician, Dr. Scipione Riva-Rocca, devised the rubber bladder as a part of the cuff of the device. The sphygmotonometer consists of an inflatable rubber cuff attached either to a mercury or an aneroid meter. Air is pumped into the cuff by squeezing a rubber bulb. An air valve prevents any leakage of air.

The mercury gravity manometer has greater reliability and accuracy than does the aneroid meter. It also does not require periodic recalibration (i.e., a rechecking for accuracy) as does the aneroid meter. But because the latter is more portable, it is used more often.

Taking blood pressure is a simple procedure; anyone can do it. The cuff is wrapped around the arm just above the elbow. It should fit snugly yet leave enough room so that it can be inflated. If the cuff has a Velcro fastening, one part of the cuff will stick securely in place over the other one. After the air valve has been shut, the cuff is inflated by squeezing the bulb. If the air valve were to be left open even a slight amount, air would be able to escape and the cuff could not be properly inflated.

The gauge or meter begins to register as the cuff is inflated. The cuff should continue to be inflated until the meter registers 30 or 40 mm. This compresses the brachial artery in the arm and allows this artery to be more clearly seen.

Next, the stethoscope is taken in the left hand and the diaphragm is placed over the brachial artery just below or just inside the edge of the cuff. The stethoscope, which was invented by a French physician, René Laënnec, consists of a piece of rubber or plastic tubing in the shape of a Y.

At the Y end of the stethoscope are the two ear pieces that fit snugly into each ear. At the lower end of the tubing there is a flat piece of metal or plastic called a diaphragm. This diaphragm is extremely sensitive and greatly magnifies sounds.

On the cuff there are usually two arrows, one marked for the left arm, the other marked for the right arm. The diaphragm is placed just below one of the arrows. There are three types of stethoscopes: those with a bell-shaped diaphragm, which are particularly useful for listening to the heart and lungs; those with a flat diaphragm, which are most often used when measuring blood pressure; and those that combine both the bell and the diaphragm. It is the diaphragm type that is described here.

With the diaphragm part of the stethoscope in place, the bulb is squeezed until the cuff is inflated to about 20 to 30 points on the guage above which it is thought the blood pressure reading is going to be. It is not necessary that the bulb be squeezed until the meter reaches its highest readings. Inflation does compress the artery, and there is no need to cause unnecessary discomfort.

By gently loosening the valve on the bulb that is being held in the right hand, the air is then gradually released in the cuff while the left hand holds the diaphragm part of the stethoscope in place over the brachial artery. The gauge should be carefully watched while the air is being released slowly and evenly. A too-rapid deflation will give an inaccurate reading.

When the air is released, the wall of the collapsed artery becomes filled with blood. When the blood resumes flowing through the artery, a thudding sound can be heard through the ear pieces of the stethoscope. The first clear sound that is heard is the systolic pressure. More air is released from the cuff until the thudding sound is no longer heard. The reading on the gauge at the moment the thudding sound ceases to be heard is the diastolic pressure. The blood pressure reading is expressed, for example, as 120/80—120 being the systolic pressure, 80 being the diastolic.

Sphygmotonometer cuffs come in various sizes, from those small enough to be used in infants to an adult size large enough to go around a thigh. The cuffs should be wide enough to cover two-thirds of the upper arm and long enough to be wrapped snugly around the arm.

Because a diagnosis of hypertension is based on a blood pressure reading, the reading must be accurate. Using a cuff of the correct size helps to assure this accuracy. Cuffs that are too small give artificially high readings; cuffs that are too large give artificially low readings. There can be an error of 10 to 15 mm in the blood pressure reading if a cuff of the wrong size is used.

Although not yet in widespread use, machines are available for measuring blood pressure. They operate on electronic sensors and make the use of a stethoscope unnecessary.

IS THERE REALLY A HYPERTENSIVE PERSONALITY?

TYPE A PATTERNS OF BEHAVIOR

Many scientific researchers, as well as physicians engaged in the practice of family medicine, believe that there is a hypertensive personality. Those persons who are hypertensive seem prone to experiencing frequent emotional upsets that tend to last longer than similar upsets would in the person with normal blood pressure. They also tend to react too quickly to stress and to respond to it with excessive irritability, anxiety, and restlessness. Hypertensives are quick to display hostility, which provokes others to anger, and this in turn only increases their own hostility. They seem to always have a defensive attitude where others are concerned.

A study conducted by the United States Air Force showed that men whose blood pressure was the most elevated were "dominant, assertive, decisive, task-oriented and made the most effective leaders." In the same study men with the lowest blood pressure were found to have "narrow ranges of interest, low thresholds for preceiving threats, challenges and hostility in other people, were overcontrolling, rigid, stereotyped and obtuse in their social relationships." This study mirrors the Type A personality.

TYPE B PATTERNS OF BEHAVIOR

The Type B person has often been described as easy-going, less aggressive, unharried, and, above all, relaxed. Because he seems to handle stress in a more casual manner, he does not experience those frequent bursts of adrenalin through his body that his Type A counterpart does, with the result that as a rule he is not troubled by hypertension.

The Type A person, on the other hand, is hard-driving, aggressive, restless, and impatient. He talks fast, eats fast, walks fast. In fact, he does everything much quicker than normal. He is constantly striving to achieve more and is never satisfied. He is extremely conscious of time, perennially in a hurry, always rushing to meet a deadline. He is constantly checking his watch and cannot tolerate tardiness. Some physicians have dubbed this type of behavior as the "hurry-up sickness." The Type A person can be found in any occupation, not just as a super salesman or a corporate president. The trait that is perhaps the hardest for this type of person to change is the feeling of guilt he experiences if and when he tries to relax. He is so accustomed to living in a pressure cooker that he does not know how to or even want to get out.

Autopsies have shown a higher rate of atherosclerosis in the Type A person who, besides having an elevated blood pressure, also tends to smoke and to eat foods that are high in cholesterol. All of these are risk factors in bringing on a stroke.

However, being a so-called Type B person is no guarantee against having a stroke or a heart attack if a low-fat diet and exercise are not part of daily living and if the blood pressure is not within normal limits.

Although it may never be possible to completely change a harried Type A to a relaxed Type B, it is still possible to modify the Type A's habits to the extent that blood pressure, diet, and exercise patterns are controlled. Perhaps then the Type A can become a Type A−, or, if you will, a Type B+. Then personality differences would not in themselves constitute so much of a risk factor as they seem to do.

METHODS OF REDUCING BLOOD PRESSURE

There are six basic methods of reducing blood pressure: salt restriction, weight reduction, exercise, drugs, rest and relaxation, and meditation or biofeedback.

SALT RESTRICTION

To lower the patient's blood pressure, the physician may decide to restrict or reduce the intake of salt in the person who has hypertension. Salt is not an essential dietary supplement, because all foods contain some sodium. Fruits, vegetables, and cereals contain less sodium than do meat, eggs, fish, and milk. A well-balanced diet will contain all the salt the average person needs.

A reduction in the amount of salt, or sodium chloride as it is chemically known, in the diet will help to alleviate the retention of fluid in the body. The buildup of fluid in the body does raise the blood pressure. When salt is either restricted or reduced, the blood pressure is lowered. Many times all that is necessary to reduce salt intake is to sprinkle less salt on food, to use a salt substitute, and not to add salt when cooking.

Using less salt can prevent hypertension. Efforts are now being made on a national scale to reduce the amount of salt in everyone's diet, including that of infants. Not only are the so-called baby foods high in salt content, but mothers are inclined to use as much salt in preparing food for their baby as the mothers themselves use in a mistaken idea that it will make the food taste better. The taste for salt is an acquired habit that is often started in infancy in just this way.

Although Americans are not alone in using excessive amounts of salt, they do tend to use anywhere from two to five times as much as they need to. Little wonder that hypertension is so prevalent in the United States. In contrast, Eskimoes and the people in some areas of China use very little if any salt and they have consistently low blood pressures. In Japan, on the other hand, where the salt intake totals more than an ounce a day, almost half the population has hypertension. In every country in which a large amount of salt is consumed, a correspondingly high proportion of the population is hypertensive.

A most interesting observation that resulted from a worldwide study on hypertension was that the natives in the small villages of

New Guinea, where modern civilization with its high salt consumption had not arrived, were virtually free of hypertension. Most remarkable of all was the fact that the blood pressures in the old men were no higher than those of the young men. This study went on to show that when these natives or their descendants moved away from their inland villages to the coastal cities, which had a more modern civilization, they invariably developed hypertension and at the same rate as those who had been living in those coastal areas for generations. Stress, of course, plays a tremendous part in hypertension, but when those who move away from their islands to the mainland and are placed on salt-restricted diets, then hypertension becomes normal.

Black Americans are especially prone to hypertension and to strokes. Recent research suggests that this may be due to the manner in which the kidneys of Blacks handle salt or, more correctly, to the way their kidneys cannot handle salt. A low-salt diet is thus a necessity for Blacks.

Along with a reduction in the use of salt as a seasoning, it is helpful to avoid those foods with a high salt content. The salt content of the following foods is considered to be high:

CANNED FOODS especially vegetables and fish.

SEASONINGS catsup, A1 sauce, mustard, relish, soy sauce, and Worcestershire sauce.

SNACK OR JUNK FOODS potato chips, salted peanuts, salted and buttered popcorn, pretzels, salted crackers, pizza, olives, french fries.

MEATS bacon, calves' liver, frankfurters, ham, sandwich meats, sausages.

FISH lobsters, oysters.

OTHERS bouillon, salted butter, cheese.

Table salt, which is used for seasoning, and sodium are not the exact same thing. Plain sodium is a mineral, whereas table salt is a combination of two minerals—sodium and chloride. Because the amount of sodium in table salt is so great, it is thought of only as a sodium, the chloride being ignored.

One gram of sodium retained in the body but not secreted through the kidneys can raise the blood pressure as much as 30 to 50 per cent. Retention of sodium takes place whenever there is a diminished flow of urine caused by kidney disease. One teaspoon of salt contains 2300 mg of sodium. One gram is equal to 1000 mg or 45 milli equivalents.

The following foods are considered to be low in salt content:

> FRUITS such as apples, apricots, avocadoes, bananas, cantaloupes, dates, grapefruit, nectarines, honeydew melons, prunes and raisins.
>
> JUICES such as apple, grapefruit, orange and prune.
>
> VEGETABLES such as asparagus, white, green and lima beans, broccoli, brussel sprouts, cooked cabbage and cauliflower, cooked eggplant, corn, peas, peppers, potatoes, both baked and boiled, radishes and cooked squash.

Like the wheels of the ancient gods, the mills of medicine at times grind torturously slow. In 1902 two French physicians, Vidal and Lemierre, first pointed out the relationship between salt and cardiovascular disease, but these findings went unnoticed until the 1940s. At that time the only way high blood pressure could be controlled was by the rice diet and Smithwick's Sympathactomy operation.

Before the advent of the antihypertensive drugs in the 1950s, the only way that blood pressure could be lowered was with the so-called rice diet, which had been introduced in the 1940s. The rice diet proved effective because of its low sodium content, but it was extremely unpalatable.

When too much salt is ingested by the body, the kidneys then have to increase their volume of urine and excrete more sodium in order to prevent too high an extracellular fluid volume (ECV). The volume of urine can be increased only by an increase in blood pressure. As the fluid increases, the blood pressure in the arteries also increases. Experiments conducted several years ago at the National Heart and Lung Association found that hypertensive persons tended to use as much as four times the amount of salt as did the average normotensive (normal pressure) person. They also drank twice as much water. Many physicians insist that their patients reduce the amount of salt they use not only to lower their elevated blood pressure but also to prevent any further rise in that blood pressure. Diets for both mild and severe sodium restriction can be obtained from your local chapter of the American Heart Association.

The other important item in an antihypertensive diet—fat, or cholesterol—is discussed in Chapter 5.

WEIGHT REDUCTION

Many centuries ago Hippocrates noticed that overweight persons were far more liable to die suddenly then those who were thin. Weight reduction is of significant importance in the treatment of hypertension, particularly in those persons considered obese. Obesity can lead to the development of hypertension and an 8 per cent increase in the risk of having a stroke.

In 1949 the City of Framingham, Massachusetts, with a population at that time of 28,000, was selected by the National Heart Institute for an ongoing health study. Framingham was chosen because its population consisted of a well-integrated cross section of people. Since then, the Framingham Study Group, as it has become known, has provided well-documented evidence of the role played by hypertension in premature deaths. Any death is considered to be premature when it occurs before the age of 70.

Out of a population of 28,000 in Framingham, 5000 volunteers were selected to participate in the study. At the beginning of this study none of the participants had any signs of cardiovascular disease. The research team conducting the investigation looked into every conceivable aspect of the volunteers' lives from their family history to their eating, drinking, recreational, and sleeping habits. Each volunteer received a complete and thorough medical examination every other year for 14 years. During this time those subjects who developed hypertension had between three to five times as many heart attacks and strokes as did those whose blood pressures had remained at normal levels.

The research team also discovered that obesity, cigarette smoking, inadequate physical exercise, and an elevation in the levels of cholesterol and triglyceride in the blood were evident in many of the subjects who developed some form of cardiovascular disease. These findings led the team to classify these factors as definite risk factors. This was the first time that an association between these risk factors and heart attacks and strokes had been documented.

As the study continued, evidence accumulated showing that even mild hypertension had to be considered a significant risk factor. Among the volunteers who became hypertensive, the incidences of stroke were four times greater than in those whose blood pressure remained at normal levels.

After extensive investigation, the Framingham Study Group concluded that for each 10 per cent in excess weight, blood pressure rose about 6.5 mm Hg and that in those who were overweight, a 10 per cent decrease in weight resulted in a 6.5 mm Hg drop in blood pressure. Other studies with an even greater number of participants have shown that weight reduction can, over a period of time, result in an average drop of 37 mm Hg in the systolic blood pressure and 22 mm Hg in the diastolic blood pressure.

Many of those persons who took part in the Framingham study and eliminated the known risk factors had a decrease in their blood pressure sufficient to place them in the normotensive group—that is, the group whose blood pressure was within normal limits.

One great advantage of weight reduction as a method of controlling blood pressure is that there are no annoying side effects, such as one experiences with many of the antihypertensive drugs. Overweight and an elevation in blood pressure seem to go hand in hand. Statistics gathered over many years show that the person who is overweight and who also has hypertension has a shorter life expectancy than would be true if the weight were normal. For men there is an 11 per cent shorter life expectancy, and for women a 6 per cent shorter life expectancy.

Extra weight also puts an additional burden on the heart. The average person's heart pumps the equivalent of 4,000 gallons of blood through the body every day. For each pound of excess weight, the heart is forced to pump that blood through the equivalent of several hundred extra miles of blood vessels a day. Taking this one step further, 10 pounds of excess weight gives the heart a workout equal to an extra 200 miles a day.

In 1979 the Pacific Mutual Life Insurance Company initiated a study of approximately 1,500 Americans. The study was conducted by Louis Harris and Associates to determine what weight was the healthiest. The evidence showed that in order to live longer, one's weight should be 10 per cent less that that considered to be the average.

Also in 1979, the Association of Life Insurance Medical Directors and the Society of Actuaries released the findings of their study on 4 million people of the relationship between blood pressure and weight. The results showed that when men had systolic blood pressures of 138 to 147 mm Hg, their risk of dying increased by 36 per cent, and when the pressure rose to 148 to 157, the risk of dying increased by 68 per cent. However, when hypertension was controlled, these risks dropped drastically to less than 13 per cent.

Women who have systolic blood pressures of 138 to 147 mm Hg have a 22 per cent increase in deaths. With systolic blood pressure readings of 148 to 157 mm Hg, the risk for women becomes 35 per cent greater than normal. Because the person who is overweight cannot move around too easily, he or she also tends to get less exercise, which also contributes to the weight problem.

Ideally, what you weighed at 21 years of age should be what you weigh for the rest of your life. Practically, this is not always possible. The addition of a few pounds with the passing years is a normal pattern and is taken into consideration when determining the normal weight for your age and height. Your own physician will advise you as to what your weight should be and will also prescribe a weight-losing diet should one be needed. This diet will not only provide for a reduction in calories but will be designed for you personally, taking into account any other health problems you may have, such as diabetes, hypoglycemia, ulcers, gall bladder disease, and so on.

The saying "He who is his own physician has a fool for a doctor," is no more true than in the matter of dieting, an area in which we have been swamped with suggestions and ideas, some from physicians and some from health faddists. Although each diet may have many excellent features to recommend it, no one diet can possibly take into account all the health problems any one individual may have. Not all people fit neatly into the same mold. Because this is so, it is the advice of your own physician who knows your medical history that should be sought and followed if you wish to lose weight.

EXERCISE

Exercise and weight reduction go hand in hand because as you exercise you use up some of those extra calories. If done regularly, exercise will go a long way toward helping to control a weight problem. Regular exercise may also help to prevent hypertension, and certainly exercise is a necessity once you have developed hypertension.

A daily walk for a mile or so, adjusted to the tempo that is most comfortable for you, be it brisk or leisurely, or sports such as golf or tennis or swimming in season, done in a relaxed rather than a competitive manner and with the knowledge and approval of your physician, should be part of each and every day's activity.

The American Medical Association has pointed out that a walk of just one mile a day for 36 days is a simple and pleasant way to lose one pound of fat, which in a year amounts to 10 pounds.

One of the first things Pope John Paul II, the most athletic pope in memory, did upon ascending to the throne of Peter was to have swimming pools constructed both at the Vatican and at the Papal Summer Palace at Castel Gondolfo. When chided for the expenditure he commented: "It's a lot cheaper than another conclave," showing the value he places on exercise as a means of leading a healthy, long, and productive life.

You can always walk indoors in a shopping mall when severe weather prevents your walking outside. Walking, as well as other sports activities, makes use of the leg muscles. These muscles contract as they are being used and in so doing squeeze the veins. This prevents blood from settling in the legs and causing them to swell. This muscle activity also aids in pumping the blood up toward the heart and then on to the brain. It was Dr. Paul Dudley White who first compared the leg muscles to a pump, and he considered them to be extremely important in maintaining good blood circulation. A constant free-flowing circulation of blood can prevent the formation of blood clots.

When you exercise, your heart works more efficiently and blood is distributed more evenly to all the blood vessels, even to the tiny capillaries. This aids in the development of good collateral circulation that may one day be called upon to take over for any blood vessels that have become diseased or injured and that cannot continue to supply blood, as happens when a stroke occurs. Adequate collateral circulation in this instance can spell the difference between recovery or invalidism, between life or death.

Exercise should always be at a steady and moderate pace, with no spurts of strenuous activity followed by long periods of inactivity. Exercise has a pleasant, relaxing, soothing effect on both the mind and the body and will do much to relieve the tension that contributes in no small measure to an increase in blood pressure.

Competitive sports are not for everyone. The tension, anxiety, and just plain anger at losing can raise havoc with some people's blood pressure. But walking is for everyone.

Using a stationary bicycle two or three times a week is another way to reduce blood pressure. Again, it is the leg muscles that are being used. Walking or bicycling outdoors, however, does have several advantages over using a stationary bicycle. Being able to breathe the fresh outdoor air and to see the constantly changing scenery can of itself be both restful and relaxing. Former President Gerald R. Ford, who used to exercise on a stationary bicycle in the White House, was heard to remark that "riding that bicycle is the most boring thing in the world." Most people would tend to agree with him.

The most important thing to remember about exercise is that whatever form it takes, it should be done on a regular basis. Walking several miles every day is infinitely better than a pressured round of golf or tennis just one day a week. Obviously such activities as snow shovelling and jogging are out of the question unless you are in superb physical condition.

If at any time, not just when exercising, but if at any time you feel any discomfort or pain in your chest, arms, back, or legs, notify your physician about it at once. Your physician will determine the reasons for this discomfort or pain. If it is necessary, an exercise stress test can be performed to see just how much exercise you can tolerate without bringing on pain.

Several types of stress tests are in use, such as a bicycle ergometer and the more commonly used multistage exercise test done on a treadmill where the work load is progressively increased by increasing the speed at which the apparatus treads. During an exercise stress test you are constantly monitored on an electrocardiogram (ECG) machine, and your blood pressure is taken at frequent intervals. The latter is extremely important for the person who already has hypertension because there may be an elevation in blood pressure while the test is being conducted. Any sign of angina (pain in the chest) or tachycardia (a rapid heart beat) will be instantly noted and, if need be, the test will be stopped.

The amount of stress your heart can tolerate without any adverse effects determines the amount and kind of exercise you can do. Stress testing is highly individualized, designed to set up an exercise program for only one person—you. Not every person of the same age has the same weight or even the same level of blood pressure and cannot, therefore, tolerate the same amount of exercise.

There are two types of exercise. The first is known as *isotonic,* which comes from the Greek words *iso* (equal) and *tonos* (tension). In this form of exercise there is no pulling or straining of the muscles. Walking, swimming, and jogging are examples of isotonic exercise. The other type of exercise is known as *isometric,* which consists of pitting one set of muscles against another set of muscles, as is done in weight lifting, water skiing, or in any pushing and pulling activity.

Isometric exercise can increase instead of decrease the blood pressure because of the tensing of the muscles of the arms or legs, thus causing a restriction of the blood vessels and a reduction in the flow of blood. If conditions were right for it to occur, isometric exercise could conceivably bring about an aneurysm. Most physicians advise anyone with any form of cardiovascular disease against doing isometric exercises.

PSYCHOTHERAPY AND PSYCHOTHERAPEUTIC DRUGS

Many people who have a mild or moderate form of hypertension also suffer from depression. For them, some form of psychotherapy, be it in talking their problems over with their physician, a member of their family, or a counsellor, may prove to be quite helpful, along with an antihypertensive drug.

The feelings of fatigue, irritability, self-accusation, and dissatisfaction that accompany depression always make the hypertension worse. Many depressed hypertensives are restless, dissatisfied people who have feelings of failure and of hopelessness and who blame themselves for their real or imagined failures. These feelings are hardly conducive to the calmness and positive thinking that are so essential in keeping hypertension under control.

If the physician feels there is a need to treat the depression along with the hypertension, many drugs are available—the so-called antidepressant drugs.

Some of the antihypertensive drugs have side effects that may include depression and a loss of libido. When the symptoms of depression are drug-related, either stopping the drug altogether or adjusting the dosage is usually all that is needed to eliminate the side effects. Those persons whose symptoms of depression are not drug-related are the ones who may benefit the most from some form of psychotherapy.

Although some of the antidepressant drugs do tend to cause an elevation in blood pressure, many others do not, and it is these that are used in hypertensive depression. In most cases, when the depression is alleviated so is the elevated blood pressure.

ANTIHYPERTENSIVE DRUGS

The use of antihypertensive drugs has become so common that we sometimes forget that they came into existence only after World War II. Prior to this time, attempts were made to control an elevated blood pressure by a variety of dietary means such as the Kempner rice diet, rutin (a substance derived from buckwheat), garlic, cucumber seeds, and even mistletoe.

In the late 1940s, the first real breakthrough in drug therapy occurred when an antimalaria drug called pentaquine was found to be effective in reducing blood pressure. This was the very first time that hypertension had been successfully treated with a drug. The side effects of pentaquine, however, prevented its continued use.

In 1954 reserpine, pharmacologically known as *rauwolfia serpentina,* came into popular use. Rauwolfia comes from a climbing shrub that grows in India and surrounding countries. These plants were used in primitive Hindu medicine for a variety of diseases such as snakebite, psychoses and, interestingly enough, hypertension. Mahatma Gandhi often chewed the roots of the rauwolfia plant for its sedative effects. Rauwolfia does have a remarkably calming effect, and its use could be considered as the first real breakthrough in the control of hypertension in modern times.

Through the use of rauwolfia and its successors in the drug field, the physician is now at long last able to control hypertension. Before the advent of these drugs, hypertension was inevitably a fatal disease. The discovery of rauwolfia was followed in 1957 by the discovery of chlorthiazide, which became the first oral diuretic. Prior to this time the major diuretic in use was a compound of mercury that had to be injected. The discovery of a diuretic that could be taken orally represented a great advance in medicine.

Today there is a veritable arsenal of antihypertensive drugs that provide safe and effective control of hypertension. These drugs can be divided into four broad categories: (1) the diuretics, (2) the adrenergic blocking agents (so-called because they block the release of epinephrine from the sympathetic nervous system), (3) the peripheral dilators, and the tranquilizers. All these drugs lower both the systolic and diastolic blood pressure.

DIURETICS

With the development of chlorthiazide in 1957, a whole new field in the treatment of hypertension opened up. The purpose of a diuretic is to prevent the retention of both salt and water by the kidneys. This is accomplished by bringing about an increase in urination. Diuretics are probably the most widely used of all the antihypertensive drugs and are the first choice in the so-called "stepped care" approach to therapy. Stepped care involves starting with a drug with the least degree of toxicity (such as a diuretic). If that does not work, the next step is to go to a more powerful drug, which although more effective may also have more side effects. Diuretics are Step One in stepped care of hypertension.

Diuretics, unfortunately, are not completely without some side effects, the principal one being a depletion of potassium. This problem can be overcome by taking a potassium supplement, by eating foods known to be rich in potassium, or by using potassium chloride instead of sodium chloride as a table salt.

Foods rich in potassium include the following:

FRUIT JUICES Grapefruit, orange, prune and tomato

FRUITS Apricots, bananas, cantaloupe, dates, grapefruit, oranges, raisins, watermelon

DAIRY PRODUCTS Milk and buttermilk

NUTS Almonds, brazil nuts, cashews, peanuts

VEGETABLES Baked beans, carrots, celery, lima beans, tomatoes, spinach. Most vegetables are rich in potassium when they are raw. Cooking causes a significant loss in the potassium content.

The level of potassium in the body tends to fall slightly in everyone during the first month or so of taking diuretics. The loss then tapers off, usually returning to a level that is just a bit lower than it was before the start of diuretic therapy. Because of the increased amount of fluid removed from the body by a diuretic, there can be an increase in the level of glucose, or blood sugar. Any of these side effects can be either eliminated or reduced in intensity by adjusting the dosage of the diuretic. So many different types of antihypertensive drugs are available that it is not difficult to find one whose side effects do not make the patient uncomfortable.

One of the great conveniences of diuretics is that they come in tablet form and often have to be taken only once a day.

TYPES OF DIURETICS

Three types of diuretics are currently used to control hypertension: the thiazides, the loop diuretics, and the potassium-sparing diuretics.

THIAZIDE DIURETICS Diuretics such as the chlorothiazides, notably diuril trichlormethiazide, whose trade names are Hygroton, Enduron, and Hydromax, work mainly because they reduce body fluid. They enable the kidneys to secrete more salt in the urine, which in turn brings about a decrease in blood pressure. Their action is relatively quick, bringing about an increase in the flow of urine within a couple of hours. A good reduction in blood pressure with these drugs is usually achieved within two or three weeks. There are two main types of thiazide diuretic, the regular and the so-called long-lasting thiazides. If thiazide diuretics are taken with other antihypertensive drugs, they tend to increase the effectiveness of the other drugs.

Some of the side effects that may be experienced include weakness, dryness of the mouth, nausea, an increase in the BUN (blood urea nitrogen), too little potassium (hypokalemia), too much calcium in the blood (hypercalcemia), too much uric acid in the blood (hyperuricemia), and an elevated level of blood sugar.

LOOP DIURETICS The loop diuretics exert a much stronger effect on the kidneys than do the thiazides. Because they act on the loop of Henle, which is located in the kidneys, they are called loop diuretics. Furosemide, known by the trade names of Lasix and Edecrin, are two such drugs. These drugs have the advantage of being available in injectible form for emergency use, as well as in tablet form for regular use. Although their action is rapid, they are effective for only a short period of time, because they are dissipated through the kidneys rather quickly. The side effects are the same as those of the thiazides. Loop diuretics are especially useful when there is any kidney insufficiency.

POTASSIUM-SPARING DIURETICS Spironolactone, known by the trade name of Aldactone, and triamterine, known as Dyrenium, are examples of drugs which, although they work by a different mechanism, still exert the same effects as the other diuretics. The difference is that these diuretics reduce the volume of fluid without depleting the body's store of potassium. A potassium determination test enables the physician to monitor the level of potassium in the blood.

The side effects of these diuretics can include nausea and vomiting along with weakness and headache.

URICOSURIC DIURETICS All these diuretics—the thiazides, the loop diuretics, and the potassium-sparing diuretics—can cause hyperuricemia or an elevation in the level of uric acid. This can be particularly hazardous in those persons who have gout. (A recently introduced diuretic, ticrynofen, known commercially as Selacryn, both controls hypertension and lowers the levels of uric acid.) Unicosuoic drugs have been developed that promote the urinary secretion of uric acid.

Urates, which are the salts of uric acid, can become deposited on the walls of the blood vessels where they act in such a way as to facilitate the deposit of lipids (fats) on the walls of the blood vessels, resulting in atherosclerosis, a known risk factor for a stroke.

When the serum uric acid level is elevated, the triglyceride level is also elevated.

VASODILATING AGENTS

Of themselves, vasodilating agents are somewhat limited in the control of hypertension, which is why they are prescribed along with diuretics or adrenergic blocking agents. The word *vasodilate* comes from the Latin words *vas* (blood vessel) and *dilatare* to widen), and their function is to widen the blood vessels.

Apresoline, Minipress, Hydralazine, Nitroprusside-D, Papaverine, and Minoxidel are some of the more widely used drugs in this category. They reduce blood pressure by relaxing the smooth muscles of the arterioles, which results in reduced peripheral resistance. These drugs were quite popular during the 1950s, but because of such side effects as headache, palpitation, and tachycardia, they fell into disfavor and in any event were superseded in 1960 by the beta adrenergic blocking agents (see page 77).

Still this class of drugs has not been totally abandoned. Nitroprusside and Hyperstat, both of which are vasodilating agents, are two of the most important drugs used in the treatment of hypertensive emergencies.

MONOAMINE OXIDASE INHIBITORS

The monoamine oxidase (MAO) inhibitors are still another class of drugs. They are not used as frequently as they once were, mainly because of the severe adverse reactions that can occur if processed cheese, yeast extract, chicken livers, or chocolate are eaten by the patient taking such drugs.

Pargyline, known as Eutonyl, is an example of an MAO that achieves its antihypertensive effect by inhibiting the release of norepinephrine. However, the effect of an MAO may be more that of bringing on a state of hypotension (i.e., low blood pressure) than in attacking the hypertension itself. The MAOs are considered to be excellent antianxiety agents as well, so they are often used for depression and related psychic illnesses.

ADRENERGIC BLOCKING AGENTS

The word *adrenergic* comes from the Latin words *ad* (to) and *ren* (kidney) and from the Greek word *ergon* (work). Adrenegic blocking agents depress an adrenergic or stimulating activity. By reducing this activity, blood pressure is lowered as a result of a reduction in cardiac output and vascular resistance. Examples of such drugs are rauwolfia and its derivatives such as reserpine; guanethedine, whose trade name is Ismelin; methyeldopa, known as Aldomet; clonidine, known as Catapres; and propranolol known as Inderal.

The ganglionic and postganglionic blockers belong to this category of antihypertensive drugs. Ganglion is a Greek word that refers to a mass of nerve tissue which both receives and sends our nerve impulses; in this case the ganglionic masses from the sympathetic nervous system.

Arfonod is an example of a ganglionic blocker, and guanethedine (known as Ismelin) and guanadrile are examples of postganglionic blockers. These drugs act by taking the place of norepinephrine, which is a hormone similar to but not the same as epinephrine. Norepinephrine, like epinephrine, raises the blood pressure. If this hormone is displaced, the blood pressure can be lowered.

Another group of adrenergic inhibitor drugs are those that inhibit both the alpha and beta adrenergic receptors on the smooth vascular muscles. Alpha and beta refer to two brain wave patterns. The alpha pattern is associated with passivity and a lack of anxiety. The beta pattern is associated with concentration and problem solving. Clonidine (Catapres) is an example of a drug that directly stimulates the alpha adrenergic neceptons.

The beta blockers help to block the anxiety, tenseness, and uneasiness that often accompany the drive and force displayed by those persons engaged in demanding jobs. The drive and force are not muted by these drugs: only the associated anxiety and tenseness are reduced.

The beta blockers help to relax the smooth muscles of the arteries and veins. In addition, they achieve an antihypertensive effect by reducing cardiac output and the volume of blood plasma by bringing about an increased sensitivity of the baroceptors and by affecting the central nervous system itself. They also decrease the excretion of renin by the kidneys.

The beta blockers are frequently used in the so-called Step Two Process of controlling hypertension, the diuretics being Step One. Stepped care requires treating hypertension at first with a small dose, then increasing the dosage, and perhaps adding other drugs as needed. It also involves matching the drug to the kind of hypertension the patient has.

Propranalol hydrochloride, known as Inderal, is one of the most frequently used of this class of drugs. Metaprolol (Lopressor) and Practolol are others. Like most drugs, they too have side effects that can include nausea, vomiting, diarrhea, constipation, rash, and depression. These reactions do not occur in all patients. These drugs are not recommended for anyone who has asthma because they can cause bronchoconstriction, nor are they recommended for persons with diabetes because they can mask the symptoms of low blood sugar (hypoglycemia), which must be carefully guarded against while taking insulin. Above all, when it is necessary to stop taking these drugs, their withdrawal must be done gradually over an extended period lest a myocardial infarction (heart attack) occur due to the sudden withdrawal of the drug.

Along with the diuretics and the alpha and beta blockers, the physician may add a vasodilator to the drug regimen, if it is indicated.

Drug therapy is always individually tailored to the needs of each person, and in this way the optimum results can be achieved.

TRANQUILIZERS

Tranquilizers such as Meprobamate, Librium, Valium, along with a host of others, have proven to be most effective in reducing tension and anxiety in persons who cannot escape from the pressures of their daily lives. The sedative effect of a tranquilizer can bring about peace of mind, which in itself lowers the blood pressure. However, tranquilizers are not a cure-all for all kinds of hypertension, nor are they a substitute for drugs whose main purpose is the lowering of blood pressure. They are effective against only hypertension that is caused by anxiety.

IN THE COMING YEARS

On the horizon is a whole new group of drugs, some only in the testing stage, others are in only limited use. Some of these new drugs will be enzyme-inhibiting compounds. There are new angiotensin antagonists. Angiotensin is a stimulating hormone secreted by the kidneys that causes a rise in blood pressure. These drugs will be able to block either the formation of or an action of angiotensin and thus be able to reduce blood pressure significantly.

Soon to be marketed is Catapril, which interferes with the renin-angiotensin aldosterone mechanism by specifically inhibiting the conversion of angiotensin.

Newer beta blocking drugs such as Metropol have recently been introduced into the United States.

COMPLIANCE WITH MEDICATION PROGRAM

In many instances hypertension has no readily discernible symptoms, such as would cause a feeling of being uncomfortable, distressed, or even of feeling pain. Because of this, many people find it difficult to understand the seriousness of the problem. Because hypertension presents no annoying symptoms, they cannot understand why they should keep on taking their prescribed medication, especially so when the medication itself has unpleasant side effects. And no one reacts well to taking any medication with the possible side effects of impotence and a decreased libido.

Feeling worse while taking medication than one does without taking it is hardly conducive to securing patient compliance. It is fortunate that so many different drugs are now available and that not all of them have the same side effects. A drug with which the patient can feel comfortable is now relatively easy to find.

Once you become hypertensive you will remain hypertensive unless and until your blood pressure has been brought down to a normal or near normal level and is kept there. In most cases achieving this becomes a lifelong endeavor. Medication and visits to your physician must become an accepted part of your life style. How well you feel is no indication of the level of your blood pressure.

Motivations for following a program designed to reduce your blood pressure are many and important. After all, lowering an elevated blood pressure can prevent a stroke or a heart attack. It can also reduce the premiums you pay on life and health insurance. Many insurance companies do charge a much higher premium for persons with hypertension, and there are even some insurance companies that will not provide insurance at all for anyone whose blood pressure is above the normal limits.

Studies by insurance companies, notably Aetna Life and Casualty and Connecticut General Life Insurance Company reveal that since 1959 the mortality rate among those who have hypertension has been drastically reduced, due in large measure to early recognition of the disease and to prompt and effective treatment.

The presence of even mild hypertension is an unacceptable risk to life and health. Even for persons whose hypertension is considered to be only mild the risk of dying from a stroke or a heart attack is four times greater than it is for those whose blood pressure is normal.

Young men in their thirties who allow themselves to become hypertensive risk an extremely unfavorable long-term effect on their health.

REST AND RELAXATION

For years the military has recognized the wisdom of scheduling periods of rest and relaxation—R and R—preferably in warm climates where those hazy, lazy days of summerlike temperatures can bathe the body and mind in peace and tranquility.

For persons with hypertension, vacation periods are of equally great importance. They should be part of a regular health program and life style. A change in scene, in the tempo of life, and having freedom from the stress and strain of daily living go a long way toward lowering blood pressure. And if this same relaxed, tranquil attitude can carry over into the post-vacation period, so much the better. Whatever relaxes you is what is important, be it fishing, reading a good book, seeing a play or a movie, or having a warm, relaxing bath. Whatever it is, that is for you. The body cannot and will not tolerate constant stress and strain.

Getting plenty of sleep is always important because it aids in relaxation, and, as we have seen, blood pressure is at its lowest level while you are asleep. An afternoon nap of a half hour to an hour is not a luxury, for it can make a great difference in helping to lower your blood pressure, in reducing tension and anxiety, and thus contributing to a longer life. Dwight Eisenhower, John F. Kennedy, and Winston Churchill all found the daily nap a source of renewed strength.

MEDITATIVE RESPONSE

The fight-or-flight response to stressful situations has fascinated scientists and medical researchers for a long time. There has never been any question that situations that give rise to anxiety or fear do cause a marked elevation in blood pressure. If these situations continue unchecked over a long period of time, what was a transitory rise in blood pressure as a response to a specific stressful situation then becomes a permanent elevation.

New methods for reducing blood pressure are constantly being sought. And in the search it was only natural that, as the interest in ancient Eastern religions and in Yoga began to have an impact on modern society, the correlation between meditation, which is so much a part of those religions, with its resulting decrease in anxiety and in blood pressure would become apparent.

Every culture down through the ages has had some technique for eliciting relaxation, usually in a religious context. In the fourteenth century, Gregory of Sinai described a meditation technique for the use of Christians. He suggested that what he described as a small prayer, such as "Lord Jesus Christ, have mercy on me" be repeated over and over while breathing in and breathing out.

In the first century BC, there was a Jewish form of mysticism called Merhabalism, which suggested that persons relax with the head between the knees and constantly repeat certain hymns or songs. Even prior to this time, in the ancient scriptures of India, meditation with its inherent relaxation was prescribed as a means of attaining a unified state with the Deity. In more recent times, hypnosis and autogenic training have come into vogue as means of elicting the relaxation response.

In the 1970s, with the support of the U.S. Public Health Service, Dr. Herbert Benson, a distinguished member of the Harvard Medical School faculty and the Director of the Hypertensive section of Beth Israel Hospital in Boston, Massachusetts, experimented with the use of the relaxation response in some of his hypertensive patients. What prompted Dr. Benson to try meditation was his observation that meditation seemed to bring about significant changes in the body's alarm system. It reduced the level of the so-called arousal response.

The technique Dr. Benson used to elicit the relaxation response was based on that used in Transcendental Meditation, or TM, and devised by Maharishi Mahesh Yogi. The word *transcendental* is derived from the Latin words *trans* (across, or over) and *scandere* (to climb). Transcendence is a state of mind that is achieved through meditation, and it enables you to rise above all fears, doubts, and negative ideas into a blissful, relaxing, peaceful state. It is not a sleeping or even a dreaming state but rather one of wakefulness in which the rate of the body's metabolism is low. During sleep, oxygen consumption is usually reduced about 8 per cent; during meditation it is reduced from 10 to 20 per cent.

The meditation technique developed by Dr. Benson is nonreligious and noncultist. The person who is to meditate sits quietly in a comfortable position in a quiet environment with eyes closed. All the muscles are consciously relaxed, beginning with the feet and going on up to the top of the head. Breathing is done through the nose, not the mouth. As you breathe in and out, instead of repeating a mantra (a special sound usually of one or two syllables, whose only purpose is to steady the mind to the point of stillness essential for meditation), Dr. Benson recommended that "One" be silently repeated, dragging the word out slowly as you breathe in, and repeating the word slowly as you breathe out. The use of a mantra or a special sound gives better results than relaxation alone because the repetition of a word tends to inhibit the drowsiness that relaxation alone brings about.

Some people find that it is easier when breathing in to say "One, two, three, four," and then when breathing out to repeat "One, two, three, four." It seems to match the rhythm of breathing in and out. This word, or words, is constantly repeated for a period of 20 minutes. During this time the slow, rhythmic breathing is relaxing the whole body and the busy, busy mind. Because meditation should not be continued beyond a period of 20 minutes at any one time, the eyes should be opened occasionally to check the time. The reason for imposing this time limit is that if meditation were to be continued for a longer period, say, several hours a day, there would be a danger of experiencing hallucinations. These incidents do not occur when meditation is confined to 20-minute periods, not more than twice a day.

When meditating, you are apt to find it difficult to keep from becoming distracted. When distractions do occur, immediately redirect your mind back to repeating the word or sound chosen; the mind will then relax and the meditation can proceed.

The best times for meditation are in the morning upon arising and before eating breakfast and again in the evening before dinner or just before retiring. It is not advisable to meditate within two hours after having eaten because the digestive processes appear to interfere with deep relaxation. Dr. Benson's patients showed an average drop of 10 mm Hg in their systolic blood pressure and about 5 mm Hg in their diastolic blood pressure. This finding suggests that the regular and faithful practice of the meditative technique does bring about a reduction in blood pressure. Blood pressure was reduced both in those patients who were taking antihypertensive medication and in those who were not taking medication.

During meditation there is a definite decrease in oxygen consumption and carbon dioxide elimination. The rate of respiration slows down to as few as four to six breaths a minute. There are even changes in the rectal temperature while one is meditating. The decrease in blood pressure that occurs while meditating carries over to those times when you are not meditating, assuring a long-lasting effect in blood pressure reduction.

Although the relaxation response admittedly may not be for everyone, those who have tried it feel it has improved their sense of well-being and that it has enabled them to develop a much more relaxed and positive mental outlook. Certainly all your problems do not disappear as the result of meditating, but you are less disturbed by those problems and consequently are better able to cope with them.

Meditation requires no complex machines or monitors. All it costs is time. It is available to all, rich or poor, sick or well.

BIOFEEDBACK

The term *biofeedback* was coined in 1969 at the initial meeting of the group that was to become known as the Biofeedback Research Society. It refers to a technique that uses an instrument called a biofeedback machine which emits continuous signals based on changes in bodily functions, particularly those changes of which you are not conscious. Blood pressure and brain waves are examples of two such functions. Biofeedback is used as a form of therapy in many functional disorders, the most frequent of which are migraine headaches and hypertension.

The human body gives off energy that can be measured. For example, when your hand is warm, that warmth can be measured in much the same way as a stethoscope picks up and amplifies the sound of the heart beat. The biofeedback machines are so constructed that any increase or decrease in energy, no matter how small, is immediately translated into flashes of light or beeps of sound.

One type of machine is equipped with lights similar to traffic lights. They are set to flash green when there is a need to speed up the rate of energy being given off by the body, to flash yellow to indicate that the rate of energy being monitored is the correct amount, and to flash red to indicate that there is a need to slow down the rate of energy being emitted. The purpose of the lights is to let you know when the correct response has been achieved.

The person who is being monitored, in this instance someone who has hypertension, sits comfortably in a chair. A blood pressure cuff is attached to an arm. Inside the cuff is a microphone that rests against the brachial artery in the arm. The microphone will amplify any fluctuations in blood pressure that occur.

The machine is set to flash a red light or give out a beeping sound when the blood pressure is too high. As the person makes a conscious effort to relax and the blood pressure is then lowered, the light turns to yellow. As the person learns to control his thoughts, be they anxious, fearful or whatever, he is able to arrive at a state where the light is almost always yellow. What he has to do to get that yellow signal serves as a guide as to what he should do to lower his blood pressure when he is under stress. Thoughts go in and out of the mind at alarming speed. As he thinks about something irritating, the light will turn red, indicating that such an irritating thought is indeed causing a rise in his blood pressure. It doesn't take long for him to begin to see all the little as well as big things in his thought processes that are causing his blood pressure to rise. Most importantly, he realizes that in a sense he can control his own blood pressure by eliminating from his consciousness all those aggravating and irritating thoughts. The biofeedback machine can also help to train the muscles to relax and in so doing can lower the blood pressure.

Waiting for a stroke to occur before doing something about controlling blood pressure is like locking the barn door after the horse has been stolen. However, even after one stroke has occurred, the risk of further strokes can be prevented by controlling the blood pressure and by keeping your blood pressure within acceptable normal limits.

SPECIFIC STROKE-CAUSING EFFECTS OF BLOOD PRESSURE ON THE BRAIN

Blood pressure that is either too high (hypertension) or too low (hypotension) may cause a stroke. The term *hypertensive stroke* is used to describe the stroke that occurs when blood pressure is extremely elevated.

The person whose blood pressure is kept within normal limits seldom has a stroke unless there are other risk factors present such as heart disease or diabetes. Repeated studies have shown that the survival rate after a stroke is lowest in those whose systolic pressure is immoderately high.

A cerebral hemorrhage is an example of a hypertensive stroke. And like a vicious circle, the severity of the hypertension increases after the cerebral hemorrhage has occurred because of the resulting increase in intracranial pressure. The risk of having a cerebral hemorrhage can be drastically reduced when the hypertension is controlled.

Hypertension adversely affects the brain, causing changes in the arteries and the arterioles, which are the smallest arterial vessels that conduct blood from the arteries to the capillaries. Generalized constriction of these blood vessels is a direct result of hypertension. This constriction leads to an acceleration of atherosclerosis in the larger arteries of the brain, which in turn causes them to become clogged, thus preventing a free flow of blood. Hypertension also contributes to impaired cardiac function, which can cause impaired cerebral function.

When blood pressure rises to a dangerously high level in the blood vessels of the brain, a vasospasm (i.e., a spasm or constriction of a blood vessel) occurs that can lead to ischemia. Autoregulation is the term used to describe the manner in which the blood vessels in the brain respond to any quick change in blood pressure. The blood vessels constrict (become narrow) or dilate (widen) in order to assure that there will be a constant, even flow of blood in the brain regardless of the changes in blood pressure. When hypertension is treated and controlled, the incidence of cerebral infarction is lowered, and hemorrhagic strokes can be prevented.

Hypertension is both the cause and the result of atherosclerosis, a condition in which the formation of plaque on the walls of the arteries causes them to become narrowed, thus interfering with the free flow of blood through those arteries. This narrowing can result in an inadequate supply of blood to the brain, which can be the cause of a transient ischemic attack (TIA) or, if the loss of blood is severe enough, a stroke.

If the pieces of plaque break off, they may clog one or more of the arteries and thus completely stop the flow of blood through those arteries, resulting in a stroke caused by a thrombosis or clot.

When the blood vessels have become overly stretched as a result of hypertension, they are unable to constrict once again. Often there is a breakthrough in the walls of the blood vessels, which allows an increased amount of blood to flow into the brain.

Sustained hypertension can cause these blood vessels to rupture and cause a hemorrhage. Hypertension that persists over a long period of time always weakens the wall of any artery so that any increase in blood pressure on that wall could cause it to break open, resulting in a cerebral hemorrhage.

Malignant hypertension can bring on many neurological symptoms that can be the result of a spasm of the blood vessel due to its inability to handle an extreme elevation in blood pressure. There can be signs of encephalopathy, which comes from the Greek words *enkephalos* (brain) and *pathos* (disease), including edema, a condition in which the tissues of the brain contain an excess amount of fluid.

The brain damage that results from a stroke is serious. Because hypertension is the number one risk factor in causing a stroke, prevention and control of hypertension deserve the highest priority.

CHAPTER FOUR
ATHEROSCLEROSIS

The second most important risk factor causing a stroke is atherosclerosis, commonly known as hardening of the arteries. By itself it is responsible for more deaths than any other disease and is a major factor in the shortened life expectancy of far too many people.

The word *arteriosclerosis*, which is sometimes used, is the general scientific term for a number of diseases of the arteries, including hardening of the arteries. The term *atherosclerosis*, on the other hand, refers primarily to the hardening and blocking of the larger arteries of the body, and the word itself describes the disease perfectly. *Athero* comes from the Greek word *athērī* (porridge), denoting a fatty material, and *sclerosis* comes from the Greek word *skērōsis* (hardness), describing the condition of the fibrous tissues of the artery.

As a rule atherosclerosis has no clearly defined symptoms until such time as an artery, being clogged by a buildup of plaque, becomes severely narrowed, which interferes with blood circulation. The presence of connective tissue that grows between these deposits of plaque makes them rapidly increase in size. At least half of an artery's width has to be blocked or narrowed before atherosclerosis can be detected by clinical means.

Dr. Paul Dudley White many times remarked on how stealthily and steadily atherosclerosis developed, with the person so affected having no knowledge of it. In fact, he found that his patients usually had felt extremely well until just before experiencing some angina (chest) pain when they were walking quickly or climbing stairs. Many times it took a heart attack or a stroke to make the extent of the atherosclerosis known.

During a physical examination, the physician invariably examines the eyes with an ophthalmoscope, an instrument equipped with a light that shines directly into the eyes. With this instrument the physician can look through the pupils of the eyes into the blood vessels located at the back of the eyes. Any constriction of the arteries, or any small hemorrhages, can be indicators of the condition of the arteries in the rest of the body. This is an invaluable, direct way of assessing the presence and extent of atherosclerosis and underscores the importance of the annual or semiannual physical examination.

An atherosclerotic artery has been compared to a tube or a piece of plumbing pipe whose insides have become filled with rust and grease to such an extent that the amount of water that can flow through it is reduced. The pipe finally becomes completely clogged so that water cannot flow through it at all. And like the buildup of rust or cooking grease in a pipe, atherosclerosis in the arteries develops not suddenly, but over a period of many years.

The inner layer of the wall of an artery becomes thickened by an accumulation of lipids, or fats. The word *lipid* comes from the Greek word *lipos* (fat) and refers chiefly to cholesterol and triglyceride. These fatty substances become embedded in the arterial walls through the course of many years. As these deposits of fats (plaque) increase in size, they gradually cause a narrowing of the artery, making it more and more difficult for blood to flow freely through that artery.

Plaques are fatty-looking, grayish-white or yellow patches or streaks in the walls of the blood vessels. The discovery that plaques contain some cholesterol led researchers onto a trail that ended in the discovery of the important part cholesterol plays in the buildup of plaques and, ultimately, to the role it plays in the development of atherosclerosis.

Plaques also contain triglycerides and fibrin. Fibrin is a whitish substance deposited as fine threads that form a jellylike substance needed in order for blood to clot. Because fibrin is often referred to as nature's glue, it may eventually be proved to be an important culprit in the development of atherosclerosis. Fibrin forms a crust inside an artery, and many researchers and pathologists are beginning to believe that this crust is the place where the buildup of plaque begins. The area of plaque does not have to be extensive in order to cause serious problems. A single piece of plaque, if it is strategically located in a place where it will completely shut off the flow of blood, can lead to a fatal stroke or heart attack.

It is reasonable to expect that those people who have a high concentration of fat in their blood will develop atherosclerosis at a much earlier age than those whose blood contains less fat. The types of fat, the conditions that cause fats to occur in the blood, and the treatments available to deal with them are discussed in Chapter 5.

Plaque may also cause a roughening of the lining of the arterial wall, and as the blood tries to flow through a somewhat clogged artery, and finds it cannot, a thrombosis or a clot develops. The clot may then increase in size so that the artery becomes completely plugged up. The part of the body in which the blocked artery is located is deprived of its blood supply, and damage to that area results.

Dr. Earl Benditt, a researcher from Seattle, evolved a theory on atherosclerosis that was supported by the renowned cardiac surgeon, Dr. Michael DeBakey. Benditt theorized that a cell in the arterial wall becomes mutated and then migrates to the inner wall of the artery where it proliferates and forms plaque. The intriguing part of this theory is that the process is quite similar to the proliferation of cells in cancer.

Although every artery in the body is subject to hardening, the arteries most often affected are the larger ones—the aorta, and the arteries that supply the heart, the brain, and the kidneys.

The buildup of plaque that leads to atherosclerosis tends to occur at those areas where the arteries fork, branch, curve, or split into smaller arteries. It is at these locations that we find evidence of the greatest degree of stress on the artery itself. The faster the blood flows through the artery, the greater the stress at those points where there are turns or bends. Stress tends to cause injury to the artery, and a buildup of plaque takes place at those injured areas. In the case of injury, atherosclerosis will develop regardless of the level of cholesterol and fat in the blood.

Plaque can also weaken an artery so that an aneurysm may develop. The word *aneurysm* comes from the Greek word *aneurysma* (widening) and is frequently described as the ballooning out of an artery.

ROLE OF ATHEROSCLEROSIS IN STROKES

When a blood vessel in the brain becomes clogged and the blood supply to that part of the brain is then shut off, a stroke occurs. This type of stroke is known as a *cerebral thrombosis* or *occlusion*.

We have seen the role atherosclerosis plays in the formation of a thrombosis. It is also implicated in the occurrence of a cerebral hemorrhage because the hemorrhage can occur as the result of the rupture of a blood vessel seriously damaged by atherosclerosis. The pressure on an artery already scarred by and filled with plaque because of an increase in blood pressure becomes something of a last straw for the artery.

The clogged artery may be located in the brain itself or in the neck where the important carotid arteries are found. The nerve cells in that part of the brain where the arteries are clogged are unable to function. This in turn causes paralysis, possibly a loss of memory, difficulty in speaking and communicating, and often an impairment in vision.

By depriving the brain of needed blood and oxygen, numerous plaques or lesions (small or large) can result in paralysis and that nemesis of old age, mental deterioration. The deterioration can encompass a lessening in intellectual capacity, an impairment of memory (especially as it relates to recent events and the names of people who are seen regularly), emotional instability, a tendency to live in the past and to reminisce constantly. In severe cases, when atherosclerosis is well advanced and present in many of the arteries of the brain, attitudes of self-centeredness and hostility that sometimes progress to a state of paranoia and delusion are not uncommon.

ATHEROSCLEROSIS OCCURS AT ALL AGES

As a rule, atherosclerosis does not begin in either middle or old age. It begins very early in life, possibly at birth or perhaps even before. This fact was brought to worldwide attention during the Korean and Vietnamese Wars when autopsies performed on American soldiers killed in battle showed that the majority of these young men had some degree of atherosclerosis. In some instances, it was an advanced degree. And remember, these were young men averaging about 22 years of age.

Fatty deposits of plaque have been found in the arteries of many, but not all, children and adolescents throughout the world. For example, they are not found in the Yemenite children whose diet is strictly vegetarian. The arteries of these children are perfectly clear. Contrast this to the condition of the arteries of the nearby Jewish children whose diet is not vegetarian and whose arteries show definite signs of atherosclerosis.

Race does appear to play a part in the development of atherosclerosis. For example, the natives of Africa and Southern India have less atherosclerosis than do the whites of the United States and Northern Europe. There are, however, difficulties in attempting to assign race as a risk factor because other factors, such as eating habits and the overall longevity of each of these races in the geographical areas in which they live, must be taken into account. Obviously, no matter where you reside, the longer your lifespan the more atherosclerosis you will tend to have.

Although there is some evidence of atherosclerosis in the Japanese people, any serious complications arising from it are rare as long as they continue to live in Japan. Let them move to Hawaii or to the continental United States, and the picture changes. They then seem to be on a par with the natives of these new places in the development of atherosclerosis.

At the age of 20 the rate of atherosclerosis is about the same in an American, Japanese, or black African. But after the age of 20, atherosclerosis tends to increase in the American, while in the black African and Japanese it does not. Atherosclerosis is the underlying reason for the increase in the number of strokes occurring in men in their early twenties and thirties.

Women are not immune to this disease although the symptoms of hardening of the arteries tend to show up some 10 to 20 years later in women than it does in men. Before the onset of menopause, women seldom have any complications from atherosclerosis. After menopause, they lose this advantage, and the incidence of complications from atherosclerosis becomes about equal for both sexes.

The tendency toward atherosclerosis rapidly increases with age, so that by the time the fourth and fifth decades of life are reached, almost everyone has some degree of cerebral artery disease. The mortality rate for atherosclerotic-related disease, such as strokes and heart attacks in males, nearly doubles with each 10-year advance in age, whereas for women it triples with each 10-year advance in age after the menopause.

Interestingly, atherosclerosis seems to be associated only with man; other species of mammals do not develop spontaneous atherosclerosis. It can be induced in them in a laboratory setting, but they do not develop it on their own.

The incidence of atherosclerosis has been on the increase in recent years, so much so that it is now considered to be one of our major health problems. The fact that the lifespan is increasing may be a factor in this increase, assuming that the longer you live the greater is your risk of having plaque build up in your arteries. But there is also a clear indication that the way we live may have to bear some of the responsibility. Rich diets, high in both calories and fat, sedentary living habits, too little exercise, cigarette smoking, and a hard-driving Type A personality are all factors that play a role in the development of hardening of the arteries. Environment thus becomes as much of a factor as does genetics, even greater perhaps in the sense that environmental factors can be eliminated.

Hypertension that derives from both genetic and environmental causes seems to accelerate the onset of atherosclerosis sometimes by as much as 20 years.

CAUSES OF ATHEROSCLEROSIS

There is still much to learn about the buildup of plaque inside the walls of an artery. So far, researchers have determined that of itself aging is an important part of the process, mainly because of the fact that the longer you live, the longer your heart and blood vessels have to work, and like the plumbing pipe that becomes clogged as it ages, so too do the arteries.

We have already discussed hypertension and the manner in which it causes the inner lining of the arteries to become damaged by the elevation in blood pressure, thus setting the stage for that lining to be more receptive to a buildup of plaque. The deposit of plaque on the arterial wall is greatest at those areas of the wall where the pressure of the blood is the greatest, indicating the critical role played by hypertension.

The role of collateral circulation in helping to take over the role of the plaque-filled arteries has already been discussed, as has the role of exercise in helping to strengthen the arteries and to keep them as clear of plaque buildup as possible.

When some of the arteries become clogged, the reserve or collateral arteries are called on to take over and supply a sufficient amount of blood to that area of the body being deprived of blood.

When an area of the brain has been deprived of blood, a stroke results. The important roles of cholesterol and triglyceride in atherosclerosis are discussed in Chapter 5, but suffice it to say that rarely is there a problem with atherosclerosis among those whose diet is largely vegetarian and low in calories, cholesterol, and saturated fats.

Atherosclerosis, which many researchers believe results from a nutritional as well as a metabolic problem, appears to accompany obesity, hypertension, a lack of exercise, smoking, kidney disease, diabetes, and hypothyroidism.

THE REVERSIBILITY OF ATHEROSCLEROSIS

After World War I it appeared that there was a much lower incidence of atherosclerosis among the people of Europe than there was before the war. Researchers felt that there was a distinct possibility that this was the result of the low-fat diet that had been a part of war-time living. Studies were undertaken in experimental animals in which one group was fed a high-fat diet, while the other group had a low-fat diet. In a study with rhesus monkeys, one group was fed coconut oil, butter, and an overall cholesterol-enriched diet. Within nine months, these monkeys showed marked evidence of atherosclerosis. Nine months later upon autopsy, there were not only indications of advanced atherosclerosis but a fivefold increase in the level of cholesterol in their blood.

Another group of monkeys, which had been fed the same cholesterol-enriched diet for 18 months, were then fed a low-fat, essentially cholesterol-free diet using corn oil as the main source of fat. Still another group of monkeys received a lipid- or cholesterol-lowering drug in addition to a low fat diet. Both these latter groups of monkeys showed significant signs of regression in the amount of atherosclerosis, and they also had a lower level of cholesterol in their blood. From these studies, the researchers learned that atherosclerosis was both reversible and preventable in animals. The next step was to determine if atherosclerosis could be reversed in humans.

Several drawbacks developed. By the time a human showed chemical manifestations of atherosclerosis, organ damage had occurred, as evidenced by a stroke or a heart attack. When this happened, the atherosclerosis had become so advanced that it had reached what might be called a self-perpetuating stage. Researchers found that by studying both the femoral (leg) arteries and the heart arteries by serial angiography, some idea of the progress of atherosclerosis could be obtained before a major catastrophe had had a chance to develop. It was at this time that the studies began to show the effect that eating fat-free diets, giving up smoking, and reducing hypertension have on atherosclerosis. The results obtained from the studies of humans were much the same as they had been in animals. By aggressively reducing the risk factors, the degree of atherosclerosis was also reduced, but not to the same extent in all patients.

Members of the same community, be it a village or a city, have much the same way of life. Overall, their eating and drinking habits are similar. Yet, despite these similarities, the susceptibility to atherosclerosis varies widely among individuals in the same community.

The factor causing this difference is the inherent structure of each individual person's arteries. In some individuals there is a tendency toward having a marked weakness in certain sections of their arteries, particularly where these arteries branch or divide into forks. It is at these junctions that atherosclerosis develops.

It has been suggested that a person's arteries may be as structurally different as are their faces. This might help to explain what has always been a enigma: Why, in a family in which both parents have atherosclerosis, do some members also develop atherosclerosis but others live to a ripe old age with little or no evidence of the disease?

The regression of atherosclerosis is accomplished much more easily when the disease first starts than when it has been present for a long time. There is such a significant degree of improvement once the risk factors that cause atherosclerosis are eliminated that it makes sense to eat foods that are low in fat, to lower any elevated blood pressure, to eliminate smoking, and to control stress.

PREVENTION

If not completely and absolutely preventable in all people, atherosclerosis at least can be held in abeyance by eliminating the risk factors that contribute to its development. Prevention must start in early childhood with emphasis on the low-fat diet, the control of any hypertension, however slight, and the need for adequate exercise and hobbies to reduce stress.

Dr. Paul Dudley White, in discussing the increase in heart attacks and strokes, stated, "Prevention must become our goal, and our first priority must be atherosclerosis, which has reached epidemic proportions in the United States. What is required is a widespread change in established habits of overeating, physical lethargy and heavy smoking—not an easy task."

To illustrate how physicians and researchers are constantly seeking ways of dealing with the problem of atherosclerosis, a number of years ago Dr. Ignatius J. Vondoukis, chief of the hypertension section of Detroit's Hutzel Hospital and a faculty member of Wayne State University School of Medicine, used a test that turned out to be quite successful in helping him screen patients for the presence of atherosclerosis. Although the test itself was not new, having been devised in the early 1930s in an attempt to identify persons most likely to develop hypertension, Dr. Vondoukis took the test one step further and applied it to atherosclerosis. The theory behind the test was that those who were hypertensive would show an increased response to cold. But since the test could not be confirmed in every instance, it was more or less abandoned. In most cases persons with hypertension showed the same response as those whose blood pressure was normal.

Dr. Vondoukis was trying to determine whether atherosclerosis existed by itself or only in association with hypertension. This test therefore became particularly useful when hypertension was not present in the person who was suspected of having problems caused by atherosclerosis. Dr. Vondoukis called the test the *cold pressor* test. When the test begins, the blood pressure is measured while the person being tested is lying down. Blood pressure readings are then taken every five minutes for a half hour. The lowest blood pressure reading generally occurs within 20 minutes and becomes the baseline blood pressure used for evaluation.

One of the person's hands is then immersed in a pan of ice water for one minute. The blood pressure is again taken and recorded at an interval of 30 seconds, then again at 60 seconds. The maximum rise in blood pressure is then taken as the response to cold pressor.

According to Dr. Vondoukis, persons with atherosclerosis show a much higher systolic blood pressure in response to ice water than do those who do not have atherosclerosis. When hypertension is present, along with atherosclerosis, the systolic pressure is even more elevated. He reached the conclusion that the excessive elevations in blood pressure precipitated by the ice water could parallel the stimulus given by emotional and other types of stress and could be considered an indication of the presence of atherosclerosis rather than of hypertension alone.

The implications of the test are interesting, to say the least. It is a safe test because there is no need for dyes to be injected into the veins, as is done with angiography, and no cutting, as when the arteries are examined by surgery. The test is mentioned as an example of how the fertile minds of experts in this field are constantly seeking ways of understanding atherosclerosis and, through this understanding it is hoped, will arrive at both a cure and a means of prevention.

ENVIRONMENTAL FACTORS

There are many continuing investigations to determine what, if any, effects the environment has on the development of atherosclerosis and other cardiovascular diseases.

The World Health Organization has found what it believes to be a connection between the concentration of cadmium in both the soil and the water in many areas of the world and the incidence of atherosclerosis, hypertension, and heart disease. Cadmium accumulates in both the liver and the kidneys. We have seen the role that is played by the kidneys in the development of hypertension. When it was observed that Africans who have little, if any, hypertension also have a low level of cadmium in their kidneys, and the Japanese with a high incidence of hypertension have large amounts of cadmium in their kidneys, the connection between cadmium and vascular disease became of more than passing interest. Subsequent laboratory studies further confirmed this connection. The more cadmium the laboratory rats consumed, the higher their blood pressure became.

The levels of two other metals, nickel and manganese, were also shown to be higher in the bodies of persons with vascular disease. Diets high in fats and carbohydrates usually have low mineral salts. This has led some researchers to question whether the effects of diet on atherosclerosis might not be because these foods are deficient in minerals along with being high in saturated fats. Recent studies have also shown that copper can cause an increase in atherosclerosis.

People who live in areas where the drinking water is classified as soft, (i.e., low in calcium and magnesium) tend to have more hypertension, an increase in plasma cholesterol, and more atherosclerosis and heart disease than do those who live in areas where the drinking water is hard (high in calcium and magnesium).

You can tell if you live in an area with hard water. If the water is hard, there will be annoying mineral deposits left on bathtubs, in steam irons, and in tea kettles. However, hard water does not leave deposits of minerals in the body.

In 1973 a study was made of 244 men living in areas where the water was soft and in areas where it was hard in separate English and Welch towns. Those living in the town where the water was soft had more hypertension, higher levels of cholesterol, and more strokes and heart attacks than did their counterparts living in the town where the water was hard. There also appeared to be a relationship between sudden death and soft water.

Sweden and the Netherlands have both reported a higher incidence of strokes in persons living in areas where the water is soft.

Both the World Health Organization and the International Atomic Energy Agency are currently engaged in a joint research project to analyze all the trace elements present in all areas of the world. They then will try to make a determination as to the actual role these substances play in the development of all forms of vascular disease.

TREATMENT

Drug therapy for atherosclerosis has met with variable amounts of success. Clofibrate (known as Atromid-S), Nicotinic acid, D-Thyroxine, and estrogen) all act on the principle of reducing the levels of cholesterol and triglycerides in the blood as a means of decreasing atherosclerosis. They are discussed in greater detail in Chapter 5.

In addition to these drugs, the roles of antiplatelet drugs such as aspirin have recently come into focus. In Chapter 2 we discussed the role of aspirin in the prevention of one of the early warning signs of a stroke, a transient ischemic attack (TIA).

Platelets not only contribute to the development of thrombosis but also to atherosclerosis itself. By adhering to the walls of the blood vessels, platelets form a place on which fibrin can form, and this facilitates the formation of thromboses.

So many factors are interrelated in the development of atherosclerosis that its prevention and treatment are dependent on removing and controlling the underlying causes.

With the exception of the use of angiography, which admittedly is both expensive and not without risk, you cannot actually see as a matter of practical day-to-day evaluation just how effective the treatment methods are. It is assumed though, that if the levels of cholesterol and triglyceride are kept low and the blood pressure is kept at normal levels, the rate of atherosclerosis can be slowed.

CHAPTER FIVE

CHOLESTEROL AND TRIGLYCERIDES

The blood lipids, the fats that circulate throughout the blood stream, are closely associated with atherosclerosis. They are a contributing factor in the development of atherosclerosis. In addition, of themselves they are known to precipitate strokes.

THE ROLE OF BLOOD LIPIDS IN BODY CHEMISTRY

Fats serve as a source of energy in the body and cannot, therefore, be completely eliminated from the diet. There are three main types of fat in the blood.

PHOSPHOLIPIDS

The word *phospholipid* comes from the Greek words *phōs* (light), *pherein* (to carry), and *lipos* (fat). Phospholipids are molecules of fat that contain phosphoric acid along with other organic chemicals. Their function is to transport fat to the liver and to other parts of the body. Phospholipids contain lecithin, from the Greek work *lekithos* (egg yolk). Lecithin is a fatty substance that acts as an emulsifying agent, thereby improving the absorption of fat within the body.

CHOLESTEROL

The word *cholesterol* comes from the Greek words *cholē* (bile) and *stereos* (solid). It is a waxy substance manufactured in the liver; it is also obtained from animal fat or from saturated fats in foods. The presence of cholesterol in the body was first observed by scientists around 1814.

Cholesterol is both odorless and tasteless. It is present in all animals, as well as in animal products such as eggs, milk, and meat. It constitutes about 0.3 percent of the body weight of an average person. It is found in the fatty deposits that cling to the walls of the arteries and that are known as plaque. These deposits eventually plug up the arteries.

Because neither cholesterol nor the triglycerides are soluble, and therefore cannot be dissolved in the blood, which is mostly water, there has to be some means of getting them through the blood stream. This is done by combining them with protein, which forms molecules called *lipoproteins,* or fat proteins, that can mix with the water. In this form they then are soluble.

Cholesterol has various functions. It serves as a part of the membrane surrounding a cell, as a solute for the protein that circulates in the blood and in other body fluids, and as a part of the secretions of the oil glands of the skin. Its presence helps to prevent the evaporation of water from the skin, helping to reduce the number of lines and wrinkles on the skin's surface.

Cholesterol plays a role in the formation of bile acids in the liver. It also plays a role in the production of those hormones produced both by the adrenal glands and the sex organs. Cholesterol is also necessary for the manufacture of Vitamin D within the body. Vitamin D is essential for the normal development and maintenance of bones.

Cholesterol is part of all the cells of the body, and a major component in the cells of the brain and the nerves. It is excreted from the body through the bowels.

The level of cholesterol tends to increase in men until they reach the age of 50, when it levels off and decreases somewhat. Although women tend to have a lower level of cholesterol than do men in early life, their level tends to rise after the menopause and does not level off until after the age of 60.

The dietary fats that contribute to the amount of cholesterol present in the blood are divided into three types.

SATURATED FATS

Saturated fats are solid at room temperature. They tend to raise the level of cholesterol in the blood by 5 to 10 per cent. The word *saturated* comes from the Latin word *saturāre* (to saturate, or capable of holding all of a substance). These fats are found in such animal products as whole milk, some kinds of cheese, butter, meat, cream, and also in some of the hydrogenated vegetable shortenings.

Hydrogenation, from the Greek words *hydro* (water) and *gennan* (to produce) is a process whereby liquid fats are changed to solid fats by the addition of hydrogen and the use of olein (oil), which is found in nearly all fixed oils and fats, and of stearin, from the Greek word *stear* (fat). The hydrogenated fats act in the same manner as do the saturated fats and thus should either be eliminated from the diet or used only in moderation. Coconut oil and chocolate, although derived from fruits, are classified as saturated fats.

UNSATURATED FATS

Unsaturated fats, which are sometimes referred to as polyunsaturated fats, are for the most part derived from plants. The word *unsaturated* comes from the Latin prefix *un* (not, or reversal) and the Latin word *saturāre*. Unsaturated fats, unlike the saturated, are capable of dissolving. They are the liquid oils of vegetable origin and remain liquid at room temperature. As it is not possible for humans to synthesize polyunsaturated fats, they must be obtained from the foods we eat.

The majority of vegetable fats are polyunsaturated (for example, sunflower and corn oils, cottonseed oil, soybean oil, sesame oil, and sunflower seeds). These are the fats that lower the overall level of cholesterol in the body by 5 to 10 per cent. They do this by helping the body to eliminate any of the excess saturated fats.

MONOUNSATURATED FATS

Monounsaturated fats are a third type of dietary fat. Peanut oil and olive oil are two examples of monounsaturated fats. Monounsaturated fats remain liquid when at room temperature. These fats appear to exert little effect on the overall level of cholesterol in the blood. Under no circumstances should they be used as a substitute for the polyunsaturated fats, which *do* lower the level of cholesterol in the blood.

The food you eat is never solely made up of saturated, polyunsaturated, or monounsaturated fat but is, rather, a combination of all three with one form predominating over the others.

THE DANGERS OF ELEVATED CHOLESTEROL

Not all cholesterol is bad; far from it. A certain amount is both healthful and helpful because it enables the body to use fat by moving it through the bloodstream. It is only when there is an excess of cholesterol and the body is unable to use it all that the surplus then adheres to the walls of the arteries and contributes to a buildup of plaque on those walls. It was not until the 1950s that medical science first noticed and documented the link between cholesterol and arterial plaque—a contributing factor in the development of atherosclerosis.

SOURCES OF CHOLESTEROL

Cholesterol comes from two sources:

1. Foods that contain cholesterol.
2. The cholesterol that is manufactured by the body itself through a process of internal synthesis. The main site of this process of internal synthesis is the liver, where large amounts of cholesterol are synthesized. The liver also acts as a storage place for the cholesterol that is absorbed from the intestines. There is a strong indication that most of the cholesterol in the body is synthesized rather than coming from the food we eat.

The cholesterol that circulates through the blood stream is called *serum* or *plasma cholesterol,* whereas that which is synthesized in the tissues of the body is known as *tissue cholesterol.*

Although everyone's body does manufacture cholesterol, some

tend to manufacture more than others. Therefore, even if it were possible, which it is not, to eliminate all cholesterol from one's diet, it would still be possible to have an overabundance of it in the blood stream. In this case, the cholesterol would have been manufactured in the liver and in the body tissues. The food we eat sometimes supplies less cholesterol than that made by our own bodies. What we eat can make it easy to accumulate far too much cholesterol. And because what we eat can contribute to the total amount of cholesterol in the body, it is only sensible to eat fewer cholesterol-rich foods. One can thus either prevent an excess amount of cholesterol from accumulating or, it is hoped, reduce the amount of cholesterol going through the blood stream.

Perhaps one of the most publicized studies done on this subject was the one headed by Dr. Frederick J. Stare of Harvard and Dr. William J. E. Jessup of Trinity College in Ireland. The study used 575 pairs of brothers. All had grown up together in Ireland for the first 20 years of their lives. Then one of the pair had migrated to the United States while the other had remained in Ireland.

Those who came to live and work in America had a higher rate of heart attacks and strokes and much higher levels of blood cholesterol than did their brothers who remained in Ireland. This was intriguing, to say the least, because the Irish-based brothers ingested far more animal fats and calories than did their American brothers. But they also had more physical exercise. The doctors concluded that it was the increased physical exercise that burned up the saturated fats in the foods eaten by the Irish brothers that kept the cholesterol from building up to dangerous and damaging levels.

TRIGLYCERIDES

The third main type of fats are known as triglycerides, sometimes referred to as the *neutral fats*. Triglycerides consist of those molecules of fatty acids that are linked to the glycols, those thick, colorless water-soluble liquids similar to glycerol. Triglycerides are produced by the body from the fat present in the foods that are eaten. They come predominantly from the breakdown of such starches as grain. They also come from sweets and from fat itself. They are either stored in the body or else used for energy. When the liver is unable to use all the available free fatty acids for the production of energy, it then uses them to manufacture triglycerides. Triglycerides play a role equally as important as cholesterol in the development of atherosclerosis.

Triglycerides can be found wherever our bodies are padded and rounded. In mammals triglycerides are stored in adipose (i.e., fatty) tissue until such time as they are needed, when they are then broken down into a molecule of glycerol. The word *glycerol* comes from the Greek word *glykus* (sweet). It is a clear, syrupy liquid formed by the hydrolysis of fat, and then formed into three molecules of fatty acid. The molecules of fatty acid combine with albumin, from the Latin word *albumen* (a coagulated egg white), which is a protein found in blood plasma. In this state they are then carried throughout the blood stream.

The storage of fat, mostly as triglycerides, occurs within the body more easily than does the storage of most other nutrients. The adipose or fatty tissue, besides acting as a storage place for fat, removes fat from the blood as well as making it from glucose. And like cholesterol, triglycerides are also found in the plaque that forms on the walls of the arteries.

Researchers have found that alcohol has a tendency to increase the plasma levels of triglycerides. Therefore, its use must be either restricted or eliminated if hypolipidemia (i.e., an excess amount of fat in the blood) is a problem. This finding is intriguing because it comes at a time when researchers, notably Dr. William P. Castelli of the National Heart, Lung and Blood Institute, feels that a small amount of alcohol may cause a drop in the low-density lipids and a rise in the high-density lipids of the blood. The key word here is "may." The whole question is still a long way from being solved.

TESTS FOR CHOLESTEROL AND TRIGLYCERIDES IN THE BLOOD

Testing for cholesterol and triglycerides in the blood can have many beneficial results. In seeking to determine the reasons for an elevation in blood lipids, previously undiagnosed diabetes mellitus, hypothyroidism, liver disease, pancreatitis, and even alcoholism may be discovered. Any elevation in the lipid levels can be decreased when the underlying disorder causing the elevation is brought under control.

By classifying the blood lipids according to type, it is easier to determine whether or not the elevation in lipids has been inherited or whether it has been acquired. The rationale for treatment is completely dependent on determining the cause. The tests are simple and easy to perform. That for cholesterol can be performed separately or as part of a health profile test called a Profile 12 (see Chapter 10), whereas the test for triglycerides is always performed as a separate test. Mallenkrodt Inc. recently introduced a new diagnostic kit for determining the level of serum triglyceride. Instead of relying on chemical hydrolysis, this test kit uses an enzyme system. A colorimeter is used to measure the concentration of triglycerides, which change color when they interact with the enzyme.

If the test were to be done to determine the level of cholesterol alone, only six out of every 10 persons with hyperlipidemia would be detected; whereas if the tests were done for both cholesterol and triglycerides, hyperlipidemia would be detected in nine out of every 10 persons. It is important that these tests be done routinely because the level of cholesterol, particularly in Americans, tends to rise with every 10 years of age.

NORMAL LEVELS

The normal level of total cholesterol in the blood is between 150 to 250 mg/100 ml. The normal level was formerly considered to be between 150 to 300 mg/100 ml. Many physicians today are of the opinion that even 200 to 250 mg/100 ml is too high and that it should be further reduced to 180 mg/100 ml. In any event, the level that would be considered as normal in a middle-aged adult would be far too high in a child. High levels of cholesterol or triglyceride, or both, in the blood of infants and older children may well be the first step on the road toward the development of atherosclerosis, even though the disease may not become apparent for many decades.

The normal level for triglycerides is between 45 to 150 mg/100 ml. It can fluctuate independently of the level of cholesterol, making it advisable to check it on at least three different occasions before a conclusive diagnosis can be reached. High fasting levels of triglycerides, at least in Americans, is often due to the consumption of excessive amounts of calories in the daily diet.

The higher the levels of cholesterol and triglycerides, the greater the danger of having a heart attack or a stroke. High levels of both are recognized as risk factors.

In 1951 it was discovered that high density lipids (HDL) in cholesterol seem to provide a built-in protection against heart attacks and strokes. Studies conducted by the Framingham Study Group have consistently shown that heart attacks occur less frequently in those whose levels of HDL are high, and they also have shown that when the elevated levels of HDL were caused by genetic factors, there was little evidence of atherosclerosis.

THE VARIOUS LIPOPROTEINS IN THE BLOOD

Electrophoresis is used to identify the various lipoproteins in the blood. The procedure separates the lipoproteins on the basis of the different electrical charges in their various protein components.

CHYLOMICRONS

Chylomicrons are comprised mainly of triglycerides. They are the largest as well as the lightest in weight of all the lipoproteins and are synthesized in the intestines. From here they transport the ingested triglycerides and neutral fat of dietary origin to the blood plasma and ultimately to other areas of the body to be used for energy or for storage.

Chylomicrons produce turbidity, that is, cloudiness in the blood plasma, when abnormal amounts are present. In fact, when the test tube of blood taken for testing is refrigerated overnight, chylomicrons form a creamy layer on the top, similar to the way cream does in unhomogenized milk.

It is perfectly normal for turbidity to occur in the blood at any time after a fatty meal has been eaten. But if it occurs in the blood when a person has fasted for 14 to 16 hours, as is necessary before a test of the blood lipids can be performed, it is a signal that there is something amiss in the metabolism of the chylomicrons.

VERY LOW DENSITY LIPOPROTEINS (VLDL)

Next in the classification are the very low density lipoproteins (VLDL). Their function is to transport the triglycerides that have been synthesized in the liver from glucose and free fatty acids. The VLDLs contain more cholesterol, phospholipids, and protein and far less triglycerides than do the chylomicrons. They do not form a creamy layer on top of the test tube of plasma after overnight refrigeration.

LOW DENSITY LIPOPROTEINS (LDL)

The low density lipoproteins (LDL), which are next on the scale, carry two-thirds of the total plasma cholesterol in the blood and therefore have become known as the chief cholesterol-carrying lipoproteins. The low density lipoproteins become trapped in the walls of the arteries. It is believed they get into the walls by infiltration. As the blood flows through the arteries, the fat and the LDLs penetrate the walls of the arteries and get stuck there. The fat filters through the artery walls, but the LDLs remain.

HIGH DENSITY LIPOPROTEINS (HDL)

The high density lipoproteins (HDL) contain no triglycerides but do have phospholipids, protein, and cholesterol. In size they are very small groups of lipids and proteins that circulate in the alkaline fluid found in the lymphatic vessels of the body. This fluid differs from blood in that it contains no red corpuscles and is more diluted. Since the early 1950s HDLs have been recognized as having a reverse effect on vascular disease, particularly atherosclerosis.

It has been shown that a higher percentage of women's cholesterol is composed of HDLs than is the cholesterol of men. The estrogen in a woman's body is believed to be responsible for this difference.

An HDL level of 45 mg per cent represents a standard risk factor in men. A level of 60 mg per cent cuts this risk by half, whereas an HDL level of, say, 25 mg per cent doubles the risk. The higher the level of HDL, the greater seems to be the protection against cardiovascular disease.

In women an HDL level of over 70 mg per cent reduces the risk factor by half, whereas a level below 40 mg per cent doubles the risk. On the whole, the HDL level in women is 55 mg per cent, 10 per cent higher than it is in men. This coincides with the fact that the incidence of heart attacks and strokes is noticeably higher in men than it is in women. It is also a fact that persons who are thin or who exercise regularly have a higher level of HDL than do those who are obese and sedentary.

Evidence from the Framingham Study shows that the level of HDL appears to have its greatest impact in the older age groups. One notable characteristic of those who live into their eighties and nineties and who also remain in good health is their universally high level of HDL.

Any laboratory that routinely does tests for cholesterol can also test for the levels of HDL. The test is of inestimable value in the overall assessment of hyperlipidemia. A cholesterol level of 200 to 250 mg/100 ml might be considered as normal or perhaps borderline, but if the HDL is below 45 mg per cent, then the combination of a moderately high level of cholesterol and a low level of HDL represents a decided risk factor.

Again, many times a person's level of cholesterol may be around 250 mg/100 ml, which is the recommended cutoff point. But if the HDL is high, say around 100 mg per cent, then treatment would not be necessary because in this case a substantial share of the total cholesterol in the blood would be in the HDL fraction, resulting in a relatively low risk of developing cardiovascular diseases.

Most men have an HDL–cholesterol level between 40 to 50 mg/100 ml, whereas most women have a level between 55 to 65 mg/100 ml. These are taken to be normal ranges. The Framingham Study showed that when the HDL fell below 35 mg/100 ml, in either men or women, there was an eightfold increase in the number of heart attacks over those persons whose HDL level was over 65 mg/100 ml.

Some interesting observations have been made during studies of the role that is played by HDL. Among them is the fact that cats, dogs, and minks, all of which are highly resistant to the development of atherosclerosis, have a high HDL, whereas humans, rabbits, and pigs, mammals prone to the development of atherosclerosis, have a tendency to have a high LDL.

Many medical researchers have come to believe that HDL interferes with the entry of the cholesterol-filled LDL into the arterial cells and also that it increases the rate at which the cholesterol leaves these cells. In other words, the HDL removes cholesterol from the tissues and delivers it to the liver. It also inhibits the intake of the cholesterol from the LDL, thus retarding the deposit of cholesterol in the walls of the arteries. The HDL actually gets the cholesterol out of the various parts of the body and transports it into the liver from which it is excreted. It has often been called the "good" cholesterol.

Long-distance runners have been shown to have higher levels of HDL than does the general population. Their high level of HDL is believed to be quite a protective influence whereas a low level of HDL is considered to be a major risk factor.

This is a phase of research that is currently exciting medical science and much is expected from it in years to come. Dr. William P. Castelli, the director of laboratories for the Framingham Study Group, has found in one dietary study that those who eat large quantities of fish have high levels of HDL.

Thus the total serum cholesterol and the HDL fraction taken together provide a much better indication of the lipid risk factor than does the cholesterol determination alone. This is particularly so in elderly persons.

In treating hyperlipidemia, the failure to recognize the importance of this HDL factor may perhaps explain why some people whose level of serum cholesterol is elevated appear to get along so well with a minimal amount of problems, whereas others whose level of serum cholesterol may be low and whose level of HDL is also low may do so poorly.

In analyzing the cholesterol levels of almost 5,000 men and women in the 16-to-49 age group in 1979, the Framingham Study Group found that the ratios of cholesterol to HDL was 3.4:1 for those whose body weight was at or below accepted normal standards and 5.1:1 for those who were obese. The ratio of the HDL to the LDL is much more important than simply the exact level of each. The higher the HDL and the lower the LDL the better.

Although there is no specific drug currently available that will increase the HDL level, weight reduction and decreasing the level of triglycerides, if they should be elevated, will increase the HDL in many instances, as will increased physical activity.

HYPERLIPIDEMIA

Hyperlipidemia is the term that is used to describe the condition where there is an excess amount of fat in the blood. It includes both hypercholesterolemia (an excess of cholesterol) and hypertriglycemia (an excess of triglyceride). Hyperlipoproteinemia is a term that is also used frequently. It refers to an excess concentration of one or more of the lipoproteins that carry cholesterol and triglycerides in the blood.

CAUSES OF HYPERLIPIDEMIA

As we have seen, there are three main causes that play a part in the development of hyperlipidemia—diet, heredity and acquired diseases.

KINDS OF HYPERLIPIDEMIA

There are two kinds of hyperlipidemia: primary, which is also called essential or familial, and secondary or acquired.

To determine whether or not hyperlipidemia is familial or whether it has been acquired, it is important to obtain a detailed medical history of the patient. In so doing, it is possible to rule out or to confirm the presence of the diseases known to be causative factors. It is also necessary to check the medical history of other members of the family to see if any of them have ever had hyperlipidemia. And, if need be, their blood lipid levels should be checked.

If there is an inherited tendency toward hyperlipidemia, it is only prudent to eat in moderation those foods known to contribute to an elevation in the blood lipids.

Secondary hyperlipidemia—rather than referring to a defect in the lipid metabolism itself as its name implies—results from those diseases that have an effect on the metabolism of fat, such as hypothyroidism (underactive thyroid) and diabetes mellitus.

SYMPTOMS OF HYPERLIPIDEMIA

The great majority of persons who have hyperlipidemia are asymptomatic, that is, they are without noticeable symptoms. The exception is found in those who have Type I or Type V, when there are apt to be recurrent bouts of abdominal pain. Bringing the hyperlipidemia under control also helps to control the abdominal pain. Raised, reddish skin lesions known as *eruptive xanthomas* are also seen in some people who have hyperlipidemia.

Another variety of skin lesion associated with hyperlipidemia is the so-called *tuberous lesion.* The word tuberous comes from the Latin word *tuber* (swelling). The swelling appears as a nodular lipid deposit under the skin. As the elevated lipids are brought under control with diet or drugs, these lesions usually decrease in size and eventually disappear.

Another type of xanthoma is called *tendinous,* so-called because it resembles a tendon. These xanthomas are hard nodules of fat deposits located in the tendon sheaths of the hands, forearms, and ankles. They are characteristic of a Type II hyperlipidemia, although they are also sometimes seen in Type III. As with the other types of lesions, tendinous xanthomas also are responsive to the general treatment for hyperlipidemia and will decrease in size along with becoming softer.

These lesions do not each represent a separate disease; each may occur in the same person simultaneously.

TREATMENT

DIET IN THE TREATMENT OF HYPERLIPIDEMIA

A million or so years ago our primitive ancestors began the habit of eating meat, a habit that has been continued into the present time. We have also, through the years, eaten those foods that contain large amounts of cholesterol and animal or saturated fat even though we do not have the physiological capability of handling these foods as well as do other animals.

Today, one out of five Americans has an elevated level of serum cholesterol, and most of them are completely unaware of it. The role played by what we eat in the development of hyperlipidemia was first noticed back in 1896 when Osler observed that vascular disease was rare among the poor but frequent among the more affluent.

Years later, dietary experiments on rabbits were conducted in Russia. These experiments showed that when the rabbits' food was enriched with animal fat or cholesterol, they developed a severe form of artery disease. It was also observed that the disease could be made regressive, or reversed, by feeding the rabbits a normal low-fat diet.

In more recent years, it has been seen that people who died from starvation (in prison camps, for example) have had little if any lipids in the plaque on their arterial walls. In contrasting the incidence of artery disease between the British and the American soldiers both before and during World War II—at a time when food restrictions were mandatory in the British Isles but not to the same degree in the United States—it was found that the Americans evidenced a rate as high as 23 times the number of deaths from cardiovascular disease as did the British. The British consumed few if any milkshakes, did not eat meat laden with fat, and only occasionally could get any butter or eggs to eat. Animal experiments have also borne out these conclusions. Animals fed diets high in cholesterol develop atherosclerosis, and, interestingly, they develop it even if their blood pressure is normal. When the animals' blood pressure was elevated, the same type of high cholesterol diet—as well as a diet substantially lower in cholesterol content—both caused severe atherosclerosis, further illustrating why hypertension remains the number one risk factor.

The main purpose in treating hyperlipidemia by means of a diet that reduces the levels of lipids in the blood is to halt, to reverse, and perhaps even to prevent the development of atherosclerosis. Although this may not always be possible, at least by coming to grips with hyperlipidemia and by actively treating it, there is some hope that it will not continue to worsen. Reducing the level of lipids in the blood definitely slows the rate at which the arteries become narrowed due to a buildup of plaque on their walls.

The second purpose of treatment is to mobilize the cholesterol from the body's tissues and to keep it circulating rather than letting it settle into a lump.

Once a diagnosis of hyperlipidemia has been made, the treatment to lower the levels of lipids in the blood plasma should begin promptly. The first step should always be to set up a diet, preferably with the assistance of a dietitian, that is geared toward lowering the level of fats in the blood. No one diet can suffice for everyone, if for no other reason than the fact that each person presents so many variables. For example, if the person with hyperlipidemia is also obese, eating large amounts of polyunsaturated fat oils with a high caloric content in order to lower the level of lipids in the blood would not be wise because these calories put on weight. And getting and keeping weight at a normal level is one of the most important aspects of the treatment of hyperlipidemia.

If hypertension is also a factor, the amount of salt allowed in the diet must be scrutinized carefully. Then again, if diabetes is present, the amount of carbohydrates that can be permitted in a diet also must be taken into consideration. If allergies are a problem, foods that either cause or aggravate the allergy must be completely eliminated.

Each diet, therefore, must be tailored to the needs of each individual person. Yet each diet designed for the treatment of hyperlipidemia does have one thing in common: It forbids eating fried foods, including food fried in polyunsaturated fat as well as that fried in saturated fat. Broiling, boiling, roasting, and stewing all help to remove fat from food.

Although the diet should always be tailored to the needs of the particular individual, there are general guidelines available as to which foods are high and which foods are low in both cholesterol and triglycerides. Foods low in cholesterol include the following:

- Fresh, frozen, canned, or cooked fruit or fruit juices
- Any cereal eaten with skimmed milk
- Vegetable soups made without meat stock and with skimmed milk
- Lean baked, broiled, or boiled beef, lamb, and veal; chicken, turkey (especially white meat with no skin), and fresh fish
- Liquid vegetable oils such as corn, cottonseed, soybean, and sunflower
- Margarine if it is not hydrogenated
- Egg whites
- Cottage, mozzarella, and synthetic cheeses
- Fresh or frozen vegetables—either raw or cooked
- Potatoes
- Any bread that does not contain egg yolk or dried egg, or lard, cream, or butter
- Skimmed milk, tea, coffee, and coffee substitutes
- Gelatin, Jello

- Sherbets
- Puddings made without egg yolk or cream
- Angel food cake and fruit pie made with egg whites and liquid shortening
- French salad dressing, macaroni, spaghetti, sugar
- Spices, vinegar, salt

Foods high in cholesterol include the following:

- Chicken and meat soup stocks and chicken soups
- Pork, bacon, mutton, duck, fish, roe, shrimp, oysters, lobsters, crabmeat
- Sweetbreads, brains, liver and kidneys, and stews
- Fish canned in oil, shrimp
- Egg yolks and foods prepared with eggs
- Cheese, except cottage, mozzarella, and synthetic
- Lard, butter and animal fats, coconut oil, solid margarine, and hydrogenated margarine
- Sweet potatoes, creamed or fried vegetables
- Avocados
- Frozen dinners
- All breads containing egg yolks, cream, butter, dried eggs, or lard
- Whole milk, cream, whole dried milk, malted milk, egg nog, chocolate flavored drinks
- Chocolates, cakes, pastries, puddings, doughnuts
- Any dessert containing animal fats, egg yolk, dried eggs, cream, lard, cocoa, butter
- Ice cream and whipped cream desserts
- Gravies, mayonnaise, noodles, peanut butter
- Nuts
- Any cream substitute made with coconut oil

Some foods low in triglyceride are the following:

- Diet jams, jellies, and candies
- Oatmeal, rye, barley
- Clear soups, consommés, and bouillon
- Salads

- Fish, lean meat, lamb, chicken
- Liquid oil (polyunsaturated)
- All vegetables except potatoes and lima beans
- Diet soft drinks, unsweetened fruit juices in bottles, unsweetened canned juice
- Gelatin
- Fresh fruit
- Tapioca prepared with skimmed milk
- Nuts, olives

Some foods high in triglyceride are the following:

- Jams, jellies, honey, candy
- Spaghetti, noodles, pastas
- Cream soups
- Salad dressings made with cream
- Animal fat, pork, ham, duck
- Butter, solid fat, shortening, solid margarine, coconut oil
- Bread made with egg or cheese
- Muffins, pancakes, sweet rolls, butter rolls, biscuits, cookies
- All fried vegetables
- Soft drinks, coffee, cocoa, sweetened fruit juices, alcohol
- Ice cream
- Sugar, candy, chocolate, icings

The difference in the diet designed to lower the level of lipids in the blood from a normal diet is that less fat is eaten in the lipid-lowering diet. Because 40 to 45 per cent of the calories in the diet of most Americans comes from fat, the fats are reduced so that they represent between only 20 to 30 per cent of the total diet. A much larger proportion of the fat that is eaten on the special diet is polyunsaturated instead of saturated. And the foods are those that contain less cholesterol.

Different approaches need to be taken when treating hypercholesterolemia from those taken in treating hypertriglyceremia. With the latter, it is essential that starches be either restricted or avoided altogether. Refined sugar, for example, is converted into triglyceride and then is partly stored as fat. Cereals are another product high in starch content. Whenever foods are eaten that are high in starch and in sugar content, the level of triglyceride in the blood plasma is elevated. This is the reason why the test to determine these values is done after a fast of from 14 to 16 hours.

Pectin, the fiber of fruit, has been shown to have the ability to reduce the level of cholesterol in the blood.

The evidence for the use of either Vitamin E or Vitamin C (ascorbic acid) in the reduction of lipid levels is not conclusive. The rationale for the use of absorbic acid seems to hinge on the belief that it can facilitate an increase in the amount of cholesterol excreted as bile in the feces.

With regard to Vitamin E, some researchers believe it helps to synthesize prostaglandin, but this belief has by no means been proved to be conclusive.

There are three main factors in a diet that have an effect on the cholesterol level in the blood:

- The amount of polyunsaturated fat in the diet
- The amount of saturated fat in the diet
- The amount of cholesterol in the diet

When these three factors are evaluated separately, the ratio of polyunsaturated fats (the P/S ratio) is qualitatively of more significance than the actual cholesterol content of the diet. To further illustrate this point, it has been found that adding 2 gm of polyunsaturated fat to a diet lowers the blood cholesterol to the same degree as removing 1 gm of saturated fat from the diet. The cholesterol in the blood plasma is affected more by the quality and quantity of the type of fat eaten than it is by the total intake of calories in the diet.

Another reason for adhering to a low-fat diet is to get rid of any excess weight and to try when possible to maintain the weight at what is considered to be the ideal level. The effects of a lipid-lowering diet may not be noticeable for as long as two weeks or even longer, but during subsequent months the cholesterol levels decline, providing the diet is one that proves to be effective for the particular individual.

The triglyceride level, on the other hand, falls rapidly with the reduction in weight and continues on a downward trend until the ideal weight is reached, at which time the level of the triglycerides then becomes stabilized. Attaining normal weight level also aids in lowering blood pressure, which is another risk factor, as we have seen in the incidence of strokes.

The American Heart Association has published some excellent diet booklets designed to provide menus carefully regulated as to the type and amount of fat they contain and that have 1200 to 1800 calories or 2000 to 2600 calories a day. Both the menus and the recipes for the foods included in the menus are available through your local Heart Association Chapter.

Only the physician, after evaluating the results of lipid tests and a health profile, is really in a position to determine if a diet severely restricted in the amount of fat is necessary.

Some fat is needed in almost everyone's diet and with the exception of persons already eating far too many fatty foods (in which case, eating less of these would only be an exercise in common sense), any diet that severely restricts the amount of fats that can be eaten should be prescribed only by a physician. Diets that are only moderately low in fat, on the other hand, will do almost no one any harm.

The American Medical Association, the American Heart Association, and all the federal, state, and local health organizations are in agreement that most Americans do need to alter their eating habits. The diet of the average American contains anywhere from 600 to 1500 mg of cholesterol a day. When prescribing a diet designed to lower the levels of lipids in the blood, many physicians reduce this amount to 300 mg a day. They also recommend that everyone's diet be modified to reduce the overall consumption of saturated foods and foods high in cholesterol. Dr. Jean Mayer, the noted authority on nutrition, has stated that 500 mg of cholesterol in the diet can raise the level of blood cholesterol between 25 to 30 points. This vividly shows how much the consumption of those foods high in cholesterol really do elevate the total cholesterol level.

In treating hyperlipidemia it is also recommended that protein in the diet be derived from fish rather than from red meat. The kind of fish eaten should be the kind that has fins and swims, which does not include all fish. Although most fish are particularly low in cholesterol, fresh salmon and tuna are high in cholesterol. Canned tuna, on the other hand, has had most of the fat removed from it during the processing. Shellfish such as lobsters and shrimp are high in cholesterol. Recent studies show that shellfish contain other sterols along with cholesterol. Previous techniques used to analyze sterols tended to group them all into the one category of cholesterol without differentiating among them. Because shellfish are high in sterols, it has always been considered advisable to avoid them when on a low-cholesterol diet. With the exception of shrimp, which is high in cholesterol, most other shellfish contains no more cholesterol than does fish and poultry on the basis of weight.

The noncholesterol sterols are not believed to have a definite effect on blood cholesterol. Because these noncholesterol sterols are still under investigation and study and because there is a possibility that one or more of them may prove to have a deleterious effect on the level of lipids in the blood, the best advice to follow is that of your physician. His diet instructions are important and are the ones to follow.

There is a layer of animal fat between the meat and the skin in poultry. This fat should not be eaten when a reduction in the amount of cholesterol in the diet is desired. Cholesterol is also found in the lean as well as the fatty part of chicken. Because what is left after the fatty part is removed is a smaller piece, to add an extra amount of lean meat to your portion in no way reduces the total amount of cholesterol you will be eating. The larger the portion of meat, the greater the amount of cholesterol.

One egg yolk contains 250 to 275 mg of cholesterol, and the white of the egg is free of cholesterol, yet both are high in protein. Two eggs for breakfast contain 500 mg of cholesterol. An ounce of butter has 300 mg. As you can see, it doesn't take long for the amount of cholesterol to build up. Despite the many warnings from the medical world that the American diet is too dependent on meat, bacon and eggs, carbohydrates, and starches, it is proving to be extremely difficult to get people to cut down on these traditional foods, let alone eliminate them. In an endeavor to find answers to the cholesterol problem, researchers are busily looking into altering the type of feed given to animals. They hope to be able to reduce the level of the undesirable saturated fats and increase the level of the desirable polyunsaturated fats in these animal feeds.

Because obesity increases the risk of developing hypertension, weight reduction achieved through reducing the number of calories that are consumed is essential. In addition, weight reduction also reduces the level of lipids in the blood. It soon becomes apparent just how really interconnected are all these risk factors for the vascular diseases that lead to strokes and heart attacks.

DRUGS IN THE TREATMENT OF HYPERLIPIDEMIA

In most instances, a diet that has been tailored to the individual needs brings about a reduction in the levels of cholesterol and triglyceride in the blood. There may be times however, when a physician will consider it expedient to add one of the lipid-lowering drugs, the so-called antilipemic drugs, to the diet regimen, partly because the diet may not be bringing about the desired results quickly enough and sometimes because of the presence of gastrointestinal disorders such as colitis and diverticulitis, which can be worsened by eating the fruits and raw vegetables that constitute such a large part of a low cholesterol and triglyceride diet. The antilipemic drug is taken in addition to the prescribed diet. It is not a substitute for the diet because when the drug is used alone it has proven to be much less effective in lowering the level of blood lipids than when used in combination with the diet. About six weeks are usually required for these drugs to exert their maximum effect on the levels of blood lipids.

There are four main lipid-lowering drugs currently used in the treatment of hyperlipidemia: clofibrate (Atromid-S), d-thyroxine, nicotinic acid (niacin) and cholestyramine (Questran). Each of these drugs is effective only during the period it is being taken. Once it has been discontinued, the levels of lipids in the blood then increase and return to what they were before the drug treatment started.

CLOFIBRATE

Clofibrate (Atromid-S) is particularly useful in treating hypertriglyceremia because it significantly lowers the levels of cholesterol and triglyceride. It acts by decreasing the synthesis and accelerating the breakdown of triglyceride-rich, low-density lipoproteins. The side effects are minimal, mainly in the form of stomach upsets.

NICOTINIC ACID

Nicotinic acid (niacin) is a derivative of Vitamin B and is effective in lowering the levels of both cholesterol and triglyceride. It does, however, have some drawbacks. One, it must be given in large doses that are far in excess of the minimum daily requirement for niacin. It can lower the triglyceride levels within four to eight hours and does so by inhibiting the production of VLDL. It also lowers the LDL indirectly within a few days. It decreases the concentration of serum triglyceride by preventing the mobilization of the free fatty acids from the adipose (fatty) tissues, thus lessening the liver's supply of a substrate or base that is necessary for the production of the triglycerides.

A second drawback to the use of nicotinic acid is that it can produce some rather undesirable effects on the liver albeit in very rare instances. It more commonly produces a most uncomfortable flushing sensation, which can be so annoying that many people absolutely refuse to continue taking it.

D-THYROXINE

D-thyroxine has proved to be moderately effective in reducing the levels of both cholesterol and triglyceride. This drug is contraindicated for those persons with angina, arrhythmia, or a history of heart disease, however, which rather limits its use.

CHOLESTYROMINE

Cholestyromine (Questran) may cause some degree of fat malabsorption, necessitating frequent checks of the prothrombin time, calcium determination, alkaline phosphatase, and the electrolytes. Questran is similar to a water-soluble, acid-sequestering agent. It is in powder form, and lowers the serum cholesterol by binding the bile acids as they pass through the intestinal tract. This in turn forces the body to excrete more cholesterol in the feces, thus lowering the overall level of cholesterol in the blood.

SUCROSE POLYESTER

There is a new approach to the lowering of the levels of blood lipids, although it is still in the study stage. Sucrose polyester (SPE), a synthetic agent that reduces the LDL that contributes to the development of hyperlipidemia, is the substance being studied. This drug, although reducing the LDL, leaves the level of HDL unchanged. The researchers hope that this substance can eventually be made available as a cooking oil.

THE ROLE OF CHOLESTEROL AND TRIGLYCERIDE IN STROKES

An elevation in the levels of both cholesterol and triglyceride has long been considered to be a risk factor in the development of atherosclerosis, which in itself is considered to be a major risk factor for a stroke.

During their research into the causes of strokes and heart attacks, the Framingham Study Group went a step further than had previously been done and considered the levels of the blood lipids themselves, irrespective of their connection with atherosclerosis. The results showed that persons under the age of 50 did show a definite association between the elevation of blood lipids and the risk of strokes. The Study Group did not, however, find this same association in those who were over the age of 50.

Although there is no absolute proof that reducing the amount of fat in one's diet can prevent atherosclerosis, most of the research studies do point to this conclusion. Consequently, most physicians believe in following the wise course. They recommend that the amount of cholesterol and other fatty substances be kept within strict limits in everyone's diet and that these substances be drastically reduced in the case of persons diagnosed as having hyperlipidemia. The Framingham Study Group did point out, however, that the increase in atherosclerosis did correspond to the cholesterol level of the blood.

The American Heart Association also believes that because foods such as eggs (which are high in cholesterol), meats, butter, cream, and whole milk (which are also high in animal fat, that is saturated fat) do tend to raise the level of cholesterol in the blood and because a high blood cholesterol level does lead to the development of atherosclerosis, the disease that underlies most strokes, it would benefit everyone if the intake of these foods were to be restricted.

The Stillman diet, popular a few years ago, was designed for a quick weight loss and illustrates perhaps as well as anything can the effects on the level of cholesterol in the blood of a diet that is high in fat content. The Stillman diet is noted for allowing the eating of shellfish and eggs at will, even though it did forbid the cooking of any food in oil. Dr. Frank Richman of the Harvard Medical School studied the effect of this diet on the serum lipids of a group of people who volunteered to be tested by him while on the diet. He reported that in these volunteers the average level of serum cholesterol significantly increased while they were on the diet. The change in the level of triglyceride was not significant. Dr. Richman concluded, therefore, that the total fat content of this high-fat, high-cholesterol diet did indeed have an effect on the level of cholesterol in the blood. The Stillman diet allowed 75 gm of fat per day, most of it highly saturated, but its outstanding feature was its allowance of an unlimited amount of eggs.

As we have seen, no one risk factor appears to operate by itself. The factors are all interconnected so that we find that the person with hypertension may also have an elevated blood lipid level and in turn will develop atherosclerosis. When found together, these risk factors become a much more serious problem than any one of them alone would be.

As the result of much publicity pointing out the dangers of too much cholesterol in the average diet, the level of cholesterol in the blood of Americans as a whole has declined between 5 and 10 per cent during the past 20 years. This drop parallels a drop in the incidence of deaths caused by vascular diseases—that is, heart attacks and strokes.

With all the controversy that has evolved and is still evolving regarding the pros and cons of the role of the blood lipids as a risk factor in strokes and heart disease, and with each side marshalling all its forces to support its contentions, it is well to remember the wry comment made by the noted Dr. Irvine H. Page. Dr. Page has said that, despite the controversy, he still follows a low-fat, low-cholesterol diet because he has no intention of being the smartest man in the cemetery.

The controversy that exists stems from differing opinions: whether reducing the level of fat in the diet can actually prevent atherosclerosis from developing or, if not, at least from developing rapidly.

CHAPTER SIX

DIABETES

Diabetics have two to three times as many strokes and heart attacks than do nondiabetics, making diabetes a risk factor of importance in these diseases. Although at the present time diabetes cannot be cured, it can fortunately be controlled. Because the average life expectancy of a diabetic who goes untreated is decreased as much as one-third, keeping diabetes under control can add many years to a diabetic's life.

The National Commission on Diabetes has estimated that every 60 seconds another American is diagnosed as having diabetes. This means that over 600,000 new cases of diabetes are found each year. There are at least 10,000,000 people in the United States who are receiving treatment for diabetes and another 4,000,000 who have it and who do not realize that they have it. The number of diabetics is increasing at the rate of 6 per cent a year. Therefore, the number of people with diabetes could double within the next 15 years. One newborn child out of every five will face the possibility of becoming a diabetic at some period.

Research by the Framingham Study Group has shown that the risk of having a stroke is increased by even a mild case of diabetes in which there is only a moderate elevation in the fasting blood sugar. When hypertension is also a factor, the risk of a stroke is further increased to six times what is considered to be the normal level.

Three thousand years ago the Ayurvedic physicians of ancient India described a disease in which the urine tasted sweet. The disease seemed to occur most often in those who had access to an abundance of food. The disease was also characterized by an excessively large output of urine. This is the same disease we know today as diabetes. The word diabetes comes from two Greek words *dia* (through) and *bainen* (to go).

Around the year 1500 BC, a thousand years before the birth of Hippocrates, diabetes was being described in the medical treatises of the times. One of these ancient treatises was discovered in 1862 during an archaeological expedition to the tombs in Thebes in Egypt.

These early Roman physicians referred to diabetes as the sweet siphon disease—siphon, because those who were afflicted with it urinated so copiously that the urine seemed to be siphoned out of the body, and sweet, because the urine had a sweet taste. Tasting the urine was the way these ancient men of medicine checked for the presence of sugar.

In the sixth century AD, the physicians of India used the word *modhuineka,* meaning honey urine, to describe this disease. For over 3000 years medical scientists have unceasingly searched for a cure for diabetes—a cure that has yet to be found.

The Latin word for honey, *mellitus,* was first used in connection with diabetes by Thomas Willis, a physician to Charles II, one of England's seventeenth-century kings.

In countries where people have tended over long periods of time to intermarry and where prosperity has permitted them a life of ease and a diet of rich foods, the rate of diabetes is high. During World War II, when the people of the warring nations had less food to eat, there was a decrease in the number of cases of diabetes.

Diabetes can affect animals as well as humans. There is no race that is immune and no age at which it cannot occur. It affects men, women, and children. But it is more likely to affect those who are over 40, who are overweight, and who have a history of diabetes in their family.

Black women are more likely to have diabetes than are white women. Noting this high incidence of diabetes in Black women, researchers have pointed a finger at the high carbohydrate diet of Blacks as a possible cause.

KINDS OF DIABETES
DIABETES INSIPIDUS

There are two kinds of diabetes. The first, known as diabetes insipidus because the urine is tasteless or insipid in contrast to diabetes mellitus in which the urine is sweet tasting, is a disease in which the kidneys secrete almost all the fluid they contain because of a deficiency in vasopressin, an antidiuretic hormone of the pituitary gland.

Some of the symptoms of diabetes insipidus are a severe, unquenchable thirst known as polydipsia and the excretion of copious amounts of urine, a condition known as polyuria. Headaches, dizziness, loss of weight, and sexual impotence can also occur. Diabetes insipidus is a relatively rare condition that can be either inherited or acquired, and it can occur at any age. An injury to the hypothalamus or to the pituitary system can be a triggering mechanism. The disease can also occur as one of the secondary effects of a brain tumor, of syphilis, or in the post-encephalitic phase of Parkinson's disease. It has also been seen for a short period in some women during pregnancy.

Usually the onset of diabetes insipidus is quite rapid, yet there are times when its progress is gradual. This form of diabetes is not fatal even when it is not treated. Unlike diabetes mellitus, it has no effect on nutrition (i.e., the way the body utilizes food), and it does not interfere either with mental or physical activity.

The diagnosis of diabetes insipidus is made by a test that determines the specific gravity of the urine. The specific gravity of a liquid is the ratio of the density of the substance, in this case urine, to the density of water at a specific temperature. The instrument used in the test is called a urinometer, which is actually a hydrometer having scale graduations that correspond to the minimum and maximum ranges of the specific gravity of urine.

The hydrometer itself has a weighted float whose stem will sink into the urine to a depth that is in proportion to the specific gravity of the urine. The specific gravity reading is taken at that graduation on the scale where the hydrometer remains. The normal reading for the specific gravity of urine ranges from 1.003 to 1.030. If the specific gravity of the urine is 1.010 or above, then there is no diabetes insipidus. When diabetes insipidus is present, the specific gravity of the urine is usually between 1.000 and 1.003, and may be even lower.

The administration of pituitary extract or pitressin tannate in oil is the usual mode of treatment for this form of diabetes. The excessive amounts of water consumed by persons with this disease have not been shown to have any effect on the cardiovascular system. No doubt this is because this excess fluid is not retained in the body.

DIABETES MELLITUS

The second, more familiar, and more common form of diabetes is known as diabetes mellitus, or sugar diabetes. This is a disease that occurs when the body is unable to utilize carbohydrates (i.e., sugars and starches) in a normal manner. It is characterized by an elevation in the amount of glucose or sugar in the blood and many times by the presence of sugar in the urine as well.

Diabetes mellitus is considered to be an inherited disease. Not all the offspring of a diabetic will develop this disease, but they will always have a susceptibility to its development. It is caused by there being too little insulin in the body or by some defect in the way in which the body's insulin acts, resulting in the insulin being unable to get into the body's cells. Some researchers believe that the defect is in the beta cells of the islets of Langerhans in the pancreas. Others believe that rather than being a disease solely of the pancreas, diabetes mellitus is also a vascular disease, a disease of the blood vessels. They believe that when these blood vessels become thickened due to a faulty metabolism, fatty substances become deposited on their walls much sooner and at a much faster rate than would occur in persons not diabetic.

The older a person gets the greater will be the chance of developing diabetes. In fact, the chances of developing it actually double with the passing of each decade. Any increase in weight over and above that which is considered to be normal for a particular age also increases the risk of the development of diabetes. And women have diabetes much more often than do men; married women develop it more often than do single women.

Insulin, the hormone produced in the pancreas (the gland situated behind the stomach between the duodenum and the spleen), regulates the body's metabolism of food. Two kinds of substances are produced by the pancreas. First, there is insulin, which is released directly into the blood stream and which regulates the amount of glucose (sugar) in the blood. The second is a pancreatic juice, which contains enzymes released by the pancreas into the duodenum, where it aids in the digestion of food. The end product of the digestion of carbohydrates is sugar or glucose, which supplies the energy needed to sustain life.

The nondiabetic person with a normally functioning pancreas experiences a slight rise in blood sugar for a short time after eating. It is then that the pancreas releases its insulin, which then acts on the glucose so that it can enter the liver where it can be stored. The insulin released by the pancreas regulates the amount of glucose that is then distributed to all the other organs of the body.

However, the diabetic does not have a normally functioning pancreas. Consequently, his or her body cannot get enough insulin in some instances because there is none, and what there is is not produced in a form that can be utilized, or there is simply not enough. As a result, glucose cannot be stored in the body for future use. Instead, it enters the blood stream directly or spills over into the urine. Because glucose is a source of energy, the body is then deprived of energy as a result of its inability to use glucose in the normal way. The levels of blood cholesterol and other fats then tend to rise, contributing to the development of atherosclerosis, which is a major risk factor in the development of a stroke. Glucose that is stored in the liver is known as glycogen. Glycogen can be quickly converted back to glucose or sugar whenever it is needed and released back into the bloodstream.

Indications are emerging that diabetes may not be simply a genetic or inherited disease. It has been known to occur after an infection, particularly from one of the Coxsackie viruses when these affect the pancreas. These viruses can destroy the beta cells in the islet of Langerhans that produce insulin, resulting in there being no way for the pancreas to continue to manufacture insulin.

A clue to the connection that exists between the Coxsackie viruses and the onset of diabetes came when it became apparent that the number of cases of newly diagnosed diabetes reach a peak during the autumn months, which is the same time of year these viruses also reach their peak. Along the same lines, the first case of the onset of diabetes following a case of mumps was reported by a Norwegian scientist in 1864.

TYPES OF DIABETES MELLITUS

There are two kinds of diabetes mellitus: juvenile onset diabetes and maturity onset diabetes.

JUVENILE ONSET DIABETES Juvenile onset diabetes is a more severe form of diabetes, occurring as its name implies, mostly in children and young adults. Its onset is abrupt, and its progress is rapid. The urine contains large amounts of glucose and also acetone. Acetone is found in both the blood and urine of diabetics whenever there is faulty metabolism or after a lengthy fast. It is produced when fats are not properly oxidized due to an inability of the body to oxidize the glucose in the blood.

In juvenile onset diabetes, the pancreas has very little insulin. Most of the time there is no insulin at all, so that the diabetic who has this type of diabetes becomes completely dependent on daily injections of insulin.

Complications such as vision impairment, heart attacks, and strokes develop with great rapidity. The most frequent cause of death in this type of diabetes is diabetic kidney disease. As one might expect, there is an overall shortening of the lifespan. Before the discovery of insulin, persons with this type of diabetes lapsed into a coma and died within weeks of the onset of the disease.

MATURITY ONSET DIABETES Maturity onset diabetes is the more common type of diabetes mellitus. Its onset is gradual, and the disease itself is less severe than the juvenile onset type. The progress of the disease can be so slow that it is possible for it to go undetected for many years. As its name implies, maturity onset diabetes occurs in middle or old age. The pancreas can usually still manufacture some insulin but not in sufficient quantity to handle the metabolism of food.

Diet, exercise, and oral drugs can usually control this type of diabetes in the majority of patients. When they do not, daily injections of insulin must be given.

SYMPTOMS OF DIABETES MELLITUS

Diabetes mellitus has many times been called "the great imitator" because it can produce a great variety of symptoms in every organ of the body, symptoms that can imitate many different kinds of diseases. It has also been called a sneaky disease because its symptoms are not always apparent and may indeed be nonexistent. Although it usually develops gradually over a long period of time, there have been instances when its onset was abrupt.

The symptoms of diabetes mellitus can be many and varied—ranging from hunger, known as polyphagia, which results in an increase in appetite; thirst, known as polydipsia; frequent urination, known as polyuria; weight loss; fatigue; drowsiness; itching and irritation of the skin, particularly in the rectal and vaginal areas; slow healing of cuts, especially on the feet; and changes in vision.

There are many people who are overweight and who have mild diabetes and yet are completely unaware that they have it. It is in fact sneaking up on them.

Recurring staphylococcal infections that show up as boils and carbuncles, as well as glaucoma, coronary insufficiency, and absence of the Achilles' tendon reflex, and any indications of peripheral vascular disease can also be suggestive of diabetes. When any of these conditions occur, the blood and the urine should be tested for diabetes.

Diabetes can also occur without symptoms. This fact accentuates the importance of having urine and blood tests each year. Only then is it possible for the disease to be detected early enough so that any of the complications so often associated with diabetes can be prevented.

The American Diabetes Association recognizes four stages in the diabetic process:

1. *Pre-diabetes* is the stage that includes those persons who have inherited the diabetic gene but who show no signs of an elevation in their levels of blood sugar. This stage lasts from the moment of birth until the onset of overt diabetes.

2. *Suspected diabetes* has also been called subclinical diabetes. Although the results of both the fasting blood sugar and glucose tolerance tests may be normal much of the time, diabetes may be suspected because the glucose tolerance level becomes elevated during periods of stress and/or illness but returns to normal when stress is no longer present and the illness has been cured.

3. *Chemical diabetes or latent diabetes* is the stage in which the blood sugar can be either normal or elevated in the standard glucose test, but the glucose tolerance test is abnormal. There are no symptoms present.

There is enough insulin secreted when fasting or when not eating so that the blood sugar remains at a normal level. After eating or after injecting glucose as part of a glucose tolerance test, however, the blood sugar levels then become elevated, and sugar may also spill over into the urine. Thirty per cent of those persons who have chemical diabetes will eventually develop overt diabetes.

4. *Overt or clinical diabetes* is the stage where the fasting blood sugar is consistently above normal limits and where there are also some clinical signs of diabetes such as loss of weight, excessive thirst and increased urination.

TESTING FOR DIABETES

There are two ways of testing for diabetes: a urine test and a blood test.

URINE TEST In *most* instances in diabetes, but not all, glucose or sugar tends to spill over into the urine. Therefore, a urine test will not disclose all cases of diabetes. In many mild cases, diabetes can be detected only by a blood test to determine the level of sugar in the blood. Sugar always appears in the blood before it does in the urine.

A urine test is a very simple, inexpensive way to determine the presence of sugar in the urine. A piece of specially treated tape (for example, Testape made by Lilly) is dipped into the urine. Sugar in the urine then colors the tape. The amount of sugar present is determined by comparing the color of the tape with the colors on a chart furnished with the test packet. Each color represents a different amount of sugar. This is the method most diabetics use each day to check on how well their diabetes is being controlled. From these results they know whether the amount of insulin they are taking should be increased or decreased, or whether their diet should be altered in any way.

There is a condition known as renal glycosuria in which sugar appears only in the urine and not in the blood. Renal glycosuria is not diabetes. There are also some other instances when the sugar in the urine is not glucose but rather grape sugar or fructose, which is considered to be harmless. Milk sugar or lactose may be found in the urine of nursing mothers and this, too, is considered harmless.

In addition to the simple tape test for the presence of sugar in the urine, there is also what is known as a 24-hour urine quantitative glucose determination test, which is conducted as follows. After discarding the first urine voided, the urine is then collected over a 24-hour period. Then a specimen from the total amount of urine that has been collected is tested, usually with Clinitest (made by Ames) to determine the percentage of sugar present in the urine. The number of ounces of urine is converted to millimeters—one ounce being equal to 30 ml. The total number of millimeters of urine is then multiplied by the percentage of sugar as determined by the Clinitest. The result is the amount of sugar that has been lost from the body into the urine during a 24-hour period. If the diabetic being tested has excreted more than 5 per cent of the total amount of carbohydrates ingested in a 24-hour period, he or she is considered to be making poor use of these carbohydrates and consequently does not have a good degree of control over the diabetes.

BLOOD TEST The second method, and by far the more accurate for checking for diabetes, is a blood test for glucose or sugar. Diabetes can always be detected much sooner through a blood test than it can through a urine test. A blood test can be done either in a physician's office, a hospital clinic, or a medical diagnostic laboratory.

The blood test is usually done in the morning after an overnight fast and before breakfast. Blood sugar always rises after eating, and a test for sugar done at this time is known as a postprandial blood sugar test.

For an accurate glucose assessment, it is necessary, therefore, to have fasted overnight. The normal fasting level of blood sugar is 65 to 110 mg/100 ml.

Another variation of the blood sugar test is known as the glucose tolerance test. This test is always done in the morning after an overnight fast, and the test can take from three to six hours. The first blood sample taken becomes the base fasting reading. Then the patient drinks 100 grams (3.33 ounces) of glucose in water or a somewhat smaller or larger amount if he is below or above the average in weight and height.

Blood is then taken, usually from a vein in the arm, at half-hour to one-hour intervals. The normal readings are as follows:

30 minutes	75 to 140 mg/100 ml
1 hour	140 to 160 mg/100 ml
2 hours	70 to 115 mg/100 ml
3 hours	65 to 115 mg/100 ml
4 hours	65 to 115 mg/100 ml
5 hours	65 to 115 mg/100 ml
6 hours	65 to 115 mg/100 ml

These readings are based on the values that prevail in nondiabetic, healthy persons. The blood taken from the arm at each of these intervals is analyzed for the presence of glucose, and the results are then compared to the normals in the chart and noted on the patient's record. This is the test that is given when hypoglycemia or low blood sugar, the opposite of diabetes, is suspected. In hypoglycemia, the blood sugar level drops drastically from the third hour on during testing.

Diabetes can be present without there being sugar in the urine. In fact, the blood sugar may have to be over 180 mg/100 ml before sugar does appear in the urine. The sugar that appears in the urine results from spillage. This test result emphasizes the importance of never relying solely on urine tests for a diagnosis of diabetes.

The kidneys filter approximately 45 gallons of fluid from the body each day. Normally the glucose in the fluid is reabsorbed by the kidneys and then returned to the body, but when there is a higher amount of glucose than normal and it then exceeds the limits of what the kidneys can reabsorb, this glucose is then excreted by the kidneys into the urine. This is the sugar that shows up when a test for sugar in the urine is made.

DIABETES AND HYPERTENSION

As a group, diabetics have more hypertension than do nondiabetics. In fact, a third of all diabetics are hypertensive.

Thus, having diabetes and having hypertension presents a double risk factor in the development of strokes.

DIABETES AND ATHEROSCLEROSIS

Diabetes contributes to the development of atherosclerosis. The control of diabetes is therefore of vital concern in the prevention of strokes.

Atherosclerosis tends to develop about 10 years earlier in the diabetic than it does in the nondiabetic. Death from atherosclerotic-related heart disease and strokes in the diabetic is five times greater than it is in the general population. Atherosclerotic complications can be lessened if the diabetic diet makes use of polyunsaturated fats in place of the saturated fats. A myocardial infarction (a heart attack brought on by a thrombosis or clot,) is the main cause of death in those persons whose diabetes developed after the age of 30.

Vascular disease that develops in diabetics is much more severe than it is in nondiabetics. It is the inability of the body to make use of sugar that brings on many of these vascular problems because of a deficiency in insulin in the body that allows fats to accumulate in the blood of a diabetic.

Two out of every three diabetics develop some form of cardio- or cerebrovascular disease. The Framingham Study Group showed that the instances of coronary disease, congestive heart failure, and atherothrombotic brain infarction (a stroke caused by the plugging up of an artery in the brain) were directly related to the amount of glucose present in the blood. The higher the level of blood sugar, the greater the risk of vascular disease. The men who took part in this study had twice as many heart attacks and strokes as did the women, even though the incidence of strokes and heart attacks for the women rose with age.

Diabetic women have no immunity at any age from either heart attacks or strokes.

Strokes and heart attacks occur earlier in those persons who have diabetes, and they are much more likely to be fatal than they are for the nondiabetics.

In the Framingham Study, 75 per cent of the deaths among the diabetic men who took part in the study were due to heart attacks and strokes whereas among the diabetic women it was 80 per cent.

The atherosclerosis that develops in the diabetic and at a much earlier age is very similar to that which develops with age in the nondiabetic person. This means that a diabetic could have a heart attack or a stroke at an extremely young age—when only in the twenties or thirties.

There is an overall 7 1/2 per cent increase in the mortality for a myocardial infarction in those men who are diabetic, whereas in women the increase in death rate after a myocardial infarction amounts to 14 per cent.

The plaque that adheres to the walls of the arteries of a diabetic is believed to be associated with the diabetes insofar as it is the diabetes that has hastened the formation of the plaque on the walls of the arteries. When the blood vessels of the heart become clogged with plaque, the circulation of blood to and in the heart is severely affected. The result can be a heart attack.

When plaque clogs up the arteries of the brain, a stroke can occur. In persons who have had diabetes for a long time, the blood vessels have a tendency to become thickened and roughened. We have already seen in Chapter 4 with what ease plaque adheres to these roughened surfaces.

Many studies conducted throughout the world confirm those made at the Royal Victoria Hospital in Belfast, Northern Ireland.

These studies showed that the majority of diabetics who have maturity onset diabetes also have abnormally low levels of HDL (high density lipoproteins), which is considered to be a risk factor in the development of heart attacks and strokes. Physicians at Flenders Medical Centre in Bedford Park, South Australia, also found that as the diabetes was brought under better control, the HDL levels rose significantly.

Xanthomas, which are small, raised reddish-yellow skin lesions composed of plaque, can develop in persons whose diabetes is untreated because of the excessively high levels of lipids (fats) in their blood.

Along with the blood vessels in the heart and brain, the blood vessels in the eyes and the kidneys are also affected by diabetes.

DIABETES AND AGING

Atherosclerosis is not the only sign of senescence or old age that comes earlier to the diabetic than to the nondiabetic. The pancreas of a diabetic at 50 years of age resembles that of a nondiabetic who is 100 years of age. Cataracts normally associated with the aging process also develop at a much earlier age in the diabetic.

DIABETIC RETINOPATHY

Eye damage as a result of diabetes is most frequently seen in the retina. It is called diabetic retinopathy. The retina is that part of the eye that is sensitive to light. Any damage to the retina affects the ability to see. Diabetes has become the third leading cause of blindness. The cells of the retina are supplied with blood and oxygen by tiny capillaries that also remove any waste material. It is when these capillaries lose their ability to supply blood and oxygen and to remove waste material because they have become clogged up because the body is unable to metabolize sugar properly that the retina is damaged. Some of the fatty molecules from the insulin itself, which is a fat-producing hormone, can remain in the walls of these capillaries and prevent blood from flowing through them. These capillaries can also lose their elasticity and balloon out so that they may in fact be bringing too much blood to one part of the retina and not enough to another part. The tiny blood vessels in the eye can burst, resulting in the appearance of blind spots when you are looking at something or someone. When a physician examines the eyes of a diabetic, he does so to see if there are any changes in the blood vessels in the eyes.

As we saw in Chapter 1, the retina of the eye is the one place in the human body where a physician can actually see the condition of a blood vessel simply by looking at it. The blood vessels in the retina give an excellent indication of the condition of the other blood vessels throughout the rest of the body.

The severity of the retinopathy is directly related to the length of time that diabetes has been present. It is also more severe in diabetics who are taking very large doses of insulin.

DIABETES AND STRESS

Severe emotional stress has been known to be the triggering mechanism for the development of diabetes in those who have an inherited tendency toward it.

Stress does not have to be only emotional. It can also be physical, such as the stress of obesity, which is seen in over 80 per cent of all adult diabetics. Other stress factors are the aging process, when the chances of developing diabetes increases with every year of life; physical trauma, which can include not only accidents such as in automobiles but also serious illnesses and surgery; some medications such as cortisone; and some conditions, like pregnancy. Any one can be the triggering mechanism for bringing on maturity onset diabetes mellitus.

The stress caused to the body when excessive amounts of hormones are secreted by the thyroid, pituitary, and adrenal glands can also bring on diabetes.

Diuretics that are taken to reduce the retention of the fluid in the body, which in excess is so damaging to the heart, can also cause a temporary increase in the levels of blood sugar. This, however, is not indicative of true diabetes.

SMOKING AND DIABETES

Diabetes increases the risk of having a heart attack or a stroke by at least five times the normal rate. Smoking adds an additional 2 per cent to this risk factor. Therefore, the diabetic who also smokes considerably increases the risk of having either a heart attack or a stroke. We have seen how smoking which causes a constriction of the blood vessels, reduces the supply of blood to the legs and feet, resulting in poor circulation. Because diabetics already have clogged and restricted arteries, any further restriction and clogging caused by smoking only worsens an already seriously impaired circulation.

The diabetic is prone to developing atherosclerosis as part of his disease, and anything that might contribute to or further accelerate this process should be avoided. The interrelationship of all the many risk factors in strokes with one another gives an added impetus to our efforts to eliminate these risk factors from our lives.

METHODS OF CONTROLLING DIABETES

From the earliest times, physicians have recognized diabetes as a distinct disease and have known and written about its symptoms. Yet they have had no successful way to treat it or even bring it under control until the discovery of insulin. Persons who had diabetes were doomed to an early death.

Thomas Willis discovered that a diabetic's urine tasted sweet like honey and added the designation *mellitus* to the name of the disease in the seventeenth century. In the eighteenth century, Matthew Dobson proved that the sweet taste was due to the presence of sugar in the urine. John Rollo went on to become the first physician to try to treat diabetes with a controlled diet consisting of meat and vegetables.

Finally, in the nineteenth century, Bouchardat of France and Nikowski and von Nering of Germany proved that diabetes was associated with a malfunctioning pancreas. From then on it became possible to understand the disease better and in so doing to find a way to control it and to prolong life.

INSULIN

As part of the ongoing study of diabetes, Dr. Frederick G. Banting and his research assistant, Charles H. Best, in 1922 discovered that when an extract of the cells of the pancreas were injected into a diabetic, the level of blood sugar was lowered and the disease could be controlled. The work on this far-reaching project was done in Toronto, Canada, in the laboratory of Professor J. J. R. MacLeod. The cells used in the extract were taken from the tissue of that part of the pancreas that had first been described in 1869 by Langerhans in Germany—the islets of Langerhans.

For their discovery, Dr. Banting and Professor MacLeod were awarded the Nobel Prize in Medicine in 1923. The extract they used for the injections was named insulin. Today we take so much for granted in medicine that it is hard to realize what a tremendous impact this discovery had on the world. It has saved literally millions of lives.

Before the discovery of insulin, diabetic children seldom lived longer than two years after their disease had been diagnosed. The young adult who become diabetic had such a short life span that he never lived long enough to develop the complications of the heart, kidneys, eyes, and other organs that today's better controlled diabetic does. In effect, the discovery of insulin opened the door to hitherto unknown complications in diabetes and brought about a whole new outlook on the disease.

Today the juvenile onset diabetic who must take insulin to keep alive can expect to live an average of 35 years from the time his disease is first diagnosed. The diabetic with maturity onset diabetes that remains well controlled can live to within a few years of his anticipated life expectancy.

Uncontrolled diabetes leads to the development of all manner of complications. The complications associated with diabetes, rather than the diabetes alone, have become of extreme importance to researchers and scientists alike.

The American Diabetes Association estimates that in the United States alone there are 1.25 million diabetics who are dependent on insulin. The effects of the original insulin of Banting and Best, although miraculous in its results, lasted only a few hours. Therefore, experiments continued with other types of insulin, such as protamine, which was first discovered in fish sperm and the nuclei of cells. Then came the addition of zinc to the protamine, creating PZI insulin with effects that could last for almost 24 hours.

Globin, Lente and NPH, which is a modification of PZI, are the so-called intermediate insulins—that is, they act over a longer period of time than does the regular insulin (RI) discovered by Banting and Best.

Today's insulin comes mostly from the pancreas of cattle and pigs, although in those countries where sheep predominate it is made from the pancreas of sheep. Most of the commercial insulin is about 70 per cent beef and 30 per cent pork in origin. If a person has allergies to one or the other, it is possible to obtain a pure pork or a pure beef insulin. Current research is being conducted on a laboratory-produced human insulin made from recombinant DNA. This type of insulin is expected to decrease the resistance to insulin that continues to occur in some diabetics. This resistance to insulin makes the use of the oral drugs a necessity in some patients.

The dosage of insulin is carefully regulated and coordinated with the diet to assure the best possible control of the diabetes. Too much insulin, or the same amount of insulin with less food, can bring on hypoglycemia (low blood sugar), a diabetic shock, or insulin reaction. Too little insulin, or the same amount of insulin with too much food, can result in a diabetic coma. Both are serious complications that can occur with the use of insulin.

Insulin lowers the blood sugar because it supplies the body with the hormone needed for the normal metabolism of glucose, thus preventing an accumulation of sugar in the blood and a spillage of sugar into the urine. Despite the advent of the oral drugs, insulin still remains the basic medication for the treatment of diabetes.

ORAL DRUGS

There are 1.25 million diabetics in the United States who are taking one of the oral antidiabetic drugs.

Because of the inconveniences many diabetics experienced in having to give themselves a daily injection of insulin, researchers were constantly seeking some way either to administer the insulin orally, which so far has not been possible, or to find another method of controlling diabetes without the need for daily injections of insulin.

Like so many other medical discoveries, a solution came about quite by accident. In 1942 Jambon and Laboutatieres of France discovered that a derivative of one of the sulfa drugs produced a low blood sugar in a patient who was being treated with sulfonylurea for typhoid fever. But it was not until 1954 when two German researchers, Franke and Fuchs, used the sulfa drug in an actual case of diabetes that the drug's properties for lowering blood sugar were confirmed. However, the drug did not lower the blood sugar in all diabetics. It proved to be most useful in those diabetics over 40 who had had diabetes for only a short time. It was believed that these patients still retained some capacity for producing insulin in their own pancreas. This was an important theory because, if true, it showed that sulfonylureas stimulated the release of insulin already present in the beta cells of the pancreas, in the islets of Langerhans. There had to be some insulin present in the body for these drugs to be able to work. The oral drugs are consequently useful only in maturity onset diabetes. Juvenile onset diabetes, when no insulin is manufactured, can be controlled only by injections of insulin.

The oral drugs are not insulin; they only stimulate the release of insulin that is already present in the pancreas. They also increase the potency of the natural insulin that is available, making less natural insulin do the work of more. They may also act on the liver, preventing it from releasing too much of its stored-up glucose. And although they are related to the sulfa drugs, the sulfonylureas are not effective against infections.

The first oral drug was called Corbutamide (BZ55) and proved as effective as insulin in those patients whose pancreas was still capable of manufacturing some insulin. Because of such side effects as skin rashes, occasional jaundice, and a possibly harmful effect on the liver, however, the search for other oral drugs with fewer side effects continued. In 1957 another oral drug, Tolbutamide, which became familiarly known as Orinase, was released for use in the United States.

Both Corbutamide and Tolbutamide lower the blood sugar gradually and therefore cut down on the extreme reactions that sometimes occur with insulin. However, they are not without drawbacks. In addition to not being effective for all diabetics, they cannot be used at the time of surgery, during pregnancy, or in the presence of infections. In these instances, a return to insulin is required. But they do last for 24 hours and do away with the daily injections of insulin.

Yet another sulfonylurea called chlorpropamine and known familiarly as Diabenese, was developed. It has three times the strength of Orinase and, because it is secreted more slowly by the kidneys, it remains in the body for a longer time. Only 60 per cent of diabinese is secreted by the kidneys in 24 hours. It also tends to accumulate in the body, thus requiring extreme care in its use. Diabinese, Tolazamide (Tolinase), and Acetohexamine (Dymelor) are considered to be an intermediate type of oral drug because of the length of time they remain in the body.

Biguanide, known as Phenformin (DBI), is a completely different type of oral drug. It acts not by stimulating a release of the insulin already present in the pancreas but by affecting the absorption of the glucose in the gut so that no new glucose is made in and released from the liver. In recent years the FDA has severely restricted the use of this drug and has classified it as an "imminent hazard" because of its serious side effect, lactic acidosis, which results from an accumulation of lactic acid in the body. Lactic acid is a substance that is normally found in the body. Any excessive amounts are usually removed by the kidneys and the liver. However, any accumulation of lactic acid can result in death. Because some deaths from lactic acidosis did occur in diabetics who were taking Phenformin, the FDA felt the risks from taking the drug outweighed its usefulness and were consequently not warranted.

The only way a physician can still prescribe Phenformin is by obtaining a certificate for the use of an Investigative New Drug—a certificate known as an IND—and to prescribe it only for those few patients who either cannot give themselves insulin or whose line of work is such that the danger from an insulin shock from too much insulin is greater than the dangers from Phenformin.

In 1970 investigators for the University Group Diabetic Program (UGDP) released a report that caused a furor in the medical world. The Natural Institutes of Health (NIH) funded the UGDP study because it was felt it was necessary to secure a review of the evidence that was accumulating showing that over 75 per cent of Americans with diabetes were dying of cardiovascular causes (heart attacks) or of cerebrovascular disease (strokes). Of this number, over 1.25 million were being treated with oral drugs. The UGDP set out to determine just what was causing this increase in deaths from heart attacks and strokes and, in addition, to find out if one form of treatment resulted in fewer heart attacks, angina, claudication (i.e., pain or lameness caused by impaired circulation in the legs), and strokes than another. The participants in this test were chosen nationwide. All had maturity onset diabetes that was nonketatic (i.e., acetonic). Women outnumbered men in the test group.

The persons taking part in the test were divided into four groups:

1. Those who were given variable amounts of insulin—that is, an amount of insulin that was needed to attain a normal level of blood sugar, an amount that constantly changed.
2. Those who were given a fixed dose of insulin.
3. Those who were given Tolbutamide (Orinase).
4. Those who were given a placebo (an inactive substance).

The conclusions reached from the study showed that the group treated with Tolbutamide (Orinase) had a significantly higher proportion of deaths from cardiovascular causes—in fact, over twice as many as did the placebo group. It was also found that a combination of diet and Orinase was no more effective than diet alone or diet and insulin in prolonging the life of a diabetic. It was the increase noted in the number of deaths in patients who were taking Orinase that brought about the complete reevaluation of the effectiveness of all the oral drugs, however.

Many physicians, realizing that diabetics are prone to having a higher incidence of strokes and heart attacks than are nondiabetics, and realizing that there is a relationship between the use of Orinase and an increased risk of having a stroke or a heart attack, are reluctant to prescribe it. Other physicians are just as positive that, despite the results obtained from the UGDP study, no such connection exists. They vehemently protest the study findings and continue to prescribe the drug for their patients. This controversy continues to be hotly debated within the medical profession and is a cause of great concern to the 1.25 million diabetics who take one or another of these drugs.

DIET AND WEIGHT REDUCTION

Whether a diabetic takes insulin or takes an oral drug, part of the basic treatment for diabetes always includes a carefully prepared diet designed to balance the intake of food with the quantity of insulin available. Up until 1922 when insulin was discovered, a specially designed diet was the only method known to be effective in the treatment of diabetes.

The Papyrus Ebera, which dates from 1500 BC and contains the oldest known references to diabetes, indicates there was the same concern then as now for the role played by diet in the control of diabetes. There has always been great emphasis placed on the carbohydrate and fat content of the diet. During the 1960s it was recognized that diabetics have a greater-than-average risk of dying from heart attacks and strokes. It became apparent that the high-fat diet that was being prescribed could very well be contributing to the buildup of fatty deposits on the walls of the blood vessels, thus contributing to these deaths. The old idea of fats in the diet was reevaluated.

As a result, today the restriction of carbohydrates is not considered to be as important as was once thought, but the amount of fat in the diet has been reduced. Greater emphasis is placed on the use of polyunsaturated fats. The emphasis now is on having nourishing, well-balanced meals. In 1971 the American Diabetes Association issued some sorely needed guidelines, which stated that there was no need "to disproportionately restrict the intake of carbohydrates in the diet of most diabetic patients."

One of the purposes of a diabetic diet is to help the patient attain the ideal body weight because weight reduction has a beneficial effect on the body's ability to control carbohydrate or sugar tolerance.

For some still unknown reason the tissues of an obese person's body are insensitive to insulin. Diabetes in the obese may be the result of a defect that keeps the natural insulin in the pancreas from functioning as it should. Actually, in the obese person the islets of Langerhans may secrete an excess of insulin, but the body's tissues act in such a way as to prevent this insulin from working. Those who are overweight seem to need more insulin than do those whose weight is within normal limits, so much so that consuming an excessive amount of calories is considered to be the most important risk factor in the development of diabetes mellitus and a contributing factor in the development of the atherosclerosis that is associated with diabetes.

One method used to determine what constitutes ideal weight suggests the following formula:

HEIGHT	IDEAL WEIGHT
Males: 5 feet	106 pounds
(add 6 pounds for each additional inch in height)	
Females: 5 feet	100 pounds
(add 5 pounds for each additional inch in height)	

In both males and females, 10 per cent can be subtracted for those with a small frame and 10 per cent added for those with a large frame.

To determine the number of calories needed each day, the ideal weight is then multiplied by 10 and adjusted to take into consideration the extent of the diabetic's daily activities, whether the lifestyle is sedentary or active.

To attain a reduction in weight, the physician reduces the caloric intake. The American Diabetes Association recommends that the composition of the weight-reducing diet should consist of 20 per cent protein and 80 per cent nonprotein food, of which 60 per cent of these nonprotein foods would be carbohydrates and 20 per cent fats.

Only a physician knowledgeable in nutrition or who has the assistance of a trained dietitian should prescribe any kind of diet for a diabetic. Diabetic diets are highly individualized, based on the individual's own levels of blood sugar. The number of calories seldom remains the same indefinitely but, rather, is subject to change as the diabetes improves or worsens.

Because the diabetic is unable to secrete a sufficient amount of insulin to metabolize the food eaten, a large amount of food consumed all at one time places a severe strain on the pancreas and the whole system and could, if there were insufficient insulin, result in a diabetic coma. To help avoid this, diabetics are advised to eat at least four meals daily, or more ideally to eat three meals and three snacks spaced so that the number of calories is evenly divided among the meals and snacks. Therefore, large amounts of food are never ingested at one time.

Formerly, great emphasis was placed on the proportion of carbohydrate to fats and the proportion of both of these to protein in the diet. Today's studies have indicated that as long as the calories and calorie distribution are constant and the diet is well balanced, the percentage of carbohydrates does not seem to have much effect on the diabetes.

The American Diabetic Association recommends a diet composed of normal proportions of carbohydrates, protein, and fat. This diet enables a physician to use a low-fat and low-cholesterol diet in an effort to prevent the rapid development of atherosclerosis, which is so characteristic of diabetes.

Hyperlipidemia (see Chapter 5) occurs frequently in diabetics and, because it is a risk factor for heart attacks and strokes, it must be brought and kept under control.

There is a tendency in diabetics toward having an increase in VLDL (very low density lipids) and an elevation in triglycerides—both considered as risk factors in themselves for strokes and heart attacks. When a diabetic is overweight, a reduction in the number of calories consumed each day can result in a dramatic decrease in hyperlipidemia.

Although the obese person who has only mild diabetes can many times gain control of diabetes with only a weight reduction, the brittle diabetic (i.e., the diabetic who has wide and rapid variations in blood glucose) may need insulin twice a day and must maintain a rigid control over the quantity and type of food eaten.

A LOOK INTO THE FUTURE

Pancreas transplants and the cloning of human insulin are some of the newer methods by which it is hoped that diabetes can be controlled to an even greater degree than it is now. The pioneer research into heart transplants and the current recombinant DNA research in gene splicing offer hope that in time diabetes can be eliminated, thus removing another risk factor in strokes.

CHAPTER SEVEN
SMOKING

Without exception every health agency, along with every physician, agrees that smoking, particularly cigarette smoking, increases the risk of having a stroke. Smoking contributes to and aggravates atherosclerosis and hypertension and causes an elevation in blood lipids, each one of which by itself is a major contributing factor in the development of a stroke.

HOW IT ALL BEGAN

Although smoking for its social enjoyment was unknown in ancient and medieval times, tobacco has been known to the modern world since America was discovered by Columbus in 1492. Smoking originated in the ancient cultures of the New World as the outgrowth of religious rites when it was customary for the priests to burn incense as an offering to the gods. In an attempt to overcome the irritation the burning incense caused to their nasal passages, the priests began to burn various herbs along with the incense. Later they began to smoke this combination of incense and herbs in makeshift pipes, successfully keeping this privilege exclusively for themselves for many years before it gradually spread to the populace.

When the most ancient of the New World civilizations—that of the Mayans—came to an end, the people from these devastated lands fled to the Yucatan peninsula, taking with them the custom of smoking. Before long the custom spread to the native Yucatan Indians. By the time Columbus made his journey, smoking had become a fully entrenched custom throughout the New World.

Columbus found the native Indians smoking not a mixture of incense and herbs but tobacco, which they smoked for religious and ceremonial purposes and also as a symbol of peace and goodwill in the now famous peace pipes. Luis de Torres and Rodrigo de Perez, who accompanied Columbus on his voyage, went on to explore the land now known as Cuba. They found that there, too, the native Indian tribes were smoking tobacco. These tribal Indians believed that tobacco had great medicinal powers to help or to cure everything from wounds to sores. It was chiefly for these medicinal powers that Columbus took tobacco back to Europe on his return voyage.

Tobacco, or *nicotiana* as it is known botanically, was originally a subtropical plant flourishing throughout the Antilles and in most of Central America. It belongs to the same family of plants as does the potato and nightshade. The plant was named *nicotiana* in honor of Jean Nicot, a French ambassador to Portugal, who had dispatched some of its seeds to Catherine de Medici to be used as a remedy for headaches.

The name tobacco was subsequently given to the *nicotiana* plant because the pipe in which it was smoked was called a *tobaco.* In addition to these pipes, the Indians frequently smoked their tobacco rolled up in corn husks. They also crushed the leaves of the plants and then enclosed them in a kind of envelope made from a single large leaf of the tobacco plant. In addition to being smoked, tobacco was used for snuff, was chewed, and was drunk as a juice.

The Mayans who fled to the Yucatan peninsula have the dubious distinction of having created the first cigarettes by making paperlike tubes about three or four inches in length and filling these tubes with tobacco. They called the tubes *cigarros* or *papeletos.*

Many other explorers followed Columbus to the New World. Notable among them was Sir Walter Raleigh, who has been credited with introducing the smoking of tobacco into England. Another great explorer of the time, the old sea dog, Sir Francis Drake, made pipe smoking an important part of the Englishman's way of life when he took this custom back from the Virginia Colony and introduced it into court circles.

Although tobacco originally was closely associated with religious rites, not all religions throughout the years have viewed the use of tobacco with approval. The Roman Catholic Church, for example, condemned the use of tobacco in 1642 in the days of Pope Urban VIII, decreeing excommunication as punishment for anyone who used it. This drastic action was taken as the result of widespread complaints about tobacco stains on the hands of the priests and the smell of tobacco on their breath. The fact that the priests were leaving the sacristy either for a smoke or a pinch of snuff during the services aroused scandal and disgust in the congregation. The Muftis in Turkey, from whence some of the world's best tobacco comes, believed its use to be contrary to the teachings of the Koran. In Russia, Tsar Michael prohibited smoking in his country on pain of death. In more recent times, smoking has been banned by the religious sect of Mormons, known as the Church of the Latter Day Saints.

Smoking tobacco in the form of small cigars or cigarettes became extremely popular in Spain during the seventeenth century. From there it spread eastward through one country after another until it finally reached Russia. It was the soldiers fighting in the Crimean War in Eastern Europe who first took cigarettes back to England and France. In succeeding years, smoking continued to spread throughout the world. During the second decade of this century, it became a national custom of people in the United States.

Known for their great inventive capabilities, Americans produced the first cigarette-making machine in the 1870s. It was this machine that made it possible to produce cigarettes both abundantly and cheaply. In fact, the year the machine was invented, when the population of the United States was 50 million, 1.3 billion cigarettes were smoked. Contrast this with the 1970s, when the population increased to over 205 million and 536.4 billion cigarettes were smoked—an increase of over 40,000 per cent!

During World War I cigarettes were distributed free to soldiers and sailors on all the fighting fronts as a gesture of good will. More than anything else this helped to entrench cigarette smoking as a habit and resulted in a tremendous increase in the number of people who became smokers.

When governments realized that their revenues could be increased by taxing tobacco, they both legalized and encouraged its use. Smoking as a major risk factor in the development of vascular disease, which results in heart attacks and strokes, dates from this time.

It is ironic that tobacco first came into use because it was considered to have great medicinal value when one realizes that in recent years physicians and medical scientists alike have come to view it as extremely hazardous to health. It contributes to or is the cause of many illnesses ranging from asthma, bronchitis, emphysema, ulcers, and cancer to heart attacks and strokes.

EFFECTS OF SMOKING ON THE BODY

Beyond a doubt one of the most important health issues we face today is the problem of cigarette smoking. It is considered to be so hazardous that by an Act of Congress the following statement must appear on all packages of cigarettes manufactured for sale within the United States: "Warning: the Surgeon General has determined that cigarette smoking is dangerous to your health."

A definite association between cigarette smoking and heart disease, strokes, and cancer has been established, particularly in the United States and the United Kingdom. Tobacco smoking in some areas of the world—notably the Soviet Union, Poland, and South Africa—does not seem to have this same cause-and-effect relationship to lung cancer and vascular diseases. One theory holds that this difference can be attributed to the way in which tobacco is cured in these countries.

Up until the beginning of this century, tobacco was processed or cured in all parts of the world by means of natural enzymatic fermentation in the process of which there was a free access to airborne oxygen. In 1905 a procedure known as *redrying* was introduced into the United States and a decade or so later into the United Kingdom. In this process the tobacco leaf is exposed to extremely high temperatures, 175°F (80°C), destroying the enzyme in the tobacco and preventing any enzymatic fermentation from taking place. This redrying process has never been used in the Soviet Union, Poland, or South Africa. In these countries cigarettes are made only from tobacco leaves that are cured by enzymatic fermentation.

The process of enzymatic fermentation produces an alkaline tobacco whereas the redrying process produces an acid tobacco. Repeated laboratory tests have shown that when the smoke from an alkaline tobacco is dissolved in water there is no residue of tar, whereas smoke from an acid tobacco has a definite tar residue.

It takes about 25 years for lung cancer to develop in a cigarette smoker. The redrying process was first used in the United States in 1905, and a marked increase in lung cancer showed up 25 years later in 1930. The same story holds true for the United Kingdom where the redrying process that began in the 1940s resulted in the same marked increase in the incidence of lung cancer 25 years later.

The dangers from smoking, and particularly from smoking cigarettes, did not come under close medical scrutiny until after World War II. It is interesting that in those European countries where cigarettes were next to impossible to buy because of the war, deaths from heart attacks and strokes decreased substantially.

Even before the dangers to the heart and brain from smoking were brought into public focus, the American Cancer Society had exposed the dangers of smoking to the lungs in the 1950s. In a well-remembered statement the Society announced that anyone who smoked two packs of cigarettes a day had a premature death rate 90 times that of the person who did not smoke. And it was not lung cancer only that was involved. Deaths from all forms of cancer were higher among smokers than among nonsmokers.

The smoke from a burning cigarette emits a mixture of particles that include tar, which is linked to cancer; nicotine, which is both a potent drug and a poison; and small amounts of arsenic, which is also a poison. It also emits various gases such as carbon monoxide, one of the most lethal of all poisons, along with formaldehyde gas, nitrous dioxide, and phenol, all of which can cause serious damage to the tissues of the body. Taken together, these particles and gases cause irritation to every single part of the body's respiratory, vascular, and nervous systems because as smoke is inhaled these poisons are absorbed throughout the body.

Tobacco is actually quite bitter tasting, so bitter in fact that cigarette and cigar manufacturers resort to blending various types of tobacco in an effort to reduce the bitterness. Various flavors are also added to the tobacco in order to give it a distinctive taste, which is reminiscent of those ancient priests who added herbs to their incense for the same reason.

EFFECTS ON THE HEART AND BRAIN

Cigarette smokers have a 70 per cent higher rate of death from heart attack than do nonsmokers. The following paragraphs give some of the reasons why.

The nicotine in tobacco is a colorless, liquid alkaloid that has a tendency to turn brown when exposed to air. It is one of the most fatal of all known poisons. If taken orally, just 1 grain, or about 50 mg, constitutes a fatal dose. It acts as a stimulant to the nervous system and to the adrenal glands. This stimulation causes these glands to release hormones which, in turn, release free fatty acids into the bloodstream within minutes.

Nicotine also causes the adrenal glands to secrete an increased amount of epinephrine into the bloodstream, causing a rise in blood pressure. Smoking raises the blood pressure of those who are already hypertensive to even higher levels, and the blood pressure tends to remain at these higher levels as long as the smoking is continued. This increases the risk of a heart attack or a stroke. An increase in the heart rate and the blood pressure results in a feeling of stimulation. The stimulation causes an increase in the work load of the heart, which can be quite serious for anyone who has heart disease.

When the heart has to work harder, it increases its need for oxygen and for blood. Because smoking interferes with normal lung function, however, it is impossible for either the heart or the brain to receive the extra blood and oxygen that are needed. Once carbon monoxide gets into the bloodstream, it actually reduces the amount of oxygen in the blood. A cigarette smoker has a continuing level of carbon monoxide in the bloodstream.

For the moderate smoker the hemoglobin (red cells) in the blood is decreased by about 5 per cent by the carbon monoxide present in the smoke. In the case of a heavy smoker, the red cells can be further decreased by as much as 8 per cent. It is the red blood cells that carry oxygen throughout the bloodstream. Therefore, any reduction in their number results in a lessened ability to engage in strenuous work or activity. The shortness of breath so many smokers experience is the result. In addition, the blood vessels of a smoker, particularly those in the arms and legs, become narrowed and constricted, reducing the amount of blood that can flow through them.

Nicotine also stimulates the production of glycogen, (i.e., blood sugar). Between this and the increase in epinephrine, the smoker gets a feeling of increased energy. Every time a cigarette is puffed, the brain gets a shot of nicotine within 7 seconds. A pack of cigarettes gives the brain 200 shots of nicotine.

Along with being a stimulant nicotine is also a depressant. It can actually cause the heart to beat as much as 20 extra beats a minute. Smokers sometimes develop irregular heart beats, which pose the danger of sudden death. The effect of smoking on the heart's rhythm and conduction results in most cases from a secondary cause brought on by smoking, such as hypertension and fibrillation. Irregular heart beats signify that the heart is out of normal rhythm. The heart can beat so slowly as to bring on cardiac arrest or so swiftly as to cause the heart to stop beating, just as a clock does when it is wound too tightly.

Smoking a pack of cigarettes a day classifies a person as a heavy smoker. If from 10 to 19 cigarettes are smoked in a day, the person is considered to be a moderate smoker. A light smoker is one who smokes less than 10 cigarettes a day.

Switching from cigarettes to pipes and cigars is not the answer to cigarette smoking. Some pipe smokers every day take into their bodies the same amount of nicotine as would be present in two packs of cigarettes. One cigar is equal to at least 5 or 6 cigarettes in its nicotine content. Heavy smokers of pipe tobacco or cigars will therefore always have a higher death rate than do the nonsmokers.

Nicotine can also cause a drop in the temperature of the skin of the fingers and the toes. A constriction of the tiny blood vessels in the skin of the extremities prevents the blood from flowing through them at a normal rate, resulting in a drop in temperature that can be as much as 6° F (3.3° C) lower than the temperature in the rest of the body. Research done at the Mayo Clinic showed that when a person smokes two standard size cigarettes, the average decrease in temperature in the fingers and toes is from 4° to 5° F (2.2° to 2.8° C) and takes from a half to one hour to return to normal.

Besides constricting the larger arteries and blood vessels, smoking can also cause a spasm of the arterioles—the small arteries. Such a spasm causes a further reduction in blood flow. A thrombosis, or clot, may also develop within the spastic blood vessel. At first the spasm reduces and then finally cuts off the flow of blood through the affected blood vessel. This condition is known as Buerger's disease and is found almost exclusively in those who smoke cigarettes. In fact, over 80 per cent of all persons with Buerger's disease are heavy smokers. The American Heart Association has concluded that "the use of tobacco in all its forms is a definite cause of peripheral vascular disease."

Ninety per cent of the nicotine in a cigarette is absorbed in the body when the smoke is inhaled. The inhalation of cigarette smoke can theoretically bring enough nicotine into the body to cause death, but this catastrophe is prevented by the swift action of the enzymes within the body, which provide a rapid and extremely effective detoxification process. And in time the body does build up a tolerance to nicotine.

Sixty-five to 75 per cent of the total amount of nicotine is absorbed in the body quite rapidly if the smoke is held in the mouth for only two seconds. When the smoke is inhaled, however, the amount absorbed is increased to 90 per cent. During cigarette smoking, the smoke is drawn in through the butt and is concentrated there, which makes the last inch of a cigarette the most dangerous.

Even just puffing a cigarette results in a 10 per cent absorption of nicotine. By not inhaling the smoke, the amount of nicotine that is absorbed can be reduced, which in turn may result in a lessened risk of a heart attack or a stroke. However, it by no means suggests that there is no risk at all in smoking if the smoke is not inhaled; pipe and cigar smokers who generally do not inhale still have the risk of having a heart attack or a stroke.

Laboratory tests have failed to show that there is any significant effect in the rate at which blood flows through the arteries of those who have no arterial disease and who smoke. Nevertheless, in persons who do have any coronary or cerebral artery disease, ECGs have shown definite indications that the flow of blood in their arteries is reduced. And who among us can be that sure that our arteries have no signs of atherosclerosis when even newborn babies have been shown to have it?

Smoking may also cause a speed-up in the time it takes for blood to clot, because it increases the tendency of the platelets in the blood to clot. This can lead to the formation of a thrombosis, which can result in a stroke.

Many studies, including those conducted by the Framingham Heart Study Group have shown a definite link between cigarette smoking and coronary heart disease and strokes. In the same way as the arteries leading to the heart can be damaged so also can the other arteries in the body, including those in the brain. All these arteries are part of a network. When one part of the network is compromised, the rest of the network suffers.

A decrease in the flow of blood can result in there being an insufficient amount of blood and oxygen to reach all parts of the body. When the arteries in the brain are deprived of blood and oxygen, the result can be a stroke.

Smokers on the average have more than twice as many strokes as do nonsmokers. There are also more deaths from other causes among those who smoke. The chief cause of death in cigarette smokers is coronary (heart) disease, followed by cancer and strokes.

The Framingham Heart Study Group showed that among those who had a low level of blood cholesterol, normal blood pressure, and no diabetes, and had never smoked, there were only 25 major coronary illnesses per 1000 men, and the death rate from all forms of heart disease was even less. On the other hand, if elevated blood cholesterol, diabetes, or hypertension was present and the person *also* smoked cigarettes, the number of coronary illnesses doubled. If any two of the risk factors were present, the rate rose to 100 instances per 1000 men.

The same risk factors that the Framingham Study Group found in coronary disease were also found to be present in strokes.

In 1960 the American Heart Association first made public its data showing that the death rate from heart disease, depending on age, was from 50 to 200 per cent higher in heavy smokers—that is, those who smoked more than one pack of cigarettes a day—than it was in those who did not smoke.

Three years later they urged that anyone who was considered to be in the high-risk category for a stroke or a heart attack should stop smoking. Even after a myocardial infarction has occurred, the survival rate is greatly improved in those who either do not smoke or who have given up smoking.

SMOKING AND THE KIDNEYS

Smoking also has an effect on the kidneys. Tobacco contains cadmium, which is inhaled while smoking. Cadmium has a tendency to remain in the kidneys. As we saw in Chapter 3, it can contribute to the development of hypertension. Hypertension is the main risk factor in the development of a stroke. Anything that contributes to its development also plays a role in bringing on strokes. Autopsies have shown that the kidneys and livers of smokers contained more cadmium than was seen in the kidneys of those who did not smoke.

Dr. Stanley Schacter, a professor of psychology at Columbia University, has done a great deal of work on the effects of smoking. One of his most interesting findings concerns the effect the alkalinity or acidity of the smoker's urine has on the cumulative effect of nicotine in the body and the intensity of his craving for a cigarette.

When the urine is acid, which could result from such an innocuous act as taking ascorbic acid (Vitamin C), more nicotine is excreted than when the urine is alkaline. In fact, in alkaline urine there is only a fourth as much nicotine excreted.

This finding led to the conclusion, later proven to be accurate, that on the days when a smoker's urine is acid he smokes about 20 per cent more cigarettes than he does on days when his urine is alkaline. This phenomenon also explains the close association smoking and alcohol seem to have. Alcoholic beverages make the urine more acid; therefore, smokers tend to smoke much more when they are drinking.

SMOKING AND THE LUNGS

Smoking affects the lungs by thickening and even rupturing the walls of the alveoli. The plural of the Latin word *alveolus* (a small hollow or cavity), alveoli in this case refers to the air sacs in the lungs.

Smoking contributes to and actually worsens such lung diseases as asthma, bronchitis, and emphysema. The circulatory system that supplies the heart and brain with oxygen and blood cannot function properly if the respiratory system, which is so closely interconnected with it, has been rendered inefficient by smoking. This is another example of an occasion when one part of the body is adversely affected, all parts suffer accordingly.

SMOKING AND CHOLESTEROL

At the American Heart Association's annual scientific meeting in 1979, evidence was presented that showed the tremendous adverse effect cigarette smoking has on the fats in the blood, notably cholesterol. A 10-city survey of over 5000 adults showed that smoking substantially lowers the levels of high density lipoproteins (HDL), which provide protection against clogged arteries. It has been estimated that smoking lowers the HDL level by as much as 11 per cent.

SMOKING AND ATHEROSCLEROSIS

Cigarette smoking definitely contributes to the advance of atherosclerosis, one of the most important risk factors in the development of a stroke. If for no other reason, smoking should not be part of anyone's lifestyle.

If atherosclerosis is already present, as it is in practically everyone, smoking can only aggravate it by further constricting the already narrowed and possibly damaged blood vessels. Fortunately, the damage that has been caused by smoking can be reversed if smoking is discontinued. After widespread study and testing, the International Atherosclerosis Project has confirmed beyond any doubt that atherosclerosis spreads more rapidly in anyone who smokes cigarettes.

In their report published in 1964 Drs. Knud Kjeldsen and Paul Astrup of the University of Copenhagen also pointed out that in their opinion it was the carbon monoxide even more than the nicotine in cigarette smoke that should be considered the major risk factor in the development of atherosclerosis and heart disease. Coupled with a diet rich in fat, the acceleration of both these diseases in those who smoked was quite rapid. The cells which form the inside lining of the arteries are unable to function normally when they are affected by carbon monoxide. This in turn upsets the chemical balance that controls fat. The carbon monoxide actually sets the stage for allowing the accumulation of large amounts of fat on the arterial walls. As we have seen, this results in a narrowing of the artery and in turn means that less blood can flow through that artery. If further proof were needed, autopsies have shown without exception how much more severe atherosclerosis is in those who smoke than it is in those who do not smoke. If atherosclerosis is already present and foods high in fat content are eaten *and* the person also smokes, there is a marked increase in the amount of atherosclerosis that will develop.

Experiments were conducted with two groups of laboratory animals. Each one of the animals in both groups was fed a diet high in cholesterol; all of them developed atherosclerotic lesions. When in addition to the high-fat diet one group of animals was also exposed to carbon monoxide (the same poison as in cigarette smoke), this group showed markedly larger and more severe atherosclerotic lesions than did the other group.

People who smoke also show more evidence of atherosclerosis—that is, more fatty plaque on their arterial walls. And there are more damaged areas on those walls where thrombi could easily develop than on the arterial walls of nonsmokers. A recent study at the University of Southern California showed that of those patients who had had a heart attack and who continued to smoke, two-thirds showed definite signs of a progression of atherosclerosis.

The death rate among smokers from all diseases is much higher than it is among nonsmokers. And the death rate is closely related to the number of cigarettes, cigars, or pipefuls of tobacco that are smoked, to whether or not the smoke is inhaled and, finally, to how many years the person has been smoking. The increased risk smokers have of developing all types of vascular disease is frightening, particularly when one looks at the number of crippling strokes that occur as a result of these vascular diseases.

SMOKING AND STRESS

The role played by stress in strokes is discussed later in a chapter on stress in general. In relation to cigarette smoking, stress does play a most important role. Anxiety, nervousness, restlessness, and irritability are all earmarks of stress, and all are also associated with smoking, either as an integral part of the smoker's personality or as brought on in an ever-expanding vicious circle of anxiety. Some people smoke for what they believe are smoking's relaxing effects on these conditions. They continue to smoke in an effort to relax, but all the while they are only making themselves more tense.

SMOKING AND ULCERS

Anyone who has ever had an ulcer is well aware that his or her smoking days are over. Nicotine slows the whole digestive process for up to an hour, and while the digestive process is being delayed, acidity in the stomach can increase so much that it causes heartburn. This increase in acidity contributes to causing the ulcer in the first place.

SMOKING AND WOMEN

Women are fast catching up with men in the number of cigarettes they smoke, and their death rates from smoking-related diseases are fast approaching the rates for men. As women assume more and more tension-filled positions that were previously thought to be male prerogatives, they, like men, are experiencing all the stress-induced diseases. Hypertension, elevated levels of blood cholesterol, and an acceleration in the atherosclerotic process are all made worse by smoking. Alone or together these conditions constitute risk factors in both heart disease and strokes, and these diseases are currently affecting more and more women.

Women who smoke and who become pregnant are at a greater risk of having stillbirths and also of giving birth to smaller babies. Both nicotine and carbon monoxide pass through the placenta into the fetus.

SMOKING AND ORAL CONTRACEPTIVES

Although oral contraceptives are discussed in greater detail in Chapter 8, it is well to be mindful of the fact that cigarette smoking and oral contraceptives together constitute a dangerous combination. The increase in myocardial infarctions and strokes in women who smoke and use oral contraceptives is such that many physicians will not prescribe an oral contraceptive to any woman who smokes.

Cigarette smoking is considered to be the single strongest risk factor for a myocardial infarction among women under 45 years of age. To add oral contraceptives to this risk factor increases the risk enormously. The Center for Disease Control in Atlanta did a study on the increased risk of heart attacks among women who took oral contraceptives and who also smoked, and concluded that such women had a 5.5 greater chance of developing a heart attack than did the women who took oral contraceptives but did not smoke.

And the risk of having a stroke was every bit as great. In fact, the risk of having a subarachnoid hemorrhage (see Chapter 1) is 5.7 times greater in the cigarette smoker than it is in the nonsmoker. The risk of this type of stroke for those women who smoked and also took an oral contraceptive was a whopping 21.9 times greater than it was in women who neither smoked nor took oral contraceptives.

Smoking is harmful under any circumstances, but for a woman who smokes while taking oral contraceptives it is lethal. The longer the oral contraceptives are used, the greater the risk becomes. A choice must be made—either the pill or the cigarette. It should not be both.

SMOKING AND LIFE EXPECTANCY

The number one cause of sudden death in smokers and nonsmokers alike is a heart attack. Cancer and strokes complete a deadly triumvirate.

Smoking has been proved to have a cause-and-effect relationship to both heart attacks and strokes by contributing to the development of those diseases. The death rate for the so-called light smoker is 60 per cent higher than it is for the nonsmoker. For the moderate smoker, it is 90 per cent higher, and for the heavy smoker it is 120 per cent higher.

A man who is in his mid-thirties and who is a heavy smoker has one chance in 23 of dying during the next 10 to 30 years in the prime of his life. The risk increases with the number of cigarettes smoked. It also increases with the number of years the person has been smoking. The risk drops to one chance in 90 if he doesn't smoke at all.

Further studies show that before the age of 65, one out of every six nonsmokers will have died, whereas one out of every three heavy smokers will have died. A source of wonder has always been why so many people are so willing to throw away their chances of having a longer life span that the advances in medicine have brought within the reach of everyone.

The life expectancy for the person who smokes less than a pack of cigarettes a day is reduced by 4.5 years. If the person smokes a pack a day, the length of life is further reduced by 6.5 years. Anyone who smokes over two packs of cigarettes a day can expect 8.5 years less of life than would have been the case with no smoking.

Smoking a pipe does not seem to have the drastic effect on longevity that smoking a cigarette does. Pipe smoking reduces life expectancy on the average by only two or three months. Cigars have a somewhat greater effect on length of life, causing about 1.5 years to be subtracted from the average life span.

From all these facts, one can only conclude that those who smoke simply do not live as long as those who do not smoke.

ADVANTAGES OF NOT SMOKING

The more cigarettes that are smoked, the greater is their effect on the body. If a person stops smoking, in time his body is able to reverse most, if not all, the damage that has been done to it as the result of the smoking.

Dr. Paul Dudley White repeatedly said that in order to minimize the risks that go with smoking, there would have to be a widespread change in smoking habits. And he regretfully conceded that changing these habits was no easy task.

Even if a person who has smoked most of his life were to stop right now, he would find the benefits to his heart, blood vessels, and lungs to be enormous. The risk of having either a heart attack or a stroke are greatly reduced even after just one year of not smoking. Many cardiologists believe that the risks are reduced to the level they are for someone who has never smoked at all. It is possible that after two years of not smoking the arteries can return to the condition they were in before the smoking began. The lungs that have been so abused by all that smoke are able to rejuvenate themselves, to become healthy once again, and to function normally.

The longer a person can stay away from smoking, the closer the body gets to a healthy state. In time, it reaches the same condition as that of someone who has never smoked. After 10 years of not smoking the death rate from smoking-related diseases approaches the level it is in those who do not smoke.

Mark Twain, with tongue in cheek, once said that smoking was the easiest habit in the world to break because he had done it a thousand times. Most smokers experience quite a bit of discomfort when they first stop smoking. This proves what a strong and harmful effect smoking has had on the mind and the body.

When the Surgeon General's first report on the hazards of smoking was made public in the mid-1960s, sales of tobacco decreased. The decline in sales lasted for only a short time. Sales began to rise once again and, unfortunately, they rose most among adolescents. Because smoking is started at such an early age, this group has the most to lose in terms of smoking-related illnesses and the resultant decrease in life expectancy.

The 1979 edition of *Smoking and Health: A Report of the Surgeon General* shows that despite the fact that there are 30 million exsmokers in the United States, there has been a marked increase in the number of smokers 17 years of age and older. Their number increased from 53.3 million in 1965 to 54.1 million in 1978.

Perhaps the most damaging of all the evidence collected is that despite the number of exsmokers, the number of cigarettes sold rose 16 per cent from 529 billion in 1965 to 615 billion in 1978. This ties in with the report's estimate that the number of cigarettes smoked by each individual person has risen 14 per cent during this same 13-year period.

The younger the person is when beginning to smoke, the greater are the chances of his or her having a heart attack or a stroke—not in old age but in the most productive years—the thirties or forties.

For those who find it impossible to give up cigarettes even when they realize how hazardous to health they are, some suggestions have been made—some good, some not so good—as to how to make cigarettes less harmful. One suggestion is that the tobacco industry should endeavor to come up with a truly efficient filter cigarette. The tobacco industry is trying to remove some of the harmful elements in the tobacco itself, but more still needs to be done. It has also been suggested that the person try to smoke less of each cigarette. In this way the tobacco itself acts as a filter in the case of regular cigarettes but does not hold true in the filter type, because the filter takes the place of some of the tobacco at the butt end. The filter does hold back much of the tar and nicotine when the cigarette is first smoked. But as the cigarette decreases in length, the tar and nicotine that have accumulated in the filter now get into the lungs in a greater amount and over a shorter period. So the smoker can have no sense of security in smoking a cigarette right down to the filter. Because filters do reduce, if only moderately, the amount of tar, nicotine, and various gases in the cigarette, smoking filter cigarettes is less satisfying to the addict because it is the combination of taste and nicotine that provides the sense of satisfaction. The death rate from cardiovascular diseases and lung cancer in those who smoke filter cigarettes is higher than it is for nonsmokers, even though it is lower than in those persons who smoke cigarettes containing a high level of tar and nicotine.

Filter cigarettes do not mix as much air with the smoke as do the nonfilter cigarettes, and so more carbon monoxide passes through them. Some studies have shown this increase in carbon monoxide to be as much as 28 per cent. In addition, not all the popular brands of cigarettes have the same tar and nicotine content. Actually, the tobacco industry itself has cut the tar and nicotine yield in the average cigarette by as much as 65 per cent since 1954, but this is only an average. It is not the same in all cigarettes. If a brand made with less nicotine is chosen by the smoker, it can cut down on the risk factors but only if the smoker doesn't try to compensate for the lesser amount of nicotine by smoking more of these cigarettes.

Some cigarette smokers have switched to pipes and cigars, but it is well to remember that persons who smoke cigars and pipes get higher doses of carbon monoxide when they smoke because there is so little ventilation through either the stems of the pipes or the wrappers on the cigars. At best these switching measures are only temporary. Any smoking at all constitutes a risk factor in an ever-increasing number of diseases.

Many people who stop smoking complain that they tend to gain weight because their appetites improve, and they turn to food and particularly to sweets as a substitute for smoking. The weight gain can be controlled by becoming more active. This is much easier to do than it was when the person was smoking because the tendency to become out of breath on exertion is no longer present. Weight also tends to return to the normal level when the acute phase of withdrawal from smoking has subsided.

QUITTING

Cigarette smoking claims 300,000 lives each year because of the diseases it both causes and aggravates. This is five times as many lives as are lost in automobile accidents and drug overdoses, two other preventable causes of death. Something must be done to convince people that beyond any doubt smoking is harmful and the practice should be stopped. Before the habit of cigarette smoking can be stopped, the smoker must really want to give it up. The smoker must be motivated. The United States Public Health Service Clearing House for Smoking has defined six distinct types of cigarette smokers.

THE ADDICTIVE SMOKER

The addictive smoker is both physically and psychologically dependent on cigarettes. This person is the chain smoker who lights up the next cigarette just as soon as the first one is finished.

THE CRUTCH SMOKER

The crutch smoker smokes cigarettes as a way of relieving nervousness and tension. This type of smoker always lights up a cigarette at the first sign of stress.

THE HABITUAL SMOKER

The habitual smoker smokes out of habit and many times is not even aware that he or she is smoking.

THE HANDLING SMOKER

The so-called handling smoker really doesn't enjoy smoking as much as feeling the need to hold something.

THE NEGATIVE EFFECT SMOKER

The negative effect smoker (one who has negative feelings that are overcome only by smoking) claims that cigarettes provide a lift, that they are stimulating.

THE POSITIVE EFFECT SMOKER

The positive effect smoker can be classified as the social smoker because he feels that nothing relaxes him quite as much as a cigarette.

Knowing what makes a person smoke can go a long way toward helping him to stop. The most important first step is to decide on how to quit—whether it is to be "cold turkey" or done gradually over a period of time. Compelling reasons are given for both choices. Some smokers find that they absolutely cannot cope with the withdrawal symptoms that are increased manyfold by stopping cold turkey. The Surgeon General in his 1979 report on smoking states that "partial abstinence from smoking leads to more, rather than less, discomfort in withdrawal. The result is that a partially abstinent smoker is in a chronic state of withdrawal. Typically, this chronic state of withdrawal leads to relapse and a return to the baseline rates of smoking." Whatever way is chosen, the person determined to stop smoking should start off by throwing away all the ashtrays, matches, lighters, and cigarettes so that they will not be at hand as a temptation.

Some smokers find that by putting the money they would have spent on cigarettes into a jar where it is clearly visible at all times and by watching the amount grow provides them with a most powerful incentive.

Smoking is a habit, a behavior pattern that has been learned and it is a habit that can be unlearned. In 1972 Consumer's Union in their publication "Licit & Illicit Drugs" stated that in their opinion smoking was more than a habit, it was also an addiction. The Assistant Secretary for Health in the Department of Health, Education, & Welfare, Dr. Julius B. Richmond, in his 1979 report agreed, stating that nicotine is "a powerful addictive drug." An addiction is a condition in which both physical and chemical changes have occurred in the body from a substance, usually a drug, that has been used for a long period of time. It is a condition in which ceasing to use the substance brings on definite symptoms associated with withdrawal and abstinence. The addictive substance in smoking is, of course, nicotine.

According to Dr. Steven Kopel of Rutgers University, who is also the director of the Multiple Risk Factor Intervention Trial Program for the Prevention of Heart Disease, 80 per cent of Americans who do quit smoking start smoking again within a few months. It is his belief that they do this because they have never learned how *not* to smoke.

Admittedly it is not an easy undertaking to quit smoking because it is associated with so many things that are done both at work and at home. What quitting takes is a new life style—what Dr. Kopel calls a *restructuring* of a person's life. In order to undo the effects of years of smoking, he advocates a three-stage program consisting of motivation, behavior modification, and nonsmoking maintenance procedures. All three must be adhered to in order to achieve the optimum result sought—quitting the smoking habit permanently.

Nothing can be achieved without motivation. The person who wishes to quit smoking must be convinced that the health hazards attributed to cigarette smoking actually apply to himself or herself, not just to everyone else.

Behavior modification means changing the conditions under which a person smokes—for example, smoking only at specific times during the day. Eliminating that first cigarette in the morning and having the last one at night at an earlier time breaks the pattern of smoking. Keeping cigarettes out of sight or in an inconvenient place where they cannot be easily reached also helps. Drinking frequent glasses of water or fruit juice, nibbling on celery or raw carrots, chewing gum, exercising, even brushing the teeth when one has the desire to smoke all help to change the smoking pattern.

The idea in Dr. Kopel's plan is to reduce the number of cigarettes that are smoked in a day by gradually cutting down or switching to a brand that has a lower tar and nicotine content, one that does not provide the same satisfaction, and finally smoking less and less of each cigarette. There is also what Dr. Kopel refers to as nonsmoking maintenance—in other words, preventing the person from going back to smoking. This phase is designed to change the smoker's whole attitude toward cigarettes. The smoker is taught how to handle those social situations in which smoking is so much a part of the scene—occasions such as weddings, cocktail parties, and the like. The smoker decides beforehand just how to handle these situations and then adheres strictly to the plan.

Shortness of breath, tightness in the chest area, headaches, sweating, visual disturbances, and gastrointestinal discomforts are the most common symptoms of withdrawal while the body is adjusting to being without nicotine. Constipation, frequent urination, increased coughing plus irritability and depression can also accompany the first stages of quitting. Fortunately, most of these symptoms vanish within a week or so.

OTHER METHODS OF QUITTING

ANTISMOKING PILLS

Pills are available that are designed to curb the desire to smoke. They contain a substance called *lobelin,* which produces some of the effects of nicotine. These pills coat the inside of the mouth and throat with a film that makes the cigarette smoke taste absolutely horrible.

SMOKE ENDERS

SmokeEnders is the name of an international organization started in 1967 by Jacquelyn Rogers and her husband, Dr. Jan Rogers. It has offices in most of the major cities. Its nine-week program has been found by many participants to be an excellent and relatively painless way of permanently ending the smoking habit.

SmokeEnders aims to change the smoker's dependence on and love of cigarettes to a feeling of contempt and loathing for them and, finally, to complete indifference to them. The meetings are usually held once a week and last for two hours. The teachers are all former smokers with special training in the SmokeEnders techniques.

During the first five weeks of the program, although those who are taking part do continue to smoke, their intake of nicotine is gradually reduced by means of switching to different brands of cigarettes and by reducing the number and kinds of occasions during which smoking is permitted. It is in this phase of the program that a very uncomfortable chair is dragged out. If a participant must smoke, he or she can do so only while sitting in this chair. Just sitting, no reading, no talking. Just sitting. By this time the smoker has been detoxified and psychologically geared to quit.

The last few weeks of the program are spent in group discussion, in which the now exsmoker's commitment to abstain forever more from smoking is constantly reinforced.

SmokeEnders' success rate is relatively high. About 90 per cent of those in the program stop smoking by the time the program is concluded, and about 70 per cent remain nonsmokers.

HYPNOSIS

Being hypnotized in order to stop smoking has become more and more widespread in recent years, particularly among those for whom all other methods of giving up smoking have failed. Hypnosis should be used only by a trained physician. There is always a physician–patient relationship in this type of treatment. The patient is asked to relax and to concentrate in a way that will bring on an hypnotic state. The patient is then told that from henceforth all cigarettes will have such a foul taste that he will be unable and unwilling to smoke. Hypnosis can be successful in just one session, but it usually has to be reinforced at least once more at a later time to achieve maximum benefit.

OTHER WAYS

Those methods that use rapid smoking and prolonged inhaling to help the person quit smoking are extremely dangerous to anyone with a heart or a lung problem. Their use is questionable because of the hazards inherent in them.

EFFECTS OF SMOKING ON THE NONSMOKER

Tobacco is a significant source of air pollution in both enclosed and ventilated areas. The air in a room filled with cigarette smoke has been evaluated by many scientific teams in terms of its harmful effects on the nonsmokers in that room. The results uniformly show that even persons resting and relaxing in a room full of tobacco smoke showed some evidence of having an increase in their heart rate and an elevation in their blood pressure.

In 1975 in a report by the Surgeon General on "The Health Consequences of Smoking" the term "involuntary smokers" was coined to describe those nonsmokers who were exposed to cigarette smoke. The inhalation of this smoke as well as simply breathing in a smoke-filled atmosphere exposes the nonsmoker to much the same effects from tobacco smoke to which the voluntary smoker is exposed. The chemical components of a smoke-filled atmosphere come from two sources. The first, called *sidestream smoke,* gets into the air while the smoker is puffing on the cigarette. Cigars and pipes also contribute to sidestream smoke because they burn over a longer period of time. The second source is called *mainstream smoke,* which gets into the air whenever the smoker exhales the smoke. Sidestream smoke has a higher concentration of carbon monoxide than does mainstream smoke. There is also twice as much nicotine and tar in sidestream smoke. Smoking in unventilated areas allows a dangerous level of carbon monoxide to build up, and it is breathed by the smoker and the nonsmoker alike. This carbon monoxide can be toxic enough to reduce the tolerance level for exercise in both nonsmoker and smoker, particularly so if either one has angina. In addition, carbon monoxide also reduces the amount of oxygen that can be carried in the blood, which can be crucial to the nonsmoker as well as to the smoker if either has any tendency toward coronary insufficiency.

The nicotine in the tobacco settles out of the air more easily than does the carbon monoxide. In fact the nonsmoker really absorbs very little of the nicotine present in the air compared to the amount of carbon monoxide absorbed from it.

Nonsmokers have become more assertive in demanding that special sections in restaurants and/or planes be set aside for those who smoke as one step toward protecting their own health.

CHAPTER EIGHT

ORAL CONTRACEPTIVES

The first oral contraceptive was introduced in 1961 and quickly became known to the millions of women who took it as THE PILL.

Dr. John Rock, a professor of gynecology at Harvard Medical School, had been trying for years to develop a safe, inexpensive, foolproof, and simple-to-use method of contraception. With the assistance of his associates, Drs. Pencus and Garcia, he initiated a complete and thorough investigation of the use of progesterone and its derivatives in women who, although apparently physically normal in every way, were still unable to conceive.

Dr. Rock's aim was to try to induce a pseudopregnant condition with the use of progesterone in the hope that when the progesterone was stopped, fertility might be enhanced and conception might then be possible. As with so many experiments, the results had effects other than the one sought. In these experiments progestin, a synthetic form of a derivative of progesterone, was taken orally on a sequential basis from day 5 to day 25 of the menstrual cycle. (The first day of menstruation is always considered to be day 1, and menstruation usually lasts five days.) Within a few days of completing the 25-day cycle and stopping the progestin, withdrawal bleeding occurred. Progestin was resumed when bleeding ceased, and it was continued for 20 days. The results showed that if the schedule for taking progestin was followed to the letter, no pregnancies occurred. Extensive field studies were then conducted at the Puerto Rico Family Planning Center, and the results were the same.

The sequential cycle of three weeks of taking progesterone and five days of not taking it created an artificial menstrual period. The results obtained with progesterone were a great development in the field of gynecology. It was to be of inestimable value as a means of regulating the menstrual cycle of those women who experience great irregularity in their cycle.

Among these first progestin compounds, some were found to have an estrogen-like activity owing, it was felt, either to their having been converted to estrogen by the body itselt or to the compounds themselves having become contaminated with estrogen.

The discovery of the estrogen-like activity of progestin was a real breakthrough because it proved that estrogen actually enhanced the effect of the progesterone. This discovery led to the inclusion of estrogen along with progesterone in the pill.

The first commercial product containing progesterone and mestranol, a form of estrogen, was called Enovid. As the result of experience gained in its use, the amount of progesterone was reduced and that of estrogen increased. This change resulted in no loss of contraceptive effectiveness.

Progesterone is a hormone that aids in preparing the endometrium (i.e., the inner surface of the uterus or womb) for receiving an embryo. Conversely, it also has a contraceptive effect because it causes menstrual bleeding even though it is no longer being taken. Progesterone also causes a thickening of the cervical mucus, which prevents penetration by sperm. Progesterone acts during the latter part of the menstrual cycle, whereas estrogen acts during the first part.

Progesterone also brings about some changes in the endometrium. Menstruation results when progesterone is withdrawn in the artificially created cycle or naturally when the body itself ceases to create progesterone. In large doses, progesterone suppresses ovulation. It decreases the contractibility of the myometrium (the muscular substance of the womb), raises the basal body temperature, and also promotes the secretion of sodium. Although progesterone is antiestrogenic, some of its synthesized derivatives do have estrogenic properties. The ability of both estrogen and progesterone to suppress ovulation has prompted their use in oral contraceptives.

Progesterone was first isolated from a vegetable, the Mexican yam, which was being studied for possible use in the manufacturing of steroids, particularly cortisone. The first progesterone manufactured was called norethynodrel. It had effects of both progesterone and estrogen when it was converted by the body into estrogen.

Estrogen itself is a hormone which, besides being produced in the ovaries, is also produced in the adrenal glands and in the liver.

The principal organ of the body that metabolizes estrogen is the liver. The water-soluble conjugated estrogens are excreted through the kidneys. Estrogen controls the growth and development of the uterus (i.e., the womb), the vagina (i.e., the sheathlike tube between the uterus and the body opening), and the fallopian tubes (the ducts that extend from the uterus to the ovary). Estrogen also controls the growth and development of the reproductive organs, which take place during the first part of the menstrual cycle.

In the uterus, estrogen promotes endometrial cell division and a thickening of the endometrium. Bleeding occurs in the endometrium when it has been stimulated by estrogen within 48 hours after the discontinuance of the use of estrogen. Estrogen also produces an increase in the amount of vaginal and uterine mucosa (linings). It tends to cause a retention of both sodium and water in the body, which, as we have noted elsewhere, can have many unfavorable consequences. Estrogen inhibits or prevents ovulation (i.e., the monthly discharge of the ovum or egg from the ovary). When supplemental or natural estrogen is given, it must be administered intramuscularly or subcutaneously because it is not effective when taken orally.

Ethinyl estradiol is one of the most potent of the natural estrogens. Some of the chemical or nonnatural substances used for their estrogenic effect are diethylstilbesterol, benzestral (known as Chemestrogen), dienestral (known as Synestra), and promesthestral (known as Meprone).

The so-called conjugated estrogens are composed of a mixture of various estrogens derived from the urine of pregnant mares. Horses have a tremendous amount of estrogen. A pregnant mare can excrete over 100 mg of estrogen a day whereas the stallion secretes more estrogen than any other creature.

The estrogen substances taken from horses are known as equine estrogen—equillin and equilenin. They are the only estrogens commonly used that are considered to be impure. Premarin, a form of estrogen widely used during menopause, is a conjugated estrogen (i.e., a mixture of estrogens blended to represent the material derived from the urine of pregnant mares.

The antifertility effect of estrogen first came to scientific attention when it was discovered that the blossoms of plants that grew along the Red Sea area had estrogenic properties. An estrogen substance known as estriol has also been isolated from the buds of the willow tree.

Sheep ranchers in Australia noticed that sterility developed among large flocks of sheep grazing on pasture land covered with subterranean clover. This type of clover was found to contain large amounts of genestein, which is a weak form of estrogen. Coumestrol, found in a type of clover known as ladine, is a much more powerful form of estrogen. Many of these synthetic hormones are much more powerful than are the natural hormones produced in the body.

TYPES OF ORAL CONTRACEPTIVES

There are four types of oral contraceptives, three of which are highly effective. A fourth, which is somewhat less effective, has been used in recent years in an attempt to cut down on the side effects of estrogen.

THE COMBINATION TYPE

One type of oral contraceptive is a combination of estrogen and progestogen, taken from day 5 through day 24 of the menstrual cycle, that is, 21 days on THE PILL and then 5 days off.

Ethinyl estradiol (Demulen), ethylnodial diacetate with mestranol (Ovulen), norethindrone with mestranol (Norinyl and Ortho-Novum), norethyrodrel with mestranol (Enovid), and norgestrel with ethinyl estradiol (Ovral) are among the best known of the combination type of oral contraceptive.

The combination estrogen/progesterone preparations produce changes in the mucus of the cervix that make it impassable to sperm.

THE SEQUENTIAL TYPE

The second type of oral contraceptive is known as the sequential type. It provides straight estrogen for 14 to 16 days of the menstrual cycle, followed by a combination of estrogen and progesterone for the next five to seven days, followed by five days with no pills.

Some of the sequential types are mestranol plus chlormodinone acetate with mestranol (C-Quens), ethinyl estradiol plus dimethisterone with ethinyl estradiol (Oracon), and mestranol plus norethindrone with mestranol (Norquen and Ortho-Novum SQ). The sequential preparations rely on estrogen alone for a contraceptive effect, adding the progesterone to ensure both a prompt shedding of the endometrium cells and withdrawal bleeding.

The five days of abstention from both the combination and sequential types of pills emulate the natural menstrual cycle in which bleeding occurs once a month.

In the 1960s as THE PILL became more widely used, it became apparent that the more serious side effects being experienced by women (such as headaches, weight gain, bleeding between periods, fatigue, depression, vaginal discharge, urinary tract infections, skin problems such as acne, and even loss of libido) were related to the amount of estrogen in the pill.

And as the use of THE PILL became even more widespread, neurologists began reporting incidences of stroke in healthy young women taking oral contraceptives. The first instance of this was reported in the *British Medical Journal* in 1962.

Previously, when strokes occurred in young women, there was usually a specific cause such as hypertension or diabetes. Strokes are also known to occur during pregnancy and during the first few months after delivery when a woman's hormones are changing back to their normal state. But for strokes to occur in healthy young women who had none of the risk factors associated with strokes was a cause for concern for all physicians. Of particular concern was that the women taking oral contraceptives had a risk of having strokes nine times greater than those women who did not take an oral contraceptive. Usually, most women who have strokes are middle-aged, when they have ceased to make their own hormones after the menopause. It was the increasing number of women in the child-bearing years, who were taking oral contraceptives and having strokes, that gave cause for alarm. These young women were having strokes caused by cerebral venous thrombosis and cavernous sinus thrombosis along with occlusions of the vertebrobasilar artery. Until the widespread use of THE PILL such strokes had been considered to be extremely rare in young women.

Also noted was the fact that when larger doses of estrogen were administered to males who had cancer of the prostate gland, cardiovascular disease resulting in a myocardial infarction (heart attack) and cerebral thrombosis (stroke) were not infrequent. As the number of cases of prostatic cancer being treated with estrogen increased, so did the incidence of heart attacks and strokes.

Studies conducted in the United States, the United Kingdom, and Scandinavia confirmed a correlation between the amount of estrogen in oral contraceptives and the incidence of heart attacks and strokes. This finding led to a decision to manufacture oral contraceptives containing a smaller amount of estrogen. However, too little estrogen brought on breakthrough bleeding (i.e., bleeding while taking the pill), so it was not simply a matter of reducing THE PILL's estrogen content. A correct balance between estrogen and progesterone had to be achieved.

THE USE OF TWO TYPES OF PILLS

The action of and the amount of progesterone in birth control pills became even more important because progesterone was not without its own adverse effects.

The end result was a third type of oral contraceptive that consisted of not one but two pills—one pill containing nothing but estrogen, which was to be taken for two weeks, and the other pill containing only progesterone which was to be taken for one week. This differed from the sequential pill in that there was no estrogen taken with the progesterone at any time. It was felt that this sequence more closely duplicated the woman's own natural menstrual cycle.

THE MINIPILL

Persons who believed that it was the estrogen that was still causing problems set about devising yet a fourth type of oral contraceptive—one that contained only progesterone and that became known as the minipill. In a way this was history repeating itself, because this was the type of pill first used by Dr. Rock. The minipill is believed to act on the mucosa of the cervix, either to prevent the sperm from penetrating or in some manner to cause it to be made inactive.

The minipill is not as reliable as the other types, nor is it as convenient because it must be taken every day and at the same time every day, beginning with the first day of the menstrual cycle and continuing even during the time of menstruation. Currently Orvette, Macronar, and Nor Q.D. are the most widely used of the minipills.

The minipill appeared first in the United States in 1973. Because it contains no estrogen and has few if any serious side effects, it is often the choice for women over 35.

EFFECTS OF ORAL CONTRACEPTIVES

In 1968, after the British had shown that there was a definite association between the oral contraceptive and an increase in the number of cases of disorders in blood clotting, the U.S. Federal Food and Drug Administration ordered all manufacturers of oral contraceptives to include a notice in their packages to warn users to "Be alert to the earliest manifestations of thrombotic disorders (thrombophlebetis, cerebrovascular disorders, pulmonary embolism and retinal thrombosis)."

Thrombophlebitis refers to both the formation of a clot and an inflammation in a vein; cerebrovascular disorders refer to strokes; pulmonary embolism refers to the condition that results when a blood clot has become lodged in the lungs, thus obstructing the flow of blood; and retinal thrombosis refers to a blood clot lodged in the eye. Those contraceptives containing only a small amount of estrogen are considered to be the safest and the least likely to bring on any of these disorders.

Well over 15 million women in the United States alone and over 50 million women throughout the rest of the world use some form of oral contraceptive, making it the most common form of contraception and the most popular because of both its effectiveness and convenience.

BLOOD CLOTTING AND DEEP VENOUS THROMBOSIS

Oral contraceptives tend to dilate (widen) the veins, causing the blood to flow through them at a slower than normal rate, which can lead to stasis or stagnation of the normal flow of blood. Then, because of the stagnation, it can lead to the formation of thromboses, or blood clots. The risk of deep venous thrombosis in women taking oral contraceptives is increased by 5 to 10 times over what it is in those women not taking them. Usually these clots originate in the arteries or veins in the feet, legs, or pelvic areas. From there they can break off, travel to and become lodged in the lungs, resulting in pulmonary embolism. These clots can also either form in or travel to the brain, causing a stroke. This tendency toward clotting is one of the reasons why, when possible, oral contraceptives should be discontinued several months before surgery.

The thrombotic stroke is the type of stroke most frequently associated with the use of oral contraceptives. The risk of experiencing this type of stroke while taking oral contraceptives is four times the normal rate of incidence.

In fact, a cerebrovascular accident (CVA) resulting from a thrombosis rather than resulting from a hemorrhage is a form of stroke that can occur even in women whose blood pressure is normal because of the increased coagulation effect on the blood caused by the oral contraceptives. The risk of having a stroke due to a hemorrhage in the arteries or the veins of the brain while taking oral contraceptives is twice the normal rate. The relative risk estimate for a stroke in those women who both smoke and take THE PILL is 21.9 times greater than it is for women who do neither.

As would be expected, the danger of experiencing a stroke is increased if a woman has hypertension, either as a condition brought on by other risk factors or solely by the use of THE PILL. However, unexpected findings came from autopsies that clearly showed that the strokes were caused by an occlusion of one of the major intracranial arteries, with no evidence of any underlying atherosclerosis. In other words, in these cases the arteries were not narrowed by the formation of plaque nor did they have roughened surfaces where plaque could have easily built up. These strokes were caused simply by an increased tendency of the blood to clot.

Usually, but not always, there are warnings that such blood clots have formed. Headaches, seeing flashing lights, the loss of vision, blurred vision, severe pains in the legs or the chest, and shortness of breath are all symptoms warning that something is wrong. They should be reported to a physician without delay.

Oral contraceptives increase the viscosity of the platelets in the blood, which in turn increases the tendency of these platelets to clump up. The contraceptives also increase coagulability (i.e., the clotting capability of the blood) and fibronalysis (i.e., the redissolving of a blood clot because of the presence of fibrin). These same conditions are noted in pregnant women and in women who take estrogen during the menopause. It is the estrogen component of the oral contraceptives that causes the platelets in the blood of persons taking them to resemble the platelets in the blood of women who have some form of arterial disease.

The usual clotting time of blood is 10 minutes. A prolonged clotting time of 18 minutes or even longer can mean that there is greater danger from loss of blood during surgery. Problems associated with blood clotting are less common in women with Type O blood. This is fortunate because 46 per cent of all women have Type O blood; 42 per cent have Type A; 9 per cent have Type B; and only 3 per cent have Type AB.

ATHEROSCLEROSIS

Oral contraceptives bring about changes in the walls of arteries and veins that accelerate the development of atherosclerosis. Contraceptives containing the most estrogen cause the greatest changes in the way fat is metabolized.

Biochemical studies indicate that the use of oral contraceptives leads to the formation of larger molecules of fat, which then travel through the bloodstream and stick to the arterial walls in the form of plaque. Oral contraceptives also cause an increase in serum cholesterol and in triglyceride. In its natural form estrogen has much less effect on the blood lipids than does the synthetic form used in oral contraceptives.

As seen in Chapter 5, a high level of HDL (high density lipid) concentration is a known protection against heart attacks. Levels of HDL are lowered in those women who take oral contraceptives, and they are lowered even further in women who in addition to taking the pill also smoke cigarettes.

HYPERTENSION

The type of hypertension brought on by oral contraceptives can be essential and primary and free of symptoms of malignant hypertension due to secondary causes.

The hormones in THE PILL can cause the kidneys to release substances such as angiotensinogen. They can also cause an increase in the plasma renin activity, which can lead to the development of hypertension. Oral contraceptives also have a tendency to cause the body to retain fluid, along with retaining sodium. Sodium, too, can lead to hypertension.

Many women notice that their appetites increase when they are taking THE PILL. Consequently, they begin to put on weight, which of itself can cause a rise in blood pressure. Should this increase in weight continue, yet another risk factor for heart attacks and strokes would be present—namely, obesity.

There is an elevation not only in the systolic but also the diastolic blood pressure of women taking oral contraceptives. Many physicians and researchers believe that hypertension is responsible for the strokes that occur in women who take THE PILL. At least 25 per cent of those women show a rise in blood pressure during the time they take THE PILL, even if their blood pressure was normal before they started taking THE PILL. After 35 years of age, the incidence is even higher, particularly in women with a family history of hypertension or who experienced hypertension when they were pregnant. In 1967 Dr. John Laragh was the first to report this relationship between oral contraceptives and hypertension, a relationship that was then becoming increasingly evident. The longer the period of time a woman takes an oral contraceptive the greater are her chances of developing hypertension and the greater her risk of experiencing a stroke.

Any elevation in blood pressure that occurs while a woman is taking THE PILL is in most cases transitory. It takes the blood pressure about a month to return to a normal level after the discontinuance of an oral contraceptive.

MYOCARDIAL INFARCTION (HEART ATTACK)

A myocardial infarction (i.e., a heart attack) is also associated with the use of oral contraceptives, particularly so in those women who also smoke. If a woman smokes along with taking THE PILL, the chances of her having a myocardial infarction increase more than five-fold. This rate is substantially higher in women over 40, and is greatest, as one would expect, in women who also have any of the other risk factors associated with heart attacks, such as hypertension, elevated blood lipids, diabetes, obesity, and so on.

Arteriograms performed in an effort to pinpoint the reasons for this increased incidence of myocardial infarction in women who smoke and also take THE PILL showed a most interesting development. Instead of the scattered changes in the arterial walls typically seen in most instances of atherosclerosis, there was instead just one smooth blocking lesion located in the left coronary artery. This finding led to the supposition that the oral contraceptive, in conjunction with smoking, caused an overgrowth of the wall of the blood vessel itself, which then led to the infarction, or occlusion.

SMOKING

The Center for Disease Control in Atlanta conducted a study that showed beyond a doubt that the risk of heart attacks among women who smoke and also take oral contraceptives is over five times as great as it is in women who do not smoke.

Cigarette smoking increases the risk of developing clotting disorders while taking oral contraceptives. And in those women who took oral contraceptives and had strokes, a large number were found to be cigarette smokers. Smoking also increases the blood pressure.

No woman who smokes should ever take an oral contraceptive.

Consequently, since 1977 the oral contraceptive packages have contained inserts warning women of the dangers of smoking while using oral contraceptives.

Women who take THE PILL *and* smoke are three times more apt to die from a heart attack or stroke than are those who take THE PILL but do not smoke. They are 10 times more likely to die from heart attacks and strokes than are those who neither take THE PILL nor smoke. The mortality rate for the woman who smokes rises from 1.2 to 1.4 per 100,000 in the teenage group taking THE PILL to 58.4 per 100,000 in the 40 to 44 age group taking THE PILL. Heavy smoking is considered by many as the principal reason for the increased mortality seen in women who smoke and also take THE PILL.

DIABETES

Oral contraceptives produce a significant change in the level of glucose tolerance. This change is seen most often in those women who use the combination type of oral contraceptive—that is, the pill containing both estrogen and progesterone. This change can make any existing diabetes much worse.

A chemical diabetes often occurs in women who take THE PILL, and many times this indicates that diabetes mellitus will develop later on in life, during middle or old age. Chemical diabetes is the result of problems experienced by the liver in metabolizing the body's glucose, causing the pancreas to increase its production of insulin. The pancreas can go on increasing production until it literally exhausts itself, at which time its production of insulin decreases to an extremely low level, or it even ceases. The body's glucose cannot then be metabolized, resulting eventually in diabetes mellitus.

An abnormal glucose tolerance level is seen in about 10 per cent of the women who have been taking oral contraceptives for one year or longer. This abnormal level can be reversed within a three-month period once THE PILL is discontinued.

OTHER PARTS OF THE BODY

Taken over a long period of time, an oral contraceptive can bring about changes in the pituitary gland, the liver, and the ovaries themselves. In fact, there is practically no organ or tissue in the body that is not affected by THE PILL.

The risk of developing complications from taking oral contraceptives is increased if the user is prone to having migraine headaches, has a family history of diabetes, strokes or heart attacks, is over the age of 30, and is overweight. Every woman who takes an oral contraceptive should tell her physician at once of any symptom or side effect she experiences, whether or not she believes it is associated with THE PILL.

Considering the difficulties that can develop from the use of oral contraceptives, physicians consider the following factors to be absolute contraindications for their use:

- Coronary artery disease
- Cerebrovascular accident (CVA), that is, a stroke
- Thromboembolic disorders
- Diabetes
- Hypertension
- Migraine or vascular headaches
- Abnormal liver function or liver disease
- Vaginal bleeding
- Being over 30 to 40 years of age
- Heavy smoking
- Sickle cell disease
- Mononucleosis
- Cancer of the breast or pelvic organs
- Hyperlipidemia

Women taking oral contraceptives are known to experience a tenderness and/or fullness in their breasts. Whether or not there is an increased risk of developing cancer has yet to be fully evaluated.

CHAPTER NINE

STRESS

If there is one common denominator for all the risk factors associated with a stroke it undoubtedly is stress. Very few ideas in medicine have engendered so much interest as has the concept of the role played by stress in all forms of illness. This relationship was first recognized by Dr. Hans Selye, an Austrian-born physician who became the founder and president of the International Institute of Stress in Montreal, Canada. His work in the field of stress has won him innumerable honors.

In 1956 in his book *The Stress of Life* Selye presented a new and, at that time, revolutionary concept of the role of stress in those diseases that were reaching epidemic proportions in all the technologically advanced areas of the world—namely, heart disease, hypertension, atherosclerosis, and stroke.

Throughout the centuries the idea of stress had always entailed the concept of strain, of hardship, or of the strong effort exerted on the body and the mind through something that had originated outside of the body. Selye's theory of stress was based on the idea that stress can also originate within the body as the direct result of the strain on various organs of the body brought about by illness or disease.

ORIGIN OF THE STRESS THEORY

As a young medical student, Selye embarked on what was to become a lifetime pursuit—the study of stress itself, of its damaging effects on the body and the mind, and of how to cope with it. At the first demonstration lecture on internal medicine he ever attended, he was intrigued by the fact that although each of the patients presented for evaluation had a different type of infectious disease characterized by different symptoms (e.g., a rash in measles or swollen glands in mumps), all of them had one set of symptoms in common. Each patient complained of the same kind of ache and pain, each had an upset stomach, fever, loss of appetite and weight, and each had a generalized feeling of being just plain sick.

The professor who was conducting the demonstration lecture was like every medical teacher of his time—primarily concerned with pointing out the classical signs and symptoms as they pertained to each separate disease. Hans Selye had a feeling that something was being overlooked. The fact that each patient had the same symptoms regardless of his or her disease seemed to Selye to be of great significance. He began to wonder if, in addition to the infectious diseases, there might be yet another disease, one that made each of the patients feel sick in the same way. For want of a better term Selye called it "the syndrome of being sick."

The medical textbooks define a syndrome as a group of signs or symptoms occurring together that are characteristic of a specific disease. In the case of the patients Selye had examined, the symptoms did not apply to only one specific disease but were present in every one of the diseases these patients had. Whether there might in reality be a disease called *sickness* continued to intrigue him. In searching for an answer, he set about learning all he could about the mechanisms of sickness itself, apart from its association with any specific disease. He concentrated on those feelings that were experienced by every patient regardless of the disease each had.

Time and circumstances interrupted Selye's efforts, and he became involved in endocrinology, the branch of medicine dealing with the ductless glands and their functions. Endocrinology at that time was having a huge impact on medicine because of the discovery of insulin by Dr. Frederick Banting in 1922. The fact that diabetes was caused by a hormonal deficiency and could be controlled by the hormone insulin made it conceivable that other diseases also could be controlled by hormones. Selye delved deeply into this field, specifically attempting to identify what was hoped would be a new female hormone. Accordingly he began experiments with the extracts from ovaries and stumbled not on a new female hormone but on the fact that the injection of the hormone extract always affected three distinctive parts of the body and without fail resulted in the same kinds of changes in those parts of the body. First the adrenal and thymus glands became enlarged; then the spleen and the lymph nodes shrank in size. Finally, both bleeding and evidence of deep ulcers developed in the stomach and the gut.

Selye called these changes a triad. Continuing his experiments, he found that not only did other hormones besides those from the ovaries produce these same effects but even those hormones in no way connected with the manufacture of sex hormones did so also. In addition, he found that extracts from other organs of the body, such as the kidney, the spleen, and the liver, also produced the same three symptoms. Realizing at this point that he was not on the right track toward the discovery of a new female hormone, he was near to admitting failure when he began to wonder if this triad of effects might be caused by the contaminants that got into the extracts during their processing rather than by the extracts themselves.

To pursue this idea further, Selye injected formalin, which is a toxic fluid related to formaldehyde, into his experimental rats instead of the hormonal extracts. Formalin is not manufactured by the body and could therefore, for experimental purposes, be considered a contaminant. When the formalin was injected, the very same triad of effects occurred as had been produced by the hormonal extracts and—most important—occurred to an even greater degree.

The same thought that had occurred to Selye as a medical student came back to him. What if all these hormonal extracts, which were foreign to that part of the body where they were injected (as was the formalin), set up a reaction that was similar to that of the body itself when it was affected by disease? In other words, could it be possible that the triad of symptoms was nothing more than the body's way of coping with damage to itself? Selye kept returning to the concept he had had so many years before: namely, the question of illness itself, not as it related to a specific disease but simply the feeling of being sick.

Up to this time no one had ever viewed these symptoms of sickness by themselves. The symptoms had been seen only in relation to specific diseases. As Selye further studied the subject, he reasoned that the symptoms of fear, anxiety, and general malaise were all evidence that the body was desperately trying to fight infection. This fight, so characteristic of all diseases, is the body's way of protecting itself, of trying to overcome disease and return to a healthy state.

Selye's experiments with the concept of the "syndrome of just being sick" brought him to the realization that the body fights stress and strain in the same manner that it fights sickness. The body raises up such defenses as an increase in the amount of adrenalin that is secreted, inflammation of the stomach resulting in ulcers, enlargement of the heart, and an increase in blood pressure. Selye also realized that the body's coping mechanism is ongoing. Stress occurs on a daily basis, whereas disease occurs only occasionally. Yet the body reacts to both in the same manner. Every disease also causes stress because the body has to adapt to its presence. The word *stress* was used by Selye to describe what was happening to the body. The use of the word in this sense has become international and is spelled the same in all languages. Selye proved that the triad of effects he had observed is the means used by the body to deal with and to combat stress, strain, tension, damage, and wear and tear. He proved that this triad of effects is the end result of the ways in which the body prepares itself to cope with stress.

It was Selye who gave us the famous definition of stress as being *the nonspecific response of the body to any demand made on it.* Stress is the result of the response made by every living organism to change, whether that change be from disease or tension. It is, in other words, the body's reaction to both ordinary and extraordinary pressure.

Although both are sometimes considered in the same context, there is a difference between stress and pressure. Stress causes the body to become geared up in order to meet any added strain. Pressure, on the other hand, can be a stimulus. It can prevent us from goofing off, and it can prod us into getting a job done. When pressure becomes too intense, however, it then becomes stress.

Stress is associated with all the multiple problems we face in our jobs, with our families, with environmental pollutants, heat and cold, the death of a loved one, retirement, exercise, illness, surgery, and so on. Stress does not affect everyone in the same way. There are people who seem to thrive in an atmosphere of conflict and chaos, whereas others simply fall apart at the slightest bit of stress. The latter are the unfortunate souls who through inheritance do not have the biological resources ever to be able to cope with stress in any form.

Whatever the problem or condition that leads to the stressful state, the body meets it in one of two ways: either aggressively by fighting it or passively by running away from it or tolerating it. This is known as the "fight or flight response" and is experienced by all creatures.

THE GENERAL ADAPTATIVE SYNDROME (GAS)

Selye further clarified his theory of stress by describing the three phases of stress. He called these phases the General Adaptative Syndrome (GAS) and defined the syndrome as the sum total of all the nonspecific reactions of the body resulting from long and continuous exposure to stress.

The three phases of the General Adaptative Syndrome are the following:

1. *The alarm reaction* when the body goes into action and releases hormones from the adrenal glands, which then brings about a response from the nervous system.
2. *The stage of resistance and adaptation* when the body fights back. This is also the stage when the body tries to repair any damage that has been done to it. If the body is unable to repair the damage, it will continue in the alarm stage.
3. *The stage of exhaustion* when the body's defenses are no longer able to handle stress. This stage ends in death. It is also the stage that occurs when the end of the normal lifespan has been reached.

The capacity of the body to adapt to stress has limits. The body's resources are not infinite. Continued stress during a period of exhaustion seriously depletes the body of energy and unnecessarily cuts into its lifetime store of energy. If this pattern of energy depletion were to continue, the body would lose its ability to replace energy. It would in fact become burned out and the stage of exhaustion as described by Selye would take place.

Heredity determines the amount of adaptation energy each person is born with. It is ours to use wisely or to dissipate. As we go through life, we constantly draw on this storehouse of energy, and nothing depletes this store of energy faster than stress. The more rapidly we rush through life responding to one crisis after another, with no break in routine to enable the body to recharge its store of energy, the quicker that supply of energy, which is designed to last a lifetime, will be exhausted.

There is no known way to replenish the supply of energy once it has been depleted. Every time we exceed the amount of energy that should be used at any given time in life, even though we may be able to sleep, relax, and rest, and consequently feel more energetic, the storehouse of energy has not actually been completely replenished. It cannot be for we have only so much to start with.

When we use up our adaptability reserve, we can neither replace it nor replenish it. However, if we realize that we have spent too much of our lifetime store of energy in a foolish and profligate manner and if we carefully husband what we have left, we can help to stretch it out to last through our remaining years of life. In this way we can be assured of having sufficient energy to carry on our everyday activities.

Gerontologists who study the phenomenon of old age believe that aging is the result of having used up too much of the store of adaptation energy at too fast a rate. This is the reason that as we grow older we seem to have less and less energy to expend even on the things we like to do, let alone those we must do.

To be certain that the storehouse of energy with which we were born will last as long as possible, most physicians recommend having frequent rest periods, particularly after the onset of middle age. These rest periods can be in the form of a daily nap as well as short vacations and long weekends.

GOOD AND BAD TYPES OF STRESS

It is impossible to avoid all stress. You cannot avoid it and still be alive. Even during sleep the body is under some stress. The heart continues to pump blood, the lungs continue to breathe, the brain remains active, as evidenced by the dreams and nightmares we experience. Stress is not all bad. In fact some stress in moderation is good because it presents challenges and keeps our lives from becoming dull and boring.

Difficulties with stress arise only when the stress situation is either prolonged or recurs too frequently, and when its effects are felt constantly in one particular area of the body. Selye refers to this type of stress as *distress,* which he defines as *a continuous form of tension that requires the body to continually adapt and readapt in order to cope with it.*

Emotional stress can result from joy as well as sorrow; from having had an argument to the death of a loved one; from making love to receiving a much-longed-for gift. Both types of emotion make it necessary for the body to try to adjust to a different kind of situation. Both types of adjustment result in stress.

Physical stress can result from shovelling snow in a blizzard, pushing a stalled car, overexercising—in fact from any effort that calls for the expenditure of an exceptional amount of energy.

Environmental stress can result from traffic jams, the tensions at work, and from noise and pollution. The role played in stress by noise and the quickening tempo of everyday life cannot be overlooked when assessing the amount of stress to which we are subjected.

Our bodies are constantly having to make adjustments to the demands made on them; this creates stress. When we are cold we shiver, when we are hot we perspire, when we overexert ourselves either through strenuous exercise or hard work our hearts beat faster and our blood pressure rises so that the blood vessels can dilate and allow more blood to flow through the arteries. The body then tries to bring itself back to a normal condition. It does not continue shivering or perspiring, the heart does not continue to race, nor does the blood pressure remain elevated. It is this attempt to return to a normal condition and to get out of the alarm stage that brings on the second phase of the General Adaptation Syndrome—the phase of resisting and adapting.

Trying to get too much accomplished too quickly always leads to stress, which is exacerbated by the further stress of the body's trying to adapt and to cope. It is not the one or two isolated incidents of stress that cause acceleration of the development of atherosclerosis, hypertension, and elevated blood lipids, but, rather, those periods of protracted stress and strain.

Nor is it only the type of job that carries with it an increased amount of responsibility that brings on stress. Most of the time the men and women who have achieved the highest ranking positions derive a great sense of satisfaction from their work. They thrive on the demands their jobs make on them. For them there may be stress, but there is no distress. It is those who find themselves working at lower echelon jobs that do not carry responsibility who often experience feelings of utter frustration, resentment, and boredom because of the lack of stimulus associated with their jobs. For them the job itself becomes a stress factor.

DIFFERENT RESPONSES OF MEN AND WOMEN TO STRESS

Historically, men and women have tended to respond to stress in different ways. This in great measure is due to fundamental differences in their makeup. Men, being the more practical and analytical, tend to view problems more or less on an intellectual level. They also tend to keep their feelings to themselves.

Women, whom nature has made more emotional and also more intuitive, tend to show their feelings more openly. As women take on more and more of the jobs so long associated with men, they too are finding that the marketplace is full of stress and turmoil. Their reactions result in their experiencing greater amounts of stress. They become just as prone to developing such stress-induced diseases as atherosclerosis, heart attacks, hypertension, elevated blood lipids, and strokes as do men.

The Chinese believe that a crisis is danger plus opportunity. Each age in life has its own set of crises. The manner in which we react to them, the ways we handle them, set the stage for the way we will react as each succeeding age unfolds. Coping successfully with crises builds a sense of confidence and provides a firm foundation upon which is built the ability to handle stress.

STRESS AS A RISK FACTOR IN STROKES

When we are no longer able to deal with stress in our lives, our bodies are literally forced to undergo a number of physical and emotional changes. Stress plays a major role in hypertension, in the acceleration of atherosclerosis, and in an elevation in the level of cholesterol in the blood. These are all risk factors associated with strokes.

Stress has an effect on the whole circulatory system of the body. We have seen how the so-called Type A personality, the stress-prone, hard-driving, time-conscious, goal-oriented person is so apt to become hypertensive. These same traits also accelerate the development of atherosclerosis and contribute to the elevation of blood cholesterol.

The World Health Organization in its 1971 report showed how much a serene lifestyle could do to offset the damage done by stress in causing diseases of the vascular system, either in the heart or the brain. This study was based on a group of people who lived in the small town of Roseto, Pennsylvania. Despite the fact that their diets were high in saturated fats, they had few heart attacks or strokes. Their life style was highly structured, based on the concept of the men being the unchallenged heads of the households. Each resident was imbued with a high degree of family and civic pride. They supported and encouraged one another in all their endeavors and sympathized with and consoled one another in time of sorrow. They were an extremely close community whose lives were remarkably free of stress and strain. Living in an atmosphere of harmony, they were relatively free of psychological stress.

For the rest of the world outside of Roseto, however, stress is everywhere, as are the heart attacks and strokes it causes.

HOW THE BODY REACTS TO STRESS

Fight or flight, the two ways in which we handle stress, play a significant role in the disease process.

When we decide to fight a distressful situation, the adrenal glands secrete an increased amount of adrenalin. The adrenal glands are the body's principal reactors to stress. The increase in adrenalin causes the blood pressure to rise, the heart to beat faster, and the nervous system to go into a state of alarm. Everything gears up for battle.

Fear and anxiety also cause an increase in the output of adrenalin and set off the same type of chain reaction. One important result of this increase in adrenalin is that the time blood would normally take to clot is shortened. The result is that blood clots tend to form more quickly and thus can precipitate a stroke.

Although every part of the body experiences the effects of stress, it is always the weakest part that breaks down first. The constant rise in blood pressure and the increase in the lipid levels of the blood that result from stress bring about changes in the walls of the arteries that weaken them so much that they are no longer able to function in a normal way.

If the blood pressure is already elevated, any further increase, such as a cerebral hemorrhage, could be catastrophic. Many studies in recent years have shown that in emotionally stressful situations blood pressure can rise from 50 to 80 points. The emotional problems themselves act as the stressor.

When the blood pressure is elevated, the blood pushes against the walls of the arteries with such force that the walls are damaged, paving the way for lesions to develop on them. These lesions become the basis for the scar tissue on which plaque develops, causing a narrowing of the arteries and decreasing the amount of blood that can flow through them.

Stress is known to cause an increase in the levels of both cholesterol and triglycerides. The level of cholesterol in the blood of students before and after examinations, of military men before and after periods of intense battle stress, and of patients before and after surgery has been shown to rise in direct response to the degree of stress experienced. In most cases the level of cholesterol decreased once the period of stress came to an end. However even if it does not remain elevated permanently, during the time it *is* elevated, the condition is not conducive to the maintenance of healthy, fat-free arteries.

The U.S. Air Force discovered that during periods of intense emotional stress the level of cholesterol can actually double. The level always fluctuates in response to occupational stress.

Elevated cholesterol contributes to the overall lessening of elasticity of the arteries, resulting in the arteries' loss of their ability to remain flexible enough to adjust to the various changes in the flow of blood brought about by atherosclerotic plaque.

STRESS AND DEATH

Can our emotions kill us? History is full of episodes of people dying in the throes of rage, grief, fear, and even joy and happiness. Emotions can be lethal. The surge of hormones released into the bloodstream by an intense emotional upset often brings about abnormal heart beats, which can result in sudden death. The release of hormones is the body's way of raising its defenses against pressure, tension, and stress. It is the body's way of protecting itself from harm.

The avalanche of hormones rushing through the bloodstream can so suppress the body's own immunological defense system that it can actually leave the body with little or no defense against disease because it lowers the body's resistance to infection. Current research is probing the relationship between stress and cancer and finding the same connection as with so many other diseases.

Stress is at the bottom of almost every physical and psychological illness, either as its cause or as one of the factors precipitating the onset of the disease. It can drastically reduce the healing process and at its extreme can be severe enough to bring about premature death.

Medical literature is full of examples of what has become known as the *anniversary syndrome*—that is, the anniversary of the death of a loved one. The traumatic emotional reaction that is experienced on the remembered date can be so intense that the one who grieves feels he or she simply cannot go on living, and in many instances actually does not go on living. Truly it was the emotions that were the cause of death. It is not the amount of stress that kills so much as how we respond to it.

HOW SHOULD STRESS BE HANDLED?

There will always be some stress in our lives. It behooves us, therefore, to learn how to handle it.

The decisions, anxieties, fears, and frustrations that are so much a part of modern life are never easy to eliminate nor, perhaps, should they be ever eliminated completely. However, feelings that are let rage out of control result in a sense of insecurity, of frustration, and, most damaging of all, a loss of peace of mind.

Some years ago Dr. Thomas Holmes and Dr. Minoru Masudi of the University of Seattle in Washington devised a scale of values for some of the most stressful events that frequently occur. This scale has become known as the Social Readjustment Scale. The most stressful situation encountered on this scale is the death of a spouse. Divorce and marital separation rank second and third. Further down on the list are retirement, loss of a job, and, surprisingly, Christmas and vacations. Statistics support these values shown on the Social Readjustment Scale. For example, widows and widowers have a high death rate after the loss of a spouse. Those persons who have been divorced have a greater incidence of illnesses. As the stressful situations in life accumulate, the rate of illness increases. The more stress, the more illness. This bears out Dr. Selye's theory of the General Adaptation Syndrome.

THE VALUE OF RECREATION IN OVERCOMING STRESS

Our bodies need and must have exercise; they are not designed for a life of inactivity. It is not simply physical activity that consumes our energy. Far more trying is mental stress. This is one of the reasons so many physicians advocate taking a walk each day, not only for the exercise it gives us but for the opportunity it provides for relaxation.

Some recreation each day, an annual vacation, and frequent long weekends help the unwinding process. Even when a situation that has been causing stress is corrected its effects may still be around for a long time. The body needs time to adjust to an improved environment in which there is less stress, and it cannot do this overnight. Stress can develop in minutes, but it may take years to overcome it.

LEARNING TO LIVE WITH STRESS

We must learn to accept those things we cannot change and learn to live with them. We must learn to adjust to the ever-changing panorama of stress. We must learn to solve our problems as they occur and not to agonize over them in prolonged indecision. Postponing difficult decisions in the hope that the problem will go away is foolhardy. The problem remains, simmering inside us, wearing us down and causing distress. Eventually we are going to have to reach a decision, to come to a conclusion. How much better to do it when the problem first arises and thus save all that wear and tear, all that unnecessary stress on our minds and bodies.

As John Donne reminded us that "no man is an island," so too do those persons who deal with stress as a medical problem. To talk our problems over with a professional in the field of stress often helps to put them into the proper perspective and thus make them easier to handle. When a situation becomes too much for us to handle, fatigue sets in. This is the signal that we have exceeded the limits of what our body is capable of handling and that our level of stress tolerance has been reached.

Each day must be lived with a purpose and lived as though we were going to live forever with all the time in the world to accomplish our goals. We must learn how to keep the damaging effects of stress to a minimum because these effects make our bodies vulnerable to disease.

Of all the conditions that contribute to the onset of disease or to the feeling of simply being sick, stress is the one we can do the most about. Each stressful situation should be balanced with a relaxing one so designed as to counteract the stress. There should always be a balance of work and play, of exercise and rest. Meditation, biofeedback, and the relaxation response (see Chapter 3) provide many people with excellent methods for reducing stress.

Being able to escape from a stressful situation for a while also helps. Seeing a movie, reading a book, playing a game of golf or tennis, taking a swim—all these can do wonders to relieve tension. Being a martyr and standing around suffering hurts no one but ourselves. It only increases the amount of stress we experience.

Dr. Selye is no less prone to finding himself in stressful situations than the rest of us. He has devised a most enjoyable and therapeutic way of dealing with stress. He takes what he calls minivacations in what he refers to as the "Florida room" in his home. In this room, which faces the sun, he spends part of every day with the windows opened wide, be it winter or summer, and he basks in the sun and fresh air. These minivacations allow him to work a 12-hour day, seven days a week, at the age of 72.

Another way of handling stress is to learn to do one thing at a time. No matter how large the work load, tackling it one thing at a time and then going on to the next thing can make great inroads in it.

It is most important that we find our own stress level and learn to live within it. Our own physical condition, emotional response, and even our environment play a vital role in stress. All three are conditions over which we have control.

The best way by far to avoid the harmful effects of stress is to select a place to live that we like and where we will be happy and well adjusted, to find a job that we enjoy and that has meaning for us. It is important that work bring us a sense of satisfaction, and it is important to balance the work in our life with a hobby that refreshes our mind and spirit to enable us to meet life with all its joys and sorrows with open arms, to live life to the fullest, where body, mind, and spirit are given ample opportunity to develop to the fullest extent possible.

George Bernard Shaw said, "Labor is doing what we must, leisure is doing what we like." Learning how to relax may be one of the most important lessons any of us ever has to learn. Only then will we be able to make stress work for us rather than against us. The ancient Greeks had a wise maxim, as appropriate now as then, "Nothing to excess, everything in moderation".

CHAPTER TEN

LABORATORY TESTS AND DIAGNOSTIC PROCEDURES

Today's patient is extremely fortunate that there are so many laboratory tests and diagnostic procedures available to enable the physician accurately and quickly to arrive at a diagnosis.

LABORATORY TESTS

Laboratory tests have many functions, among them detecting the presence of disease, ruling out disease when the symptoms are vague and unsubstantiated, and confirming a diagnosis that has already been made by clinical means.

The tests that are most frequently done are the ones included in the group called a Sequential Multiphastic Analysis (SMA). These tests are routinely performed as part of a patient's health profile.

In addition to this health screen profile are the specific tests associated with the diagnosis of cerebrovascular disease—a stroke. In many instances, the principal reason for an SMA is to rule out the existence of any disease or abnormality that could mimic the symptoms of a stroke.

Blood tests are done to determine the levels of hemoglobin, hematocrit, and leukocytes (white blood cells) as well as the fasting blood sugar, cholesterol, triglycerides, prothrombin time, blood gases, and thyroid function. Tests for syphillis and those infectious diseases that are known to mimic a stroke may also be included.

Tests are done on the urine to ascertain its specific gravity, sugar, ketone, and protein levels. A 24-hour vanilmandelic acid test (VMA) may be done to determine the presence of a pheochromocytoma, which can cause hypertension.

The cerebral spinal fluid is also tested for color, glucose, protein, and mononuclear cells.

Although these represent the most frequently performed laboratory tests used to confirm the diagnosis of a stroke, literally hundreds of tests are available and can be used if they are required.

DIAGNOSTIC EQUIPMENT AND PROCEDURES

The advances that have been made in diagnostic equipment in recent years have made it possible to see the inside of the brain as never before. The latest and most sophisticated equipment is available in the large teaching hospitals although many of the smaller hospitals are striving to keep abreast.

In this age of informed consent, no one has to or should undergo any test without first understanding the procedure itself, the risks that are involved, or the results that are expected.

BRAIN SCAN

The age of nuclear medicine arrived in the 1970s with the development of the scan. Nothing has so revolutionized the diagnosis of diseases of the brain as has the invention of the brain scan. The scanning procedure is variously knows as computed tomography (CT), computerized axial tomography (CAT), or computerized transaxial tomography (CTT).

The scanners map the distribution of radioactive material and take cross sectional pictures of the head. Because of the vast amount of information they are able to provide they have in many instances made it unneccesary to perform emergency angiography with its inherent risks.

THE DEVELOPMENT OF THE BRAIN SCAN

Dr. William Oldendorf of Los Angeles developed and built a model of a brain scan in 1961. This model took cross sectional images of the brain's soft tissues by scanning the brain from many angles with an X-ray beam capable of detecting the slightest variations in radio densities. Difficult as it is for us to imagine today, when the brain scan is so widely used, Oldendorf was unable to interest a single manufacturer to produce his machine.

Some years later in 1972 a British company, Electrical and Musical Industries Ltd., known all over the world for its sponsorship of the famous rock group "The Beatles," as well as for its manufacture of a wide variety of electronic products, computers, and radar, became even more famous for its development of the brain scan, which bears its name, the EMI Scan. Godfrey N. Hounsfield, who worked for EMI as an electrical engineer specializing in computers, devised a system of scanning called computerized transverse axial tomography (the CAT scanner). In 1979 he received the Nobel Prize for Medicine for this invention.

The traditional X-rays, such as those taken in a skull series, were able to provide only 1 per cent of the amount of information that actually should have been available. The EMI Scan provides 100 per cent of the information by having the X-ray source and the detectors cross the brain linearly—that is, in lines. At the end of each crossing, the scanning unit is rotated one degree around the head, and the process is repeated.

THE SCANNING PROCEDURE

In computerized tomography (CT) no contrast dye is used. The scan shows high and low density areas. High density is the term used to describe a high resistance to the penetration of X-rays. On the CT image high resistance is depicted as white or light gray. Low density is depicted as black or a dark shade of gray.

In other scanning procedures a radioactive material, an isotope, is used. This is given to the patient either by injection or by mouth as a pill. The patient lies on his or her back on a special table that is part of the scanning equipment. A rubber cap is fitted onto the head, and then the head is placed in a round, water-filled section of the equipment, which is then rotated a full 180 degrees around the head.

The water-filled section contains a combination of an X-ray emitter and a detector. As it rotates one degree at a time, a narrow X-ray beam is sent through a thin cross section or slice of the head. Readings of the amount of radiation passing through the head are sent directly to the two scintillation detectors. There are 160 readings for each degree of the brain that is scanned. Each section or slice is 13 mm thick. This information is then stored in a computer. The X-ray beam emitter and the detector are then moved one degree further along, and the process is repeated all over again. The procedure is continued one degree at a time for a full 180 degrees. Each completed 180-degree rotation is considered as one scan. This part of the procedure takes about five minutes.

Another five minutes are required for another detector to measure the intensity of the X-ray source. From this information the computer then calculates 6400 separate pieces of data on the absorptive values of the radioactive material in each part of the X-ray beam. Some 28,000 simultaneous equations are computed.

All these data are then stored on a magnetic disk. The data can be retrieved either as a numerical printout, or they can be displayed on a cathode X-ray tube. A gray scale picture is shown of each slice of the brain that has been scanned. The result is a true density map of the brain.

The conventional X-ray picture is two-dimensional, whereas the picture received from a scanner is three-dimensional. The extent of the detail of the soft tissues of the brain that emerges is almost unbelievable. For example, the brain scan shows the difference between the white and the gray matter of the brain, which is not possible with conventional X-ray equipment.

The scanning procedure itself takes comparatively little time. There may be an interval of time between the administration of the isotope and the actual start of the scan to give the isotope time to reach the brain.

ADVANTAGES OF THE BRAIN SCAN

A brain scan involves no surgery. The procedure is not toxic. It is painless and has no aftereffects. The risks are only what would be present with any form of radiation, and the exposure to X-rays is minimal. Normally, the blood brain barrier prevents the radioactive material from leaving the vascular compartments of the head. However, when the blood brain barrier is no longer intact or is weakened because of the presence of lesions, the radioactive material can become trapped in some of the extravascular areas. The images this produces have a greater density when it is viewed on the monitor.

The brain scan can easily detect the difference between an infarct and an intracerebral hemorrhage as the cause of a stroke. It can show whether there are any lesions and whether they are in a place where it would be possible to remove them surgically. It can confirm the diagnosis of atherosclerotic brain disease. It can show the size and location of any hemorrhage. It can outline a blood clot and delineate its effect on the brain tissue. It can also identify those tumors with symptoms that mimic a stroke. The overall accuracy is between 90 per cent and 98 per cent. Its accuracy in the detection of intracranial hemorrhages is 100 per cent.

The scanning procedure can be repeated as often as is necessary in following the progress of treatment and for determining whether the neurological deficits are progressing, remaining static, or perhaps regressing. The brain scan is especially useful when a person is too weak to withstand angiography.

CEREBRAL SCINTIGRAPHY

Cerebral scintigraphy, or the static brain scan, maps the route taken by the radioactive material, the isotope, through the blood vessels of the neck and head. This procedure, unlike angiography, does not involve the use of a catheter.

DYNAMIC RAPID SERIAL SCINTIGRAPHY

Dynamic rapid serial scintigraphy uses a scintillation camera called a gamma camera to depict the course of the intravenously injected radioactive material through the blood vessels of the neck and head. The results are shown as a serial display either in the form of dots or as a photograph. The procedure can provide information necessary to determine whether there is any arteriovenous malformation, cerebral infarct, or neoplasm.

Although scintigraphy provides less overall information than does angiography or the CAT scanners, it is nonetheless a valuable procedure that can be used to detect cerebral arterial lesions. There is no discomfort and no risk in using the procedure.

POSITRON EMISSION TOMOGRAPHY (PET)

The principle of the new procedure called positron emission tomography is similar to that of the CAT scan. It differs in that it involves the use of positron-emitting radionuclides of natural nutrients produced by a linear accelerator or a cyclotron.

The radionuclide FDG (F2-deoxy-2fluoro-D-glucose) is used as a tracer for evaluating the metabolism of glucose in the various areas of the brain. Thirty minutes after the FDG has been injected into the patient, the PET scanner with its computerized sensors indicates the metabolic activity in a series of sections of the brain. The results are shown as a three-dimensional image on a TV screen. The PET scan shows where the nutrient is being used, and shows how long it takes the nutrient to reach the brain and to be consumed. It thus enables the physician to discover specific areas of the brain that are active or that are malfunctioning.

The PET is important in the arsenal of diagnostic equipment because it allows matabolic scanning in place of the anatomic scanning of the CAT scanner or angiography. Whereas CAT scans locate lesions, PET scans monitor the flow of blood and glucose in all parts of the brain. It is hoped that this new procedure will eventually enable physicians to control the destructive cellular processes that occur in cerebrovascular disease.

SKULL X-RAYS

Skull X-rays are taken of the skull from various angles and are shown as a series of X-ray films. They can identify lesions in the brain, show any calcification in the arteries that would be indicative of atherosclerosis, and delineate the outline of a tumor. They are useful in showing evidence of a fracture that could have resulted from a trauma such as might occur after a fall. In many cases their greatest usefulness is in ruling out any diseases or injuries that might be causing symptoms usually associated with a stroke.

ELECTROENCEPHALOGRAM (EEG)

Whether we are asleep or awake, the brain is the source of electric potentials. The process of recording these electric potentials is called *electroencephalography.* The word comes from the Greek words *ēlektron* (amber), *egkephalos* (brain), and *graphein* (to write), and refers to electric brain writing.

The instrument used is called an electroencephalograph, and the record that is made of the test is known as an electroencephalogram, abbreviated as and referred to as an EEG. An EEG is not a routine procedure in all instances of stroke. Rather, it is used to obtain answers to specific questions most often relating to seizures.

Any focal seizure activity indicates that the symptoms are epileptic rather than ischemic.

THE EEG PROCEDURE

During electroencephalography, the patient can be either lying down or sitting up, sleeping or awake. At least a portion of the EEG, however, must be conducted while the patient is fully awake because slow mind activity and slow alpha frquencies are important in the detection of a stroke. On the other hand, readings recorded while the patient is sleeping provide information that would be impossible to obtain during waking. Quite often the person who has had a stroke tends to become drowsy during an EEG.

Electrodes are attached to the scalp with a gluelike material or by small needles inserted just under the skin of the scalp. This is an entirely painless procedure. The electrodes conduct minute electrical currents directly from the brain through the EEG machine. Each individual electrode is equipped with a pen to record its lines on a graph-like sheet of paper. The electrical currents produce wavy lines called brain waves. The pattern thus produced is then read and interpreted to give a diagnosis.

While the electroencephalograph is recording the brain waves, the technician may conduct several tests including the following:

1. The flashing of strobe lights at various speeds directly into the eyes.
2. The administration of a medication that can produce a seizure-like condition.
3. The patient is asked to hyperventilate—that is, to breathe quickly and deeply.
4. A hypnotic drug may be given to induce a sleep-like state.

ADVANTAGES OF THE EEG

An EEG can be done in a laboratory, a physician's office, or in a hospital. It is painless, noninvasive, and relatively free from any complications. It provides useful information on the electrical activity of the brain. It can detect any type of seizure the patient may be experiencing either along with or as the result of a stroke. These seizures can be grand mal, petit mal, or psychomotor. The latter most often consist of episodes of mental confusion during which the patient performs actions without being aware of doing them or even remembering doing them.

An EEG takes about one hour to perform. If a hypnotic has been given to induce sleep, the procedure is extended to approximately three hours to give the patient time to sleep off the effects of the hypnotic. And in this case, the patient will not be allowed to drive home. Other than this there are no after effects.

LUMBAR PUNCTURE (LP)

A lumbar puncture, which is also known as a spinal tap, is a procedure in which cerebrospinal fluid is withdrawn for analysis. It is more useful in the evaluation of a cerebral hemorrhage than a thrombosis. However, a lumbar puncture shows evidence only of hemorrhages that have gone into the ventricular system. Hemorrhages that bring about a decline in consciousness usually produce a bloody spinal fluid. A lumbar puncture can provide useful information in determining a mode of therapy.

The procedure is not without risk, and because there are other noninvasive methods of obtaining the needed information, an LP is done only when the information to be obtained outweighs the risks involved. For example, if a CAT scan is available, it can identify the presence of a hemorrhage, eliminating the need for an LP. If through other diagnostic procedures, however, there is a question as to whether there is a subarachnoid hemorrhage or meningitis, a lumbar puncture is then justified.

THE LP PROCEDURE

In the LP procedure the patient lies on his side with the knees drawn up toward the abdomen and the chin pushed down into the chest. In this position a larger area of flesh is available so that the physician can insert the needle with greater ease. A puncture is made in the small of the back between the two lower lumbar vertebrae. Although there is a slight sting when the local anesthesia is injected into the site, the lumbar puncture itself is not painful. The procedure takes anywhere from 10 minutes to half an hour.

AFTEREFFECTS OF AN LP

Some, but not all, patients experience a headache after a lumbar puncture because of a leakage that has occurred through a tear in one of the membranes surrounding the spinal cord. The severity of the headache depends on how much fluid has been lost. The headache does not usually last for more than one day and can be relieved if the patient lies flat on the back. Because the site of the puncture is below the end of the spinal cord, there is no risk of there being any general paralysis.

OPHTHALMODYNAMOMETRY (ODM)

Ophthalmodynamometry measures and compares the pressure of the blood in the arteries of each eye. It is a simple, noninvasive procedure that can be of invaluable assistance in the diagnosis of carotid artery disease. It provides important information about the possible occurrence of a TIA because some of the symptoms of a TIA affect the blood circulation in the eye itself. It is also useful as a diagnostic tool when there is aphasia and hemiplegia. Opthalmodynamometry has the advantage of being able to be repeated as often as needed.

THE ODM PROCEDURE

Two types of ODM instruments are used. One has a spring lock plunger that can apply pressure to the eye's globe; the other is a device that uses suction and is operated electrically.

The test can be done with the patient either lying down or sitting up. The ophthalmic artery and its branches can be seen with the ophthalmodynamometer while intraocular pressure (i.e., pressure within the eyeball) is temporarily increased. While the central artery and its branches in the eye are being observed through an ophthalmoscope, pressure within the eyeball is increased until it is equal to the diastolic pressures in the artery of the eye. When these pressures are equal, the artery and its branches begin to pulsate. This pressure is called the *diastolic end point.* As the pressure on the globe of the eye is further increased, these pulsations decrease and ultimately stop. This is known as the *systolic end point.*

Should the blood pressure in the internal carotid artery be reduced on one side only, either by occlusion or stenosis (either of which causes constriction or narrowing of the artery), the blood pressure would then be decreased in the ophthalmic artery on that side only. The amount of the decrease would depend on how adequate the collateral circulation was.

Measurements are then compared from one side to the other. If the measurements recorded by the ophthalmodynamometer are 20 per cent lower on one side than on the other, then there is likely to be an obstruction on the side with the lower measurement. It is believed that the pressures in the ophthalmic arteries reflect the pressures in the internal carotid arteries.

This procedure is ineffective whenever there is disease in both eyes or when both eyes have been affected by a stroke because in interpreting the results a comparison is made of one eye with the other.

ADVANTAGES OF ODM

Ophthalmodynamometry provides extremely useful information in a TIA and in aphasia and hemiplegia and can help to determine the mode of treatment.

FACIAL THERMOGRAPHY

Facial thermography is a noninvasive technique for measuring the temperature of the skin and recording it photographically. Dr. Ernest H. Wood of the University of North Carolina is credited with the discovery that stroke victims tend to have abnormally cold areas on their foreheads over the eyebrow on the side affected by the stroke. The first time thermography was actually used as a diagnostic procedure was in 1956 by a Canadian physician, Dr. Roy W. Lawson.

The temperature of the skin is directly related to the flow of blood, and it fluctuates in response to variations in the blood flow. This dependence of the skin temperature on blood flow can be an important factor in the clinical detection of strokes. The supraorbital area of the forehead is supplied with blood from terminal branches that originate in the internal carotid artery.

A stroke occurs when there is a shortage of or an interruption in the flow of blood to the brain. The blood flow originates in the carotid artery and follows a path up the side of the neck and into the head. When a stroke has occurred or when one is imminent, there is a decrease in the amount of blood flowing through the artery on the side of the head that has been or soon will be affected by a stroke. Consequently the forehead on the affected side of the head is cool and on a thermogram will show up as a dark area.

THE FACIAL THERMOGRAPHY TECHNIQUE

Thermistors, devices that can measure changes in electrical resistance as a result of alterations in temperature, are placed at various points across the forehead where they record the temperature at each of these points. They also measure the changes in the infrared emission from the surface of the head. The thermogram itself takes from 0.06 seconds to 3.50 seconds to record. The entire procedure takes about five minutes.

ADVANTAGES OF THE THERMOGRAM

The possibility of a stroke occurring can be determined by a thermogram because the blood flow through the carotid artery diminishes over a period of time. Any diminishing in the flow can be detected by the thermogram and serve as a warning signal.

Facial thermography can identify about 85 per cent of the incidences of stenosis or occlusion of the internal carotid artery.

Thermograms are used after surgery to determine whether the normal flow of blood has been restored to the carotid artery. If the cold spot over the forehead has disappeared, the thermogram will be normal and the surgery can be considered to have been successful.

Another advantage of this procedure is that it can be repeated as often as necessary.

ULTRASONOGRAPHY

The technique of ultrasonography came into being during World War II when sonar was first used to detect and track down submarines. It has been further refined to give us echoencephalography and the Doppler technique.

ECHOENCEPHALOGRAPHY

Echoencephalography is the ultrasonic procedure most often used in the diagnosis and evaluation of cerebral disorders. It is referred to as pulse echoencephalography or A-mode encephalography. Short pulses of ultrasonic energy are emitted in the 1 to 5 MHz frequency range. The sound is transmitted from 200 to 2000 times per second. It is spaced so that returning signals are received from areas having differing accoustical impedances. The sound is directed toward a specific area—for example, the brain. The reflected signal can then be seen on an oscilloscope, or it can be recorded on a polygraph. It is also possible to combine these signals with a scan.

Echoencephalography provides invaluable information on the position of the midline structures of the brain. These midline structures are identified by an echo that is a reflection from the walls of the third ventricle. A tumor tends to push the brain to one side, as does a hemorrhage, and this causes a midline echo to show up on the oscilloscope to one side rather than in the center as it should do. In a normal, healthy person the midline echo is equally distant from the echoes received from each side of the head.

An echoencephalogram can also show the diameter of the common carotid artery.

THE DOPPLER TECHNIQUE

The Doppler technique differs from echoencephalography in that there is a continuous source of energy used rather than short pulses. The continuous ultrasonic wave changes according to the velocity of the blood and is monitored by a Doppler flowmeter. This technique permits the blood vessels of the brain to be mapped.

The Doppler technique is extremely useful in determining whether the bruit, that is the murmur or swishing sound that is produced by the blood when it rushes through an artery that has been narrowed by a lesion, comes from the external, internal, or common carotid artery or is instead coming from the heart. It can also detect a reversal of blood flow, which would indicate a problem in the collateral circulation. While indicating the direction of the blood flow, it can also detect any blockage further up in the vessel of reverse flow through the collateral blood vessels.

The Doppler scan produces maps of the bifurcation—that is, the place where an artery branches into two divisions, as well as of the site of an occlusion and the area containing plaque.

THE DOPPLER SCAN PROCEDURE A transducer that both generates and transmits a sonic beam is placed on the head. The Doppler effect results from the shift in frequency when a wave source and the receiver are in motion relative to each other. In measuring the flow of blood, the Doppler probe transmits a sound wave of ultrasonic frequency. This wave is then reflected by the red blood cells. The direction in which the blood is flowing is determined by measuring these reflected waves.

Normally, blood flows from the ophthalmic artery into the supraorbital artery and then into the superficial temporal branch of the external carotid artery. However, when there is an occlusion in the internal carotid artery, the flow of blood in the supraorbital artery is reversed. It is this reverse flow that is detected by ultrasonography.

The transducer emits waves and picks up echoes that are then seen as visible images on an oscilloscope.

ADVANTAGES OF THE DOPPLER SCAN There is little risk and no discomfort in the Doppler scan procedure. The low level of energy used assures that there are no thermal, or heat, effects. The procedure can be repeated as often as needed. Unlike exposure to X-rays, exposure to ultrasound has no cumulative effect. The use of ultrasound has reduced the number of instances in which a lumbar puncture is needed. It also helps to pinpoint the causes of cerebrovascular disease and strokes and is of invaluable assistance in determining a mode of treatment.

ELECTROCARDIOGRAPHY (ECG OR EKG)

An electrocardiograph records the electrical impulses originating in the heart. The paper on which these impulses is recorded is known as an electrocardiogram. The dicharge of electrical activity is recorded as waves known as P, Q, R, S, and T waves. The QRS waves are grouped together and referred to as the QRS complex. When there are any abnormalities in the Q wave or the ST segment, the risk of an ischemic stroke is more pronounced. When the T wave is inverted, it signifies that there has been heart damage.

Approximately 10 per cent of those persons who have had a

stroke have also experienced a myocardial infarction (heart attack). An electrocardiograph therefore becomes an important diagnostic tool for both the evaluation and treatment of the cardiac disorder.

Abnormalities in the heart's rate and rhythm are commonly found when a stroke has been caused by an intracranial hemorrhage. The ECG can also help to determine whether these abnormalities are the source of or the result of a lesion in the brain.

THE ECG PROCEDURE

The patient can be either lying down or sitting up. A jelly- or salt-like substance is spread on those areas of the body where the chest and the limb leads will be placed. The leads are then put in position. In a 12-lead ECG six limb leads and six chest leads are used. The changes in the electrical impulses of the heart are transmitted through these leads to the machine. When the machine has been turned on, the wave pattern of each lead is usually recorded separately. Some of the ECG machines used in hospitals, however, record all 12 leads simultaneously.

Electric currents produced by the heart's beats are picked up and transmitted to the machine through the leads, which activate an inking pen that moves up and down in lines on a moving strip of paper. When the recording of all 12 leads has been completed, the ECG is finished, and the electrocardiogram is ready to be interpreted by a cardiologist.

An ECG can be done in a physician's office, in a medical laboratory, or in a hospital. The entire procedure takes less than half an hour.

Because there is no absolutely normal ECG (i.e., an ECG pattern that is common to all healthy persons), it is extremely wise to have an ECG done when you are young and healthy. Later ECGs can then be compared to this one to determine if there are any deviations that would alert the physician to a possible problem.

Evidences of a heart attack will, of course, always be seen on an ECG. When an ECG is done after the attack, it determines the severity of the attack and the extent of the damage.

ADVANTAGES OF THE ECG

The ECG is completely painless. There is no risk entailed in the procedure, and there are no aftereffects.

An ECG quickly shows the presence of any cardiac arrhythmia—

that is, any variation in the normal rhythm of the heart's beat—and confirms the diagnosis of a myocardial infarction (heart attack).

CEREBRAL ANGIOGRAPHY

Cerebral angiography is an invasive procedure in which radiopaque material that does not allow the passage of X-rays is injected into the cerebral blood circulation to permit the blood vessels of the brain to be photographed by X-rays. The pictures give a clear and an accurate visualization of the blood vessels and provide a "road map" of these blood vessels in the brain that can be of inestimable value in any contemplated surgery. The pictures are known as *angiograms*. They show the size, the location, and the type of any pathological change in the blood vessels.

Angiography can locate tumors, as well as abscesses and other kinds of lesions. It can accurately pinpoint the site of any bleeding or the presence of any blood clots lodged in the blood vessels. It can also identify any significant shift in the brain structure that may have occurred.

THE RISKS OF ANGIOGRAPHY

Angiography is not without risks to the patient. The radiopaque material is normally prevented from passing through the intact blood brain barrier, but if this barrier has been damaged by a hemorrhage, ischemia, or prolonged edema, the radiopaque material can get through. Deposits on the walls of the blood vessels can become dislodged by the radiopaque material. Blood clots can form at the end of the catheter that can possibly break loose and become lodged in one of the blood vessels. Were this to occur in a blood vessel supplying the brain, the result could be a stroke or even death. There is always a risk of a blood vessel being punctured by the catheter as it threads its way through the blood vessels. Allergic reactions to the radiopaque material can also occur, sometimes resulting in an anaphylactic shock. The carotid artery can also become irritated, which could conceivably affect the nervous system.

Angiography is always done in a hospital by highly trained personnel. The procedure takes from 45 minutes to as long as four hours. At its completion, the patient is closely monitored at frequent intervals for several hours for any adverse reactions that might occur.

All the risks entailed in this procedure are carefully explained in great detail by the physician both to the patient and also to the family before the procedure is begun. The risks and the benefits that are anticipated are weighed one against the other. Only when the benefits outweigh the risks is angiography considered as a viable diagnostic technique.

WHEN ANGIOGRAPHY IS NECESSARY

Although CAT scanning does provide an alternative procedure, there are still some instances when it is felt that angiography is essential, particularly before surgery. Not everyone who has a cerebrovascular problem needs to or should have an angiogram. It is usually considered to be necessary only when there is uncertainty as to the cause of the stroke (infarction, ischemia, or hemorrhage) or when there might be some other problem (such as a brain tumor) that could be causing the stroke-like symptoms.

THE ANGIOGRAPHY TECHNIQUE

Two techniques are used in angiography. One is known as the aortic arch catheterization technique; the other is known as the noncatheter retrograde arterial technique.

Venography is the term used to describe the X-ray study of the veins, and the pictures that are produced are called *venograms*.

Phlebography is yet another term used to describe the X-ray study of veins; in this case the pictures are called *phlebograms*.

The study of the arteries by X-ray after radiopaque material has been injected into the blood stream is called arteriography; the pictures are called *arteriograms*.

AORTIC ARCH CATHETERIZATION TECHNIQUE In the aortic arch catheterization procedure one of the carotid arteries in the neck is chosen as the site of the puncture, both for the catheter and for the radiopaque material. Without radiopaque or contrast material, many of the soft tissues could not be seen by X-ray. The patient can be either completely anesthetized or have only a local anesthetic around the puncture site.

A wire known as a guide wire is passed through a needle at the puncture site. The needle is removed and the catheter is passed over the guide wire and on into the artery. With the aid of a fluoroscope (a device used for the examination of deep structures by means of X-rays and that shows these structures on a screen) the catheter is guided to the artery to be studied. As the catheter passes through the small branching arteries, it can detect any problem in these areas at an early stage before the problem affects a major artery.

As the radiopaque material is injected through the open end of the catheter, X-ray pictures are taken in rapid sequence, showing the course of the radiopaque material. If necessary, medication can be given either to dilate or to constrict the blood vessels. Sometimes magnification instruments are used so that the small intracranial blood vessels, which are located at the base of the brain and cannot usually be seen because of the bones of the skull, can be seen in greater detail.

NONCATHETER RETROGRADE ARTERIAL TECHNIQUE The noncatheter retrograde arterial technique consists of making a puncture with a thin needle in the wall of the artery and then injecting radiopaque material into that artery. Unlike the aortic arch catheterization technique, no catheter is used. Serial pictures are taken to show the course of the radiopaque material through the blood vessels. Although there may be brief periods of discomfort, they are not severe.

THE ADVANTAGES OF ANGIOGRAPHY

Angiography has made possible the development of surgical techniques such as cerebral bypass surgery by showing the exact location of any lesions and their accessibility.

CHAPTER ELEVEN
THE COMPLETED STROKE

In contrast to the stroke in evolution, or what is sometimes referred to as the progressive stroke in which the disabilities or neurological deficits gradually or even intermittently grow more severe, the completed stroke is the stage at which the neuorological deficits have ceased to increase in scope and have become fixed. Whatever damage this particular stroke has caused has been done. Nonregenerative nerve tissues have been destroyed, and there are neurological deficits that may or may not improve.

The rehabilitation process should be started as soon as it is medically possible to do so in order to bring back some function to the disabled parts of the body and to minimize the degree of disability. This is accomplished by retraining the person to function with or around his disability.

In the aftermath of a stroke it is possible for some areas of the brain to function in a normal manner; others show signs of having sustained damage varying from slight to severe. At times the person may seem as capable as ever in dealing with intellectual tasks; at other times the person may appear to be completely unable to cope. This inconsistency is what causes some days for stroke patients to be good while others are bad.

The most obvious sign of stroke damage is paralysis. Because the left side of the brain controls the right side of the body, damage to the left side of the brain affects the right side of the body and damage to the right side of the brain affects the left side of the body.

Because each side of the brain controls separate functions of the body (see Chapter 1), the effects from this damage to each side of the body will differ.

If the person is right-handed, and the majority of people are, damage to the right side of the brain can cause a deficit in visual and spatial skills, whereas damage to the left or dominant side of the brain can cause difficulties with speech.

It is interesting to notice that about 5 per cent of those persons who are left-handed have the right side of the brain as the dominant side, which means that for them damage to the right side of the brain can cause the speech impediments normally associated with damage to the left brain. Damage to the left side of the brain of such people can cause deficits in visual and spatial skills. Because not all left-handed persons have the right side of the brain as the dominant side, those who do not will have the left side of the brain as the dominant side, as do the majority of persons.

LEFT BRAIN INJURY (RIGHT-SIDED PARALYSIS)

Damage to the left side of the brain can cause paralysis on the right side of the body that is known as right hemiplegia. Hemiplegia can be either progressive or it can be total. When it is total, it is known as catastrophic hemiplegia. Most total hemiplegia results from an embolism or a thrombosis that has formed on or slightly away from an area of plaque in an artery and that has then blocked one of the major blood vessels in the brain. Hemiplegia can also result from a progressive narrowing or stenosis of a blood vessel, particularly when the collateral circulation in the brain is inadequate. Because of being paralyzed in one arm and leg, the person with hemiplegia will to some extent become mentally, physically, and socially dependent on others.

EFFECTS ON SPEECH AND LANGUAGE

APHASIA

The left side of the brain controls the speech center; any damage to this area can cause aphasia, a condition caused by injury to the cortex and dominant hemisphere of the brain. It has been estimated that between one third and one half of all strokes that occur in the left hemisphere of the brain produce aphasia. Of the approximately 500,000 persons who have a stroke each year, 90,000 (about 20 per cent) will have aphasia. Another 10 per cent will develop severe aphasia. The person who has aphasia has lost the ability to convey ideas by the use of words.

The word *aphasia* comes from the Greek words *a* (without) and *phasia* (speaking). It is used to describe a condition in which there is interference with the understanding of and the use of language. It usually is caused by a lesion in the dominant cerebral hemisphere.

Aphasia is not a new disease. Hippocrates himself believed that speech disturbances were associated with lesions in the brain back in 400 B.C. He described this loss of speech capacity in his writings and called it *aphonia* from the Greek words *a* (without) and *phonic* (voice). Throughout Greek and Roman history difficulties associated with speaking and reading were recorded by many of the physicians of the times. The term aphasia was first used by Sextus Empiricus, a philosopher and physician in the first half of the third century, to describe these difficulties. Wernicke, the nineteenth-century Greek neurologist for whom a form of aphasia was named, was the first to locate the auditory speech center in the brain. Dejerine, the nineteenth-century French neurologist, was the first to describe the condition that we know as word blindness.

Speech is an extremely complicated process. It is composed of many different facets, each of which is located in a different and specific area of the brain. The noted surgeon and anatomist, Paul Broca, was the first to locate the speech control center of the brain for which feat he became known as the founder of modern brain surgery. His research led him to conclude that when a person loses the ability to speak as a result of brain damage, there is a lesion in the damaged area of the brain. Broca successfully proved his thesis when he removed these lesions.

Since 1945 another school of thought has emerged that rejects the idea of there being exact locations for motor and auditory speech in the brain. Proponents of this theory minimize the idea of a speech disorder being caused by damage to a specific area of the brain and emphasize the psychological aspects of speech. They divide the phases of speech into voluntary, emotional, and common.

Aphasia is characterized by a lessened ability to interpret and formulate the symbols of communication. Some of the common signs of aphasia are difficulty in naming objects, hesitancy in speech as well as stuttering and difficulties in spelling, reading, writing, and in repeating and understanding what is spoken. Not all these aspects are present in every person who has aphasia. In fact each aspect is isolated from the other in such a way that problems with any one or even with several of these aspects can completely disappear while leaving others in various nonfunctional phases.

An inability to speak or to write is called motor aphasia; an inability to understand what is spoken or what is read is called sensory or receptive aphasia.

In motor aphasia, although the person cannot express himself in words, he may be able to understand what is said to him and is often able to reply by using gestures. It is with sensory aphasia that word deafness is encountered; the person is unable to differentiate between the sounds of words and other sounds that he hears. The words, or sounds, convey no meaning to him.

The most frequent causes of motor aphasia are cerebral thromboses, emboli, or a hemorrhage from the middle cerebral artery. The treatment depends on the cause. In some cases the surgical removal of a blood clot brings relief, as does the removal of a tumor.

Although aphasia is not caused by mental deterioration, nevertheless many of its signs and symptoms are often associated with such mental deterioration as memory loss and confusion. In mental deterioration the degree of language impairment is proportional to the degree of loss of other mental functions. In aphasia it is the disturbance in language itself that predominates. If there is any doubt as to the cause, a form of testing known as psychometrics can be helpful in differentiating between the two problems. Psychometrics or psychometry measures both the degree and force of mental operations and of intelligence itself.

The components or parts of language include the following:

1. Vocabulary, that is, a group of words having special meanings.
2. A set of rules, known as grammar, used in putting words together in certain sequences in order to form sentences.
3. A retention span sufficiently long so that words can be retained and put together.
4. The ability to be able to choose words appropriate to the ideas being expressed.

Many persons who have mild to moderate aphasia do retain one or more of these components of language. Usually there is some impairment in such areas as listening, reading, speaking, and writing. The degree of impairment in each one of these areas may not be the same.

Just because the person may have difficulty in listening is no reason to assume that he is deaf. It may be that his attention span has been affected. When the aphasia is severe, however, all recognition of words, of objects, and of pictures may be lost. Less severe forms of aphasia may result in only a lessened retention span and only partial comprehension.

Words often simply elude the person, who may then substitute some other word for the correct one. The person may also utter a whole string of unconnected words because of the lost ability to put them into sentence form.

When writing, the person who has aphasia usually makes the same kinds of errors made when speaking. Misspelled words and the inability to form letters into a word are common problems.

When the aphasia is mild, the person may be able to write well but will be extremely slow in forming words and consequently will tend not to use too many words. The person will be quite brief in speech.

DYSARTHRIA

Aphasia is an inability to speak or to understand what is spoken or written. There is yet another form of speech impairment known as dysarthria, a mechanical defect in speaking caused by disturbances or injuries to the area of the brain that controls the muscles that regulate articulation. Weakness, slowness, and incoordination in the mechanics of speech are some of the signs of dysarthria. Dysarthria may be caused by lesions in either the left or right cerebral hemispheres, the cerebellum, the brain stem, or the cranial nerves.

Several motor processes are involved in speaking. Among them are respiration, in which breathing controls the sounds of speech; phonation, which is the process of uttering sounds; resonance, which refers to the clear enunciation of speech; and prosody, which refers to the melodic pattern of speech and includes the variations in pitch and volume. Prosody also includes the rate and rhythm at which words are spoken, the manner in which the syllables of a word are stressed, and the inflection in pitch.

There is a difference in meaning between speech and language. Speech refers not only to the sounds used when one person communicates with another but also to the gestures and expressions used. Speaking gives the person with aphasia the greatest difficulty. When the aphasia is severe, he may literally be speechless. In its milder forms he may simply experience some difficulty in uttering certain words or phrases.

Along with affecting the ability to speak, a stroke may also affect both comprehension and the mechanics of speech. When the person with aphasia is able to speak at all, it will be noticed that his vocabulary (i.e., his range of words) has probably shrunk considerably. The words he retains are those he was accustomed to using frequently. Those he rarely used he has forgotten.

Just because he cannot speak and therefore communicate his needs and desires verbally does not mean that he is incapable of understanding what is said to him. To isolate him to a sort of no man's land where he hears no sounds and where no effort is made to talk with him is both cruel and wrong. If he cannot speak and does not understand the words that are spoken to him, the message that you are trying to get across can be acted out as you would do in pantomime. This can become an excellent means of communication between you and the person with aphasia.

Should the person with aphasia use what you perceive to be an incorrect word when identifying an object (e.g., calling a chair a "rah"), there is no reason why you cannot be the one to learn a new language and at this stage of his illness you too can refer to the chair as "rah." It may be a first step toward starting a dialogue.

Always remember that there has been damage to the patient's brain. When, in trying to speak he groans or curses or even lets out a stream of babbling incoherent nonsense, never ever lose patience with him. He is even more frustrated than you are at not being able to speak coherently. Unless he is helped to communicate by whatever means possible, he may give up trying altogether. And this results in a needless and tragic failure.

Along with your encouragement and joy at seeing him progress, particularly in the area of nonverbal communication, in which he may appear to be quite competent, never lose sight of the fact that in your satisfaction at his progress you just might be expecting too much from him. This can be particularly true when he nods and smiles and gives all the indications of understanding, yet does not do what you ask him to do. The fault lies not with him but with you. Because of the progress he has made and your eagerness to see him progress, it is all too easy to assume that he has actually progressed further than he really has.

You can check his ability to understand what you are saying by pointing to an object and identifying it by using a word different from the one you and he have previously been using when referring to it. If he does not object and agrees with this choice of word, it is apparent that he is responding to your gesture as you point to the object rather than in identifying it in his mind by the word that is the correct one for it.

Try not to rush the understanding process. There is no doubt that it is both trying and nerve-racking, but rushing it and overestimating the patient's ability both to use and to understand speech causes him nothing but frustration, confusion, and bitter disappointment. In overestimating his understanding capability what appears as uncooperative and even irrational behavior can simply be a result of his misunderstanding of what you want plus a frustration on his part at not being able to understand.

Never shout in an effort to get your point across. Speaking loudly accomplishes nothing. Although the patient may not be able to speak, in most cases he can hear quite well. If there are any doubts as to the patient's ability to hear, this can be checked by having a hearing examination.

Always tell the patient what you want him to do in as few words as possible in order to avoid confusing him. Above all, do not talk baby talk to him, nor use the mother-knows-best tone of voice. Treat the patient as an adult; this will help him to make greater progress.

BEHAVIOR PROBLEMS

The person who has aphasia is prone to changes in behavior. It is to be expected that he will have less control over his feelings than he had before the stroke. Unusual behavior can stem from his frustration at not being able to communicate. He may become irritable, cry easily and frequently, or laugh when there is nothing to laugh about. He may act impulsively with no apparent reason for his actions. His attitudes, feelings, and abilities change from day to day—even from moment to moment.

The patient can be lethargic and withdrawn. His attention is apt to wander. He may tend to live in the present with no desire to think about the future. One moment he may be happy, the next depressed. One moment he may be cooperative, the next stubbornly defiant. He is almost always self-centered. All these actions and mood changes result from damage to his brain from the stroke. He cannot help acting the way he does. Often he has severe headaches and may at times have seizures or convulsions. Some persons with aphasia also have problems with their vision.

TYPES OF APHASIA

Broca's aphasia is named after Paul Broca. In this type of aphasia there is a pattern of speech that consists almost entirely of content words or nouns. Any verbs used are used in their simplest form. There is difficulty in finding the correct words. The speech is slow and labored. Connecting words such as "the," "an," and "a" are often omitted. Comprehension of both speech and writing is good. Any problems in writing duplicate the problems encountered in speech. This type of aphasia is usually associated with anterior lesions. Broca believed that comprehension remained intact but that spontaneous speech was impaired. Broca's aphasia is also known as ataxia.

Ataxia or *motor aphasia* is a type of aphasia in which the person knows what he wants to say but is unable to say it because of an inability to coordinate the muscles of the speech control center of his brain.

Anosmic aphasia or *nominal aphasia* is an inability to remember the names of persons or objects. The almost normal speech of those persons with this type of aphasia is marred by a difficulty in finding words. The comprehension of language and the ability to read are almost normal. There is always a groping for words along with an inability to find words of substance. However, if a word is provided that the person has obviously been searching for, he invariably will recognize it immediately and is then able to repeat it correctly. Writing ability is also affected by this type of aphasia.

Ageusic aphasia is a loss of power to express words relating to the sense of taste.

Amnesic aphasia is an inability to remember the correct word for identifying an object. The speech may, therefore be hesitant and fragmentary.

Wernicke's aphasia is named after a nineteenth-century German neurologist and refers to cortical aphasia—that is, aphasia that results from damage to the cortex of the brain. The person with this form of aphasia often speaks with excessive volubility, making the speech sound pressed and loquacious. There may be a lack of clarity in both the content and the direction of what is spoken. Many times the speech is composed of a jargon of words that attach new meanings to old familiar words. Often a loss of ability to comprehend the speech of others is found. Reading ability is also affected.

Alexia is an inability to read and is often referred to as *word blindness*. It is associated with damage to the rear part of the left optic radiation.

Agraphia is an inability to express thoughts in writing. It is caused by damage to the top part of the parietal lobe of the brain, which controls the motor skills.

Auditory aphasia is known as *word deafness*. It results from damage to the hearing center of the brain, which is located at the top part of the temporal lobe. An inability to understand the spoken word is associated with this condition.

Conduction aphasia results in the comprehension of language but the use of inappropriate words when speaking, causing a truly bizarre kind of conversation. The person may not always be able to make use of some of the verbal clues that may be given to him, but if the word he is seeking is spoken he will invariably recognize it. Reading and writing skills are not affected.

Global aphasia involves all the functions in speech and communication. It results when a lesion involves both the anterior and posterior speech areas. There is little in the way of speech, and there are problems with comprehension similar to those in Wernicke's aphasia. Global aphasia is the most frequently seen form of aphasia and is the most severe form.

Paraphasia is marked by a veritable torrent of words, all of which are inappropriate.

Agalculia is the loss of the ability to do arithmetic problems.

FLUENT AND NONFLUENT APHASIA

Lesions in the posterior distribution of the middle cerebral artery produce what is known as fluent aphasia. Lesions involving the anterior distribution of the middle cerebral artery bring on nonfluent aphasia. Among the fluent forms of aphasia are Wernicke's, anomic, and conduction aphasia. Among the nonfluent forms are Broca's and global aphasia.

EFFECTS ON THINKING AND PERCEPTION

The disturbances that occur in the thinking processes after a stroke may consist of an inability to account for thoughts and actions, of not being able to keep all aspects of a task in mind, of not being able to grasp the whole of an idea but only a small part of it. The person so afflicted seems to have no concern for the future. Everything is in the present, which can and often does lead to a withdrawal from reality and a life lived in a very narrowed and circumscribed world.

EFFECTS ON MEMORY

Memory is the mental registration of past experience. Even the slightest injury to the brain can result in memory problems. An important aspect of memory is the retention span, which refers to the amount of information that can be retained in a person's mind, then used and acted on. The person who has right hemiplegia tends to have memory difficulties associated with language. He may be unable to remember even the simplest word.

EFFECTS ON RETENTION SPAN

Persons who have had a stroke tend to have a short retention span. This effect is quite apparent when one mentions a number of subjects in a sentence but only one or two can be remembered by the patient. For example, if one asks the person who has had a stroke and who is having retention span difficulty to stand up, remove his jacket, and then put the jacket on a chair, he might not be able to proceed beyond standing up. This is all of the sentence his memory capacity will have allowed him to retain.

On the other hand, if short, concise requests are made, the patient may then be able to carry them out. He does not feel so perplexed and confused as when he is given a whole list of things to do at once.

OLD VS. NEW LEARNING

Often after a stroke there is a tendency to remember things selectively, based on whether they are new or old remembrances.

Old learning refers to the information that has been acquired throughout a person's lifetime and before the onset of the stroke. New learning refers to those areas of information and ideas the person is experiencing for the first time, such as experiences in a hospital setting or even at home when it is necessary to learn new ways of coping with disabilities.

After a stroke has occurred, there is a tendency toward experiencing some difficulty with new learning, whereas there is little if any problem with recalling old learning. Old friends and events of years ago can be recalled in minute detail, whereas there may be no memory whatsoever of what was eaten at the last meal, or even the names of the nurses and therapists who are caring for the person. These people and experiences have come into the patient's life after the stroke and represent a phase of new learning.

Problems with new learning can be lessened by trying to help the patient associate the old learning with the new. For example, when the patient is given a new room, items such as pictures, ornaments, or even some of the furnishings from the old room can be placed in the new one. The appearance of old and familiar objects then helps the patient to have a feeling of continuity, which makes it easier to accept the new.

EFFECTS ON GENERALIZATION

The application of what has been learned in one setting to another setting is referred to as *generalization*. Many times the person who has had a stroke has difficulty in carrying over what has been learned from one setting to another. The person tends to isolate and compartmentalize pieces of information. For example, while in the hospital, the patient is taught how to go from bed to wheelchair and back to bed again with no problem. However, on returning home to a setting different from that in the hospital, to a different bed, room, and wheelchair, the person becomes confused and is unable to associate these objects with those used in the hospital. The person may have to learn again how to use these items as if learning to do so for the first time, just as originally done in the hospital.

Persons who have generalization problems tend to become confused whenever there are even minor changes made in their surroundings or routine. A rigid routine, the same thing done at the same time each day with no variation, provides them with a sense of security. Because any sort of change in routine is bound to be upsetting, every effort should be made to avoid change if at all possible.

If changes have to be made, they should be made gradually, never abruptly. The changes to be made should be discussed in a calm manner, describing in advance just what the changes are going to be, why they have to be made, and what effects they will have on the patient. The new changes can actually be rehearsed to give the patient time to assimilate the proposed changes and also to practice them before they are put into effect while still having the security of the old ways to which to return. In this way adjustments can be made easier, and in time the changes become the accepted routine.

As time goes on and the person is able to get up and about, there may still be signs of generalization problems. Writing down in a notebook in consecutive order each place he will go, each thing he will do on his daily schedule, and the names of the people he will meet can be of tremendous help. The person should also be encouraged to write down items himself to use as a reference. The notebook then becomes in effect an artificial memory. It is a memory that will not fail and one that can always be relied on. This helps to build the patient's confidence and sense of security. The patient knows that the whole day is planned and that there will be no surprises that cannot be coped with.

EFFECTS ON VISION

Right hemiplegia brings on problems usually in the right field of vision. In other words, objects cannot be seen in about half of the field of vision. When this occurs, the person has to be taught to turn his head to compensate for the lack of vision. This problem is called *one-sided neglect* because the whole of an object cannot be seen. The condition often prevents the person from being able to see one whole side of his body, and he may even fail to recognize his own arm or leg. The person who has this type of vision problem should always be approached from his unimpaired side. If this is not done, he will not know that you are there.

One-sided neglect may even carry over to the way the patient eats. He may eat from one side of the plate, leaving the other side untouched. If the plate is turned around where he can see the other side, he can continue eating with no difficulty. The patient may occasionally have difficulty in trying to locate his mouth with his hand in order to get the food into his mouth.

This type of vision problem can contribute to a marked feeling of isolation, which becomes more pronounced at night. The patient's bed should be placed in such a way that he or she can look out the window at all times, even at night. This goes a long way toward lessening the feeling of isolation. It also helps to place all the objects frequently used on the patient's good side. In this way they can be seen and reached when needed, making the patient less dependent on others. Rearranging the clothes and the contents of a bureau's drawers in such a way that the items needed can be readily seen from the unimpaired side is also helpful.

BEHAVIOR IN THE RIGHT HEMIPLEGIC

A person with right hemiplegia tends to be slow and quite cautious in movement. When approaching a situation or a problem that is unfamiliar (new learning), the person can easily become disorganized and confused.

Previous to the onset of the stroke, the person might have had all the qualities we normally associate with a Type A personality—

assertive, time-oriented, and adventurous in approaching problems. A stroke brings about great changes, and all these qualities may be lost. Because of the difference in behavior and attitude after a stroke, frequent and enthusiastic encouragement at each step of the way in a new learning process must be provided. The approach to everything must be a positive one at all times.

RIGHT BRAIN INJURY (LEFT-SIDED PARALYSIS)

Damage to the right side of the brain may cause paralysis to the left side of the body. This is called left hemiplegia.

EFFECTS ON JUDGMENT—SPATIAL AND PERCEPTIVE DEFICITS

The memory problems associated with left hemiplegia, although they can be associated with language, are more apt to be associated with spatial and/or perceptual skills.

Spatial pertains to space; *perceptual* pertains to the act of receiving an impression through the senses. Both terms refer to the ability to judge distance, size, position, form, and the rate of movement. Spatial difficulties result in confusion between right and left, which makes for problems in trying to find one's way about, even in familiar surroundings. In addition, there is usually a loss of visual memory. Perceptual ability includes the ability to perceive the relationship of the parts to the whole.

Most of the tasks we associate with spatial and perceptual ability are performed automatically. Think for a moment of how automatically we bathe ourselves, eat, dress, and the like. When the ability to do these things automatically is impaired by a stroke, it is extremely difficult actually to have to learn how to do these things step by step, mainly because they have always been done without a second thought.

When those of us who have never had a stroke walk downstairs and, because of fatigue or preoccupation miss that last step and come down onto the floor with a bang, we are momentarily experiencing spatial perceptual difficulty. What the person who has had a stroke experiences is much more severe. No matter how he tries to concentrate, he still may not be able to get through a doorway in his wheelchair, for example, without bumping into the door jam. He cannot judge the amount of space that is available in the doorway. He may not be able to tell the difference between the right and the wrong side of his clothes. He may not be able to read a magazine or a newspaper, not because he does not still have the ability to read, but because his perception is impaired he is unable to keep his place on the page.

Multiply these few instances by all the things most of us do automatically and you can readily see why spatial and perceptual difficulties are among the most difficult to deal with, both for the person who has had a stroke and for those who are providing care.

BEHAVIOR IN THE LEFT HEMIPLEGIC

It is quite common for the person with left hemiplegia to behave in such a way that it is easy to overestimate his ability to handle problems and tasks. In contrast to the slowness of the right hemiplegic, the left hemiplegic tends to act too quickly, to be too impulsive.

He gives the appearance of being aware of the difficulties he is experiencing but on the other hand is constantly placing the blame for these difficulties not on himself but on the lack of the availability of correct equipment or some other factor which he feels is making it impossible for him to perform a task. That this is not so he never seems able to accept. He also has a tendency to do things that are clearly beyond his capabilities and that actually may be unsafe.

The left hemiplegic's ability to judge his own capabilities is usually quite poor. Many times the person with spatial and perceptual impairment does not have speech difficulties; this can be of great benefit in trying to teach him how to perform a task. He often talks to himself as he tries to master tasks that would be simple for healthy people but that are for him extremely difficult. This is a good sign; it shows that he is concentrating on what he is doing.

The left hemiplegic needs every bit as much encouragement as does the right hemiplegic, but in his case he must be urged to slow down and to carefully check all the procedures that are necessary to accomplish a task before he attempts it. Because of his spatial and perceptual difficulties, the movement of people or objects around him should never be rapid. Although the person with left hemiplegia may sometimes have difficulty in the left field of vision, the ability to see all or parts of an object is much greater than it is in the person who has right hemiplegia.

When a lesion in the brain cuts off the supply of blood to vital areas of the brain that control the many functions of the body, it is natural to expect that because these areas have been damaged there will be a change in the person's behavior. As a rule when the lesions are in the frontal lobes of the brain, the person may function quite well intellectually, but experience a personality change that may include being lewd and profane as well as untidy and apathetic.

When the left hemisphere of the brain, which controls both spoken and understood language has been affected, the person may show signs of realizing that he has a problem in this area, but he can and will respond in an appropriate manner in other situations that do not require speech. When the areas of the brain that control comprehension are affected, the person may appear to be completely and happily unaware that there is anything at all wrong with him.

Because of the damage the brain sustains from a stroke, the changes in mental function can range from mild to severe. A goodly number of persons return to complete mental capacity and normal emotional reactions, whereas others are left with some degree of change either in their personality or their mental capacity. It is these latter persons who have suffered the most severe brain damage.

EFFECTS OF A STROKE ON PERSONALITY

The ability of a person to control his own behavior is affected to a greater or lesser degree, depending on the extent of the damage to the brain. For example, the person who once prided himself on his neat and stylish appearance may now show no interest in his appearance and may be totally oblivious to his sloppy, unkempt appearance. He may say the wrong thing at the wrong time. His performance of everyday tasks may become inconsistent. One day he will do everything without a mistake; the next day he will make one error after another. His demeanor may change drastically. The once shy, retiring individual may now become noisy, immodest, aggressive—almost like another person. Where he might have been frugal in handling his money before the stroke, he may now have become an impulsive spender, acting as though he were the last of the big time spenders. The hitherto talkative, agressive, dynamic person may now be moody and uncommunicative. The once-engaging conversationalist may now be boring and repetitious. And most distracting of all, he may hear and respond to some things that are said to him and completely ignore others.

These personality and behavior changes do not indicate that the person is in any way psychotic. They are not caused by what are referred to as emotional or mental problems. Although the person who has had a stroke surely experiences emotional difficulty in trying to deal with his utter lack of ability to understand and to be understood, still this is not the same emotional problem that is associated with mental illness.

The best way to solve these problems is through behavior therapy. Take the case of the sloppy dresser, for example. He is physically able to dress himself, but his damaged intellect makes him unmindful of his sloppy appearance. A check list of the items to be followed while dressing can be of great help. It can be attached to a mirror. The check list can start with a clean face, brushed teeth, and combed hair and progress to appropriate items of clothing. The person usually responds to helpful feedback rather than to nagging, which only makes the problem worse.

Just because a person has had a stroke is no reason to go along blindly accepting all his outbursts. The cursing and swearing should never be tolerated. To correct this type of behavior you must act firmly yet gently. Tell the person that you are upset by the way in which he is talking. Ask him to request what he wants without cursing and give him an example of the way you expect him to speak. For example, tell him that he should say, "May I have a glass of water?" You have shown your disapproval by correcting him, and most important you have offered an alternative to the offensive type of behavior.

EFFECT OF STROKES ON EMOTIONS

To have control over your emotions you must have the ability to guide and restrain them. There is often a marked loss of emotional control in the person who has had a stroke, particularly if the stroke was recent. Crying seems to occur more frequently than does laughing. Many times the person cries simply because he is so depressed. It is not hard to realize why a person who has had a stroke may be depressed. Depression is a normal response to the loss of the ability to do even the simplest things that not so long ago were taken for granted. Speech, movement, thought, memory, family relationships, job, career—in fact every facet of the person's life has been affected by this sudden catastrophe. What the reaction to a stroke will be is in large measure based on the person's prestroke personality pattern—

whether he was an introvert or an extrovert, a pessimist or an optimist.

There are times when excessive crying can be the result of brain damage; at other times it can be the result of depression. You can tell the difference. Loss of emotional control caused by brain damage is characterized by little if any relationship between the emotional frenzy the person is experiencing and what is actually occurring around him. Emotional lability is usually only temporary and not a permanent result of a stroke. This type of emotional behavior can be stopped by diverting the person's attention toward something else. For example, if you ask him about the weather or call his name and he immediately starts crying, the crying is then a result of emotional lability caused by brain damage and not by depression.

It is not always easy to divert a person's attention when his crying is caused by depression. Above all, remember that because of the brain damage, what the person says and does may have no relationship to the way he actually feels. He may not be sad when he cries or happy when he laughs. Even when he displays anger, he may not be angry. His feelings and emotions do not always have a cause-and-effect relationship, such as is seen in everyday life. All these emotional outbursts—crying, anger, laughing—contribute to a sense of fatigue. When at all possible, if the emotional lability is caused by brain damage, try to intervene and get the person to stop this physically depleting activity by diverting his attention to something else.

The patient's anger and aggression are often very difficult to manage. At times his anger may give vent to retaliation. Hardest of all to cope with and to understand is the anger directed toward the very people who are most trying to help. Patience, sympathetic understanding, and absolutely no angry response on your part are the only ways to handle this problem. After all, what else can you do? The person has had brain damage, and that is why he acts as he does.

When a person feels cut off from the outside world because of problems with sight, hearing, touch, speech, and comprehension, it is easy to become irritable, confused, and given to having hallucinations. Add to this the fact that the patient may be confined to bed for a long period and consequently lacks the variety of environmental stimuli that we all take for granted. His behavior becomes understandable when these factors are considered.

The night hours are the most difficult. The activities of the day no longer go on around the patient. He is no longer being fed, moved about, and fussed over. He is entirely alone and, with so many of his senses impaired by the stroke, this isolation can be horrendous. It is often helpful to leave a dim light on in the patient's room and to have some music playing softly in the background.

THE PATIENT'S PSYCHOLOGICAL REACTION

A stroke is viewed by many persons as the first step on the downhill road toward death. The level of functioning has been impaired, life goals may no longer be attainable, there may be paralysis, and the person may be sexually impotent. The older a person is when a stroke occurs, the less drastic seems to be the reaction to it. To a young, vigorous person in the prime of life who is working hard and heading a family unit, the effect of a stroke can be devastating.

The person who was affable, outgoing, and optimistic before the stroke is better able to deal with its effects than is the person who was withdrawn, pessimistic, and negative in outlook. Any neurotic or psychotic tendencies that may have been present before the stroke occurred can be intensified with its onset. The fear of death, even fear of insanity, are ever present in many stroke victims.

THE PATIENT'S ATTEMPTS TO COPE

To anyone who has experienced it, a stroke will always be remembered as a catastrophe of the first magnitude—a catastrophe so sudden and so complete that there is no time for any gradual adaptation. In one fell swoop the stroke victim is reduced to being completely dependent on those around him. Because the stroke has blurred his mind, he is unable to grasp all that is happening to him. He knows he cannot walk, possibly cannot even talk, is barely able to sit up if at all, and is unable to eat normally. At first, all he is concerned about is whether he will live. After this first hurdle is passed, he becomes concerned about his family's reaction to what has happened to him. He wonders if they will stand by him. Now that he is pretty sure he is not going to die, he becomes concerned about getting well. And all the time, over and above every other consideration, is the fear that he will have yet another stroke. There is no doubt that a stroke affects every area of a person's life. His relationship with his family may trouble him as much as the probability of his ever being able to go back to work again.

These factors, complicated by the neurological deficits brought on by the stroke that impede him in so many areas of living, bring on strong emotional reactions. These reactions can run the gamut from pure rage to sullen withdrawal. The person's age has a lot to do with how he accepts his condition. One who is young is more resilient and also has a greater chance of having a full recovery than does the older person.

Regardless of the mental deterioration that has taken place, most persons who have had a stroke do regain intellectual function. There is usually no permanent intellectual disturbance. However, persons whose mental deterioration is progressive have a less hopeful outlook.

The state of crisis and personal chaos that is experienced at first and the anxiety, fear, and depression are overwhelming. Once in a while the person may try to deny the fact that he has had a stroke. This defense mechanism is his way of coping with an overwhelming situation. As he learns to accept and then to adapt to this new set of circumstances, he goes through yet another phase. For example, once he feared he would never walk again. Now that he can walk, he fears he will fall. One fear takes the place of another. But through it all, he still hangs on to his first fear of having another stroke.

Lesser illnesses allow a patient to retreat into comfortable passivity during which he is waited on hand and foot, but this is not the case with the patient who has had a stroke. There is no time for him to luxuriate in the perquisites of illness. Rather, he must as soon as possible embark on a rigorous program of rehabilitation during which he will experience even more fear and frustration. There will be fear of trying to do what at the present time seems impossible, shame that he is so inept, resentment that he of all people should have been the victim of a stroke. These negative feelings are gradually replaced by more positive ones, with pride in his achievements. This pride marks the beginning of his comeback.

Deep fear and extreme anxiety beset a stroke victim. Depression is commonplace. If the depression is so deep that suicide is a distinct possibility, the physician will have to intervene with appropriate antidepressant medication. Suicide occurs rarely among persons who have had strokes, perhaps only because they have neither the strength nor the mental capacity to plan it or carry it through. However, any indication that the person might be considering suicide should be reported to the physician at once. A delay could be fatal.

Fatigue often accompanies hemiplegia, but it seems not to be connected with the paralysis per se or the extra work load placed on the person's unaffected side. Research has shown that this fatigue has psychological roots. In other words, it can be increased by either emotional of physical failure, such as not doing as well as expected in rehabilitation or not progressing as fast as the person would like or really thinks he should. You cannot push a fatigued person. The course of treatment must be altered to allow for these periods of fatigue. The therapy may take longer but there is no other way around it.

Denial mechanisms are another way of coping with a crisis. In one type of denial, the person either refuses or is unable to acknowledge reality because the reality is so unpleasant. In another type of denial, the person acknowledges that he has a disability, but he refuses to think about what that disability entails. Above all, he refuses to consider what the consequences of the disability will be in the future. For example, the person may refuse to make any plans for the future at all until his paralyzed arm or leg returns to functioning normally. Obviously, this attitude presents a formidable hurdle to recovery. It is true, of course, that impaired vision can cause the patient not to see his paralysis, but when he knows it is there and either ignores it or simply denies it, it is a way of trying to cope. Many factors play a role in the way a person tries to cope. Among them are the family's life style, the person's work, and the severity and extent of brain damage. None of these can be overlooked.

Denial can make a person completely unaware of paralysis. It can even bring about a period of amnesia covering the time of the paralysis, and the person simply never remembers being paralyzed.

Suppression is another form of denial. The person may simply never make any reference to having had a stroke. By refusing to acknowledge it, the person can refuse to believe it ever happened.

Rationalization is yet another mechanism of coping. The person denies the very fact of the stroke by not accepting the fact of having had one. For example, the patient may refer to a headache or to some numbness in his leg or arm but will never associate these disabilities with a stroke. Still others, who have always been deeply spiritual, will often retreat into thoughts of spiritual salvation and prayer and, being so occupied, can refuse to accept the fact that they have had a stroke.

Avoidance as a means of denial brings out the worst in some people. They actually become hostile to those trying to help them. They neither want nor accept help from anyone. They loudly proclaim that they are all right. Others may need help but not they.

Displacement is another means of denial. The anxiety experienced about the stroke is directed to some tangible thing such as the person's job. The patient may keep on wondering out loud when he can get back to work.

Projection occurs when the person projects his worries onto someone else. He tries to forget his own worries by concentrating on worrying about someone else's problems or someone else's health.

Regression is by far the most difficult form of denial to handle. It can lead to excessive dependency. The patient refuses to participate in any activities designed to help him, such as therapy and rehabilitation, often simply lying in bed, sullen and helpless. Actually, this regression goes far back beyond the person's reaction to a stroke and calls for expert and experienced mental therapy.

CHAPTER TWELVE

MEDICAL AND SURGICAL TREATMENT OF A STROKE

There are four main objectives in the treatment of a stroke: first and foremost is to save the patient's life; second, to limit the amount of brain damage; third, to lessen the degree of disability and deformity that might result and increase the patient's invalidism; and finally, to prevent any recurrences. Every stroke is considered to be an emergency until a diagnosis has been made and a mode of treatment determined.

The initial period after the onset of a stroke is chiefly spent in evaluating the patient's condition to determine the severity and the extent of the neurological damage through laboratory and diagnostic tests (see Chapter 10). Both physical and neurological examinations are conducted. As a means of preventing further deformity, an appropriate range of motion exercises is started as soon as the patient's condition stabilizes.

During the acute phase of a stroke, particularly when there has been a cerebral hemorrhage, the patient is kept in bed until the symptoms of headache, stiff neck, and prostration have subsided. Sometimes the period of bed rest can be as long as four to six weeks, particularly in the case of a cerebral hemorrhage, or as short as a day or two when the neurological deficits have stabilized and the patient is beginning to improve.

MEDICAL TREATMENT
PRESERVING LIFE—MAINTENANCE OF AN OPEN AIRWAY

The maintenance of a wide open airway to enable the patient to breathe is the first step in preserving life and thus gets top priority. An oral pharyngeal tube may be inserted in the throat to assure that there will be an adequate airway.

If the patient is unconscious or if he is conscious and for some reason is unable to clear secretions from his throat, the physician may insert a cuffed oral endotracheal tube into his throat. The cuff can be deflated for 15 minutes every two hours to prevent any necrosis (i.e., death of the tissues) in the windpipe, which might occur if the cuff were to remain constantly inflated. This is also the reason the endotracheal tube is not left in place for more than a day and a half.

If the patient is pooling secretions (i.e., if his secretions are building up to a dangerous level), a tracheotomy (a cut made in the trachea, or windpipe, and through which a tube is inserted to aid breathing) may be necessary.

If the patient is hypoxic (i.e., if he has a deficiency of oxygen), oxygen can be administered by the use of a face mask or by a cannula, which consists of a main tube attached to the source of the oxygen and two branching tubes that fit into each nostril. These can be held in place by a piece of tape.

Should the patient be in a coma, he will have to be monitored constantly to assure that adequate ventilation is maintained. He will have to be turned from side to side every two hours so that hypostatic pneumonia (i.e., pneumonia caused by remaining too long in the same position) will not develop.

ADEQUATE INTAKE OF FLUIDS, CALORIES, AND ELECTROLYTES

The person who has had a stroke should be given only clear liquids until such time as he is able to swallow without difficulty or without the aid of an aspirator. The aspirator is designed to remove fluids and gases by means of suction.

The patient can then be given soft foods. In the conscious patient this feeding presents no problems. In fact, those who have any weakness in the pharynx (the tube through which air and food pass to the stomach) often find it much easier to swallow soft foods than to swallow liquids. The patient who is unconscious for a long time can still be provided nourishment by means of a nasal tube or by intravenous feeding.

Every effort must be made to keep the patient nourished so that weight loss is kept to a minimum. Ideally, the patient's weight should be kept at the same level it was before the stroke occurred, provided he was not overweight at that time. Fluids sufficient to maintain a high volume of urine output and to keep a sufficient amount of fluid in the body tissues will be needed. If warranted, fluids may have to be given either intravenously or by a gastric tube. Although fluids are a necessity, an excess amount can cause an overloading of the circulatory system and bring about hypo-osmolality, or water intoxication. The serum electrolytes are constantly checked. A decline in the concentration of sodium results in hyponatremia, whereas less than the normal amount of potassium results in hypokalemia, a sign of overhydration.

LIMITING THE AMOUNT OF BRAIN DAMAGE

MAINTAINING BLOOD PRESSURE

The circulation of blood in the brain usually is adjusted automatically to any changes in the systolic blood pressure, thus maintaining a constant level of blood flow. When a stroke has occurred, however, and areas of the brain have been damaged, this ability automatically to regulate the flow of blood can be lost. This means that not only must any hypertension (i.e., an elevation in blood pressure) be brought under control but also any hypotension (i.e., blood pressure considerably lower than normal) must also be treated.

Even though lowering the blood pressure, especially when the stroke has been caused by a thrombosis, will have no effect on the neurological deficits that have developed or may develop, still when the elevated blood pressure is eventually lowered to somewhere near normal levels, the possibility of having further thromboses is substantially reduced.

Lowering the blood pressure too rapidly can cause cerebral insufficiency, a condition that occurs when there is not enough blood flowing to the brain, or perhaps not flowing fast enough to supply the brain with oxygen. More than three-fourths of all strokes are the result of cerebral insufficiency and its resulting ischemia. By preventing further thromboses, cerebral insufficiency, or hemorrhage from developing, it is possible to limit the amount of brain damage.

Whether anticoagulants are used to prevent further thromboses from forming will depend on the cause of the stroke. If the stroke has been caused by a hemorrhage, anticoagulants are contraindicated. Anticoagulants do not dissolve existing clots, but they can help in preventing the formation of new ones.

RISK FACTORS

Any of the diseases that are risk factors in the onset of a stroke (such as diabetes mellitus, hypertension, hyperuricemia, hyperlipidemia) must be treated and brought under control as quickly as possible (see Chapters 4,5,6, and 7).

Any other diseases such as uremia (a serious disease involving the kidneys), obstructive pulmonary (lung) disease, and heart disease along with any cerebrovascular disease must also be treated.

MEDICAL PROBLEMS

Some of the pulmonary complications that might develop include pneumonia and an embolic infarction (which results when emboli are large enough to occlude or block a blood vessel in the lungs). The onset of the symptoms of pulmonary embolism are quite sudden and call for prompt treatment. Changing the patient's position at frequent intervals, the use of elastic stockings, getting the patient out of bed as soon as medically advisable, and the avoidance of leg massage can all help in preventing emboli from becoming lodged in the lungs.

If the patient has difficulty in coughing, it will be necessary to turn him from side to side every two hours. Any fluid that accumulates in the lungs will have to be suctioned out. The patient should be both encouraged and urged to breathe deeply and also to cough. This helps to relieve any congestion in the lungs. Intermittent positive breathing for 15 minutes several times a day also helps to inflate and expand the lungs.

Urinary tract infections can to a great extent be prevented when there is no need for catheterization (i.e., placing a tube through the urethra into the bladder in order to withdraw urine from the kidneys). When there is urine retention, however, catheterization can be life saving. In order to induce a flow of urine, the patient should be offered a urinal every two hours. A urinal can also be placed where the patient can reach it at will. When there is incontinence, a condom catheter or an indwelling catheter can help to keep the patient more comfortable. Frequent urinalyses should be performed to detect any developing infection as soon as possible. Appropriate antibiotics can then be prescribed to control the infection.

Constipation is another common problem, particularly in the partially or totally disabled person. A sufficient intake of fluids, especially fruit juices, helps in this situation as does that old standby, Haley's MO, which contains magnesia and mineral oil. Stool softeners such as Colace, PeriColace, and glycerine suppositories are also helpful.

It is not always advisable to give an enema either with plain water or as a Fleet's solution. The patient's general condition as well as the cause of the stroke will dictate whether an enema is advisable. For example, an enema should not be given when there has been a subarachnoid hemorrhage caused by an aneurysm because, while attempting to expel the contents of the enema, the patient could conceivably cause a more serious rupture of the aneurysm, which could result in sudden death. If there is a considerable increase in cranial pressure, the straining after an enema could herniate the brain stem. While the patient is hospitalized, all these problems are taken care of by trained personnel. Once the patient returns home, however, problems such as these point up the necessity of following the physician's instructions to the letter and not substituting other measures that you might deem appropriate.

Both restlessness and pain can make the patient very uncomfortable. The restlessness can be caused by pain; alleviating the pain with analgesics will often reduce the restlessness. Mild sedatives and tranquilizers can help and are often prescribed by the physician at this stage of the patient's illness. The sedatives used are always mild because of the importance of not depressing respiration, which in many instances is already impaired. Headache is a particular source of pain, especially when there has been a subarachnoid hemorrhage. Any fever that develops must be reduced to prevent any further damage to the brain.

The seizures and convulsions that sometimes occur usually do not last long and can be treated in the same manner as are epileptic seizures with drugs such as diazepan (Valium), phenobarbitol, or Dilantin. Convulsions and seizures occur in about 10 per cent of those persons who have had a stroke. Controlling the seizures prevents any further increase in intracranial tension.

Cerebral edema (i.e., a swelling of the tissues of the brain) can cause death during the first few days after the onset of a stroke. Edema tends to occur around the area of the infarct rather than in the infarct itself. It usually reaches a peak within three to four days after the stroke has occurred. Antiedema drugs such as Mannitol, Hydergine, and the corticosteroids help to reduce the swelling.

A breakdown in the skin can first become apparent as a small area of redness, followed in a few hours by the formation of blisters. If not treated promptly, this condition can result in necrosis or the death of the tissues in the affected area. Redness or pallor of the skin can signal skin breakdown. Massaging the areas with the fingers and relieving the pressure by supporting the affected areas with pillows can give relief.

The patient should be kept both clean and dry at all times and should be turned frequently from side to side as a means of preventing a breakdown of the skin. An alternating pressure mattress or a sheepskin fleece placed beneath the body can also help. The knee and the ankle of one leg should be kept separated from the knee and the ankle of the other leg by placing pillows or folded towels between the legs to keep the skin from becoming bruised, as it would tend to do if the two legs were close together. The affected hand and arm should be placed in what is called a *functional position* with a pillow placed beneath the armpit to prevent the arm from moving toward the center of the body and even beyond, which could result in deformity of the arm. Any of the areas where the bones stick out, such as at the elbows, should have pads placed beneath them. If the legs show signs of becoming edematous (i.e., swollen), they should be elevated at once. The sheet should be kept as smooth as possible because wrinkles can irritate delicate and weakened skin. Even when the patient can finally leave the bed and sit up for a while, he should not be allowed to sit in one position for long periods.

LESSENING THE DEGREE OF DISABILITY AND DEFORMITY

Therapy to lessen the degree of disability and deformity resulting from a stroke and the prevention of any complications that might arise while the patient is bedridden for any protracted period of time, is incontinent and weak, and is not able to do the simplest of tasks must begin as soon as all danger of the development of further neurological deficits has passed. Because many stroke patients have hemiplegia, their legs must be carefully watched for signs of any thromboembolism.

The patient should be encouraged both to bathe and to feed himself as soon as possible. The bedside table with such personal items as eyeglasses, tissues, a urinal, the telephone, and the call light button and cord should be placed where it can be easily reached by the patient's unaffected hand.

Should there be blindness in half of the field of vision in one eye (a condition known as hemianopia), everyone who comes into contact with the patient, whether it be the physician, nurse, therapist, or a member of the family, should approach the patient from his good, or unaffected, side. In this way he will not feel isolated and not be so aware of this deficit. It is a small thing, but it does help the patient's morale.

PREVENTING PRESSURE SORES AND CONTRACTURES

The prevention of pressure sores and contractures (i.e., permanent shortenings of the muscles due to paralysis) is especially important when the patient must spend a long period in bed. The bed should be equipped with a firm mattress and, if need be, a bed board for further support. Above all, the patient should be moved from side to side every two hours, and the sheets should be kept free of wrinkles. These are the best means of preventing these sores from developing. Because of spasticity (i.e., increased muscle tension that makes the muscles stiff and the movements awkward), contractures often begin within the first 10 days from the onset of a stroke. Before this, there may have been indications of flaccid paralysis (i.e., defective or absent muscle tone). Contractures are especially noticeable in the shoulder, knee, and hip. They usually occur somewhat later in the fingers and the toes. Any pain that develops in conjunction with the contractures can be relieved by heat and massage. Sandbags, pillows, and footboards are useful in preventing the shoulder and hip from turning outward or the knee from bending or the foot from dropping.

PASSIVE EXERCISES

When a patient is in a coma, all his joints must be moved for him through the full range of motion several times a day in order to prevent them from becoming stiff, painful, and perhaps deformed. Both strength and mobility must be maintained in the uninvolved as well as the paralyzed extremities. Passive exercise is the best method of accomplishing this. If the patient is conscious, both active and passive exercises (sometimes called range of motion exercises) of the affected limbs should be started as soon as possible.

In the beginning the patient will need assistance with these exercises. These exercises prevent the joints from becoming fixed and help to maintain the normal length of the muscles and tendons. If contractures are not prevented, it may be impossible to correct the damage that occurs later on in the course of recovery.

Paralyzed limbs should be moved through the full range of motion exercises at least twice a day. These exercises can be done with the assistance of a nurse or a member of the family who has been taught how to do them. The arm, for example, should be moved outward and rotated and then held upright several times a day to prevent a "frozen shoulder" or a shoulder disability caused by a gravitational pull resulting from the pulling and tugging on the shoulder as the patient is moved around in the bed or transferred out of it. A triangular bandage placed around the arm can prevent "frozen shoulder" from occurring.

The shoulder–hand syndrome is another problem that can develop. The shoulder becomes extremely painful, and the hand becomes both painful and swollen. Passive exercises followed by more active exercises and the application of heat can alleviate this condition.

RANGE-OF-MOTION EXERCISES

When members of the family are going to assist the patient in range-of-motion exercises, they should first receive instructions from the physician, nurse, or therapist who is taking care of the patient. This is extremely important because exercises done incorrectly can do more harm then good. For all the range of motion exercises, the patient should lie flat on his or her back.

SHOULDER AND FOREARM To keep the arm straight, place one hand under the patient's elbow while holding the wrist with your other hand. Then slowly lift the patient's arm over his or her head as far as possible without causing discomfort.

Next, with your hands still under the elbow and wrist, gently move the arm out away from the body. Then bend the elbow and raise the forearm up over the head. Then, gently bring the arm down to rest by the patient's side.

In rotating the forearm, one hand is placed under the patient's elbow while your other hand holds his hand. The arm is then gently turned so that the palm of the patient's hand faces the ceiling.

WRIST Place one hand under the patient's elbow for support; with your other hand, take his hand and gently move the wrist forward and backward. The palm of the patient's hand should be turned upward and then downward.

FINGERS AND THUMB Grasp the patient's wrist with one hand and cover his clenched fist with your other hand. Then, using your fingers, gently extend his fingers out straight, all the while holding onto his wrist with your other hand. Gently separate the thumb from the fingers. Holding the thumb gently, bend it backward at the knuckle as far as it can go without discomfort. The finger joints can be stretched by holding the palms of the hands together with each finger intertwined and then gently moving the wrist backward.

LEG AND KNEE While supporting the patient's ankle with one hand, gently flex the knee with your other hand. Then gently raise the knee and straighten the leg. Bend the knee backward toward the abdomen as far as it will go without causing discomfort. While the knee is still raised, gently rotate the leg away from the center of the body. Then rotate the leg toward the center of the body.

ANKLE Hold the patient's foot at the toes with one hand and place your other hand at the bottom of his foot. Gently rotate the ankle away from the body and then rotate it toward the center of the body.

TOES While holding the patient's foot with one hand, use your other hand to point his toes downward. Then gently bend the toes up as far as possible without causing discomfort. With your fingers gently separate and stretch each toe.

This regular bending and straightening of the hip, knee, and ankle should be continued until the patient is able to walk. The patient can be taught how to do these range-of-motion exercises by himself using his unaffected hand. Those patients who have a marked spasticity—that is, a stiffening and awkwardness—have a tendency toward an overextension of the spine to compensate for the full range of outward movement of the paralyzed shoulder. As soon as this becomes apparent, it must be stopped by drawing the patient's attention to what is happening.

In addition to the passive and active motion exercises that are done twice a day, the arms should be kept away from the body with pillows. The legs can also be supported by pillows. Footboards can be used to support the feet so that each foot is kept at a right angle to the shin. The footboard can also prevent any foot drop or shortening of the Achille's tendon located at the back of the heel.

To keep the pressure of the bed covers away from the legs and feet while the patient is bedridden, a cradle especially made for this purpose can be placed over them. Also during the time the patient must remain in bed, he should lie flat on his back except for those times when he is eating when he can then be propped up in a semireclining position. After eating, he should once again be placed flat on his back in the bed. If this were not done, there would be a tendency for him to slide down in the bed and not be able to pull himself back up. The paralyzed leg, which then could not be moved from where it became jammed up against the bed frame at the bottom of the bed, would then become bent at the knee. The good, unaffected leg that the patient would be able to move about could slide off the bed. This uncomfortable and hazardous position would just add to the problems of rehabilitation.

BECOMING AMBULATORY

Before the patient can be considered ready for a rehabilitation program, he must have mastered some simple maneuvers to enable him to get out of bed and move around. More than anything else, moving around helps to prevent pressure sores and contractures. The patient who has bilateral involvement—that is, who has both sides of the brain affected by the stroke and who thus is totally paralyzed—will be less able to become ambulatory than the patient who is hemiplegic—that is, paralyzed on only one side of the body.

Ambulation is started by practicing turning from side to side while still in bed. In turning to the right, the patient can grasp the right-hand edge of the mattress and pull himself toward the right with his unaffected arm while pushing against the foot of the bed with his unaffected foot. When turning to the left, he can grasp the left-hand edge of the mattress and pull himself toward the left while pushing his foot against the foot of the bed. Whichever foot is the stronger one can hook itself over the weaker one and help to pull itself toward the side.

The patient learns to come to a sitting position by first placing his weakened arm across his abdomen, then sliding his unaffected foot under the weak ankle. Because he will be getting out of bed from his strong, unaffected side, he can grasp the edge of the mattress and push himself against the bed with his unaffected elbow and forearm. If he needs assistance at this point, the person helping him should place his left hand in back of his shoulders and press forward toward his strong side. This will enable the patient to come to a half-sitting position with the weight of his body supported on his strong, unaffected forearm. As the patient goes from a half-sitting to a sitting position by moving his hand toward the back of his body, he can get enough leverage to push himself up to a full sitting position. If he feels weak after the unaccustomed effort, an aide can sit on his weakened side and support him until he feels comfortable. Once the patient is upright, his legs can be uncrossed and he should be encouraged to sit on the side of the bed for a while, with a footstool under his feet.

Sitting up unaided must be learned as if for the first time. The patient must be made to realize that most of his body is still functioning and that only a small part has been affected by the stroke. He must use those parts of his body that are still functioning in such a way as to compensate for those that are not functioning. As he gets used to the idea of sitting up on the edge of the bed and is able to retain his sense of balance, he can begin eating while sitting up.

GETTING BACK INTO BED

While sitting on the side of the bed, the patient should place his weak arm across his lap and then slide his strong foot beneath his weak ankle. Using his strong hand, he can then grasp the edge of the mattress near his hips and, while pressing himself against the bed, lower his body to the bed as his elbows bend. His legs can then be swung into the bed.

LEARNING TO STAND

The day the patient learns to stand is truly a red letter day. It may be the greatest step taken toward full recovery. He will now realize that he will not be bedridden forever and that things are truly beginning to look up. Learning to stand is quite a morale booster.

As the patient sits on the edge of the bed with his feet on the floor, he can be given some assistance in getting into a standing position. Care should be taken to be certain that the bed has been locked into place so that it will not skid. One person can stand in front while another gently braces the patient's back. Care must be taken to be sure that there is no pulling on the affected side. The person in front can use a knee to help stabilize the patient's knee on the affected side of the body. This knee will always have a tendency to buckle. The patient whose stroke was caused by a lesion in the brain stem has greater difficulty in regaining a sense of balance than does the one whose stroke was caused by an infarction or by cerebral cortex involvement. Mobilization can usually begin within a week to 10 days from the onset of the stroke. The length of stay in the hospital seldom exceeds three weeks.

BRACING

It may be necessary to provide some external support for the leg that is paralyzed; this can be done with a brace. The use of an ankle support, such as a strap, along with a foot strap can help to prevent the backward movement of the ankle. A high-laced boot and an elastic bandage around the ankle can also provide needed support. Sometimes the affected side must be elevated so that the braced leg can clear the ground when it swings forward. Bracing should be provided soon enough to prevent any injury to the joints and ligaments, which could ultimately interfere with a safe and proper gait. Because bracing, like putting a cast on a leg, is an art, it should be done only by a trained and qualified orthotist—that is, a specialist in the fitting of orthopedic braces.

AMBULATORY TRAINING

To further decrease the degree of disability and immobility, after the patient is able to stand up he is given in-hospital ambulatory training. Exercises in balancing are done. The patient learns to shift the weight from the unaffected leg to the affected one and vice versa. It should be kept in mind that a patient who does not have a fairly good degree of motor recovery (i.e., an ability to move about) will not benefit or profit from balancing exercises.

A patient will not be able to recover his balance whenever he leans toward his paralyzed side, so he must remember always to lean toward his unaffected side whenever he goes to sit, to stand, or to walk. The person assisting him should always be on his affected side because of the tendency to fall toward that side. If the paralysis is not too severe, the patient can relearn the art of walking with no special equipment. However, if the paralysis is severe, parallel bars should be used for the project of learning to walk again.

Further ambulatory techniques are discussed in Chapter 13 on Rehabilitation.

Many of the exercises done during the first few days or weeks following the stroke must be continued when the patient returns home. In the home setting it is most important that any available equipment be used to prevent those caring for the patient from becoming so fatigued from the stress of holding up dead weight that they become discouraged and disinclined to continue. This could be disastrous for the patient.

The recovery phase after a stroke not only concerns the patient and the physician; it also involves the whole family.

PREVENTING THE RECURRENCE OF STROKES

Preventing further strokes is the goal of all medical and surgical treatment. Medical treatment per se may not seem to offer the dramatic, almost miraculous cures that surgery sometimes does, but nonetheless it can and does prevent further strokes from occurring. Because the rehabilitation process (see Chapter 13) allows the patient to be mobile, it can of itself help to prevent thromboses and emboli from developing as they are likely to do when a stagnant blood circulation results from enforced inactivity.

SURGICAL TREATMENT OF STROKES

The laboratory tests and diagnostic procedures outlined in Chapter 10 provide the information that is needed before a decision can be reached as to the advisability of surgery. It is imperative that the cause of the stroke be isolated and clearly visible. Five per cent of the patients whose symptoms suggest ischemia (i.e., an obstruction in an artery) as the cause, are found when the tests are evaluated to have a tumor, an aneurysm, or some other vascular malformation.

The same kind of surgery is not performed with all types of strokes. Not so long ago, an obstruction in the vertebral basilar artery was considered to be inoperable. Now, thanks to the advances that have been made in the field of microsurgery, this is no longer the case.

The majority of strokes occur in the more surgically accessible areas of the brain, which are supplied by the carotid arteries. From 40 to 60 per cent of all strokes are caused by extracranial lesions that can be removed surgically. The intracranial lesions that are not so readily accessible can now be removed surgically by the use of a microscopic technique known as *microvascular anastomosis*.

The age of the patient must be taken into consideration before surgery is contemplated because older persons are less able to tolerate surgery. Medical treatment and good nursing care may be the best choice of treatment for those who because of advanced years have relatively few years of life remaining to them.

Because of the high rate of complications that ensue when surgery is done within the first few days after an acute stroke has occurred, most surgeons prefer to wait at least two weeks before operating unless there is an emergency situation that makes surgical intervention imperative.

Surgery is not recommended for all stroke patients. For example, the patient who has a complete occlusion or blockage of the major arteries in the neck, whose paralysis is considered to be permanent, whose speech defects developed not at the time of the stroke but after weeks or even months, and who is considered to have suffered irreversible brain damage would not benefit from surgery. The neurological deficits are fixed and would remain so even if the obstruction were removed and the circulation of the blood returned to a normal state in those arteries by the removal of the occlusion or blockage. Perhaps if the surgery had been done on an emergency basis within hours after the occurrence and completion of the stroke, the damage could have been reversed, but this is only a "perhaps" and a very chancy "perhaps" considering the surgical risks that would have been present at the time.

Surgery is also usually not indicated for persons who are experiencing what is called a "stroke in evolution," which is a stroke that is in progress and that has not reached completion, such persons are consequently at a high operative risk. In a stroke in evolution, the neurological deficits may not appear for hours or days after the onset of the stroke. These deficits may even temporarily improve, only to reappear later on after more extensive damage becomes apparent as the course of the stroke progresses. These neurological deficits may tend to come and go, varying in intensity over a period of hours or days.

The term *stroke in evolution* is used to describe those disabilities that arise from either cerebral ischemia or infarction and that gradually grow worse over a period of time in contrast to the completed stroke, which is sudden in onset and in which the damage is immediate and the deficits fixed in moments.

In strokes resulting from a cerebral hemorrhage, surgery is seldom indicated except in those instances when there is a definite hematoma. Even in these instances, consideration is given to the size and location of the hematoma as well as to whether the patient will be able to withstand the necessary angiography as well as the surgery. Many times all evidence of the origin of the bleeding has been destroyed by the hemorrhage.

Most parenchymal hematomas (i.e., hematomas located in the very essence of the brain) involve the basal ganglion and capsular areas and are so destructive that surgery would be pointless. A hemorrhage in the pons area of the brain also results in great damage to the surrounding area.

Those hematomas located in the cerebellum or the subdural region are amenable to surgical removal, and in such cases removal is often a life-saving procedure. A hematoma occurring in the outer third of the putamen (i.e., the shell of the brain) can be removed with good results because the innermost part of the brain will not have been affected. Surgical removal of a hematoma in no way alleviates extensive brain damage that might have occurred.

However, surgery is recommended for those obstructive lesions that are well localized, for ulcerated lesions occurring in the carotid artery, for obstructive lesions at the point of origin of the vertebral arteries, and for obstructive lesions in the arteries that rise from the aortic arch.

Ulcerated lesions occur in the walls of the arteries either from atherosclerotic deposits or from a clot. The flow of blood is not completely obstructed as is the case with an occlusion, but nevertheless these ulcerated lesions can produce stroke like symptoms.

TYPES OF SURGERY

Five types of surgical procedures are currently used in the treatment of strokes: endarterectomy, thromboendarterectomy, cerebral bypass, microvascular bypass, and ultramicrovascular bypass.

The purpose of all surgery is to restore normal blood circulation by removing the lesions that are blocking normal flow. Taken into consideration before proceeding with surgery are such factors as what the course of the neurological deficits would be if the lesions were not removed, whether these lesions are accessible by current surgical techniques, what if any risks there would be, what long-term benefits could be expected, and, finally, the certainty that all forms of suitable medical therapy have been ruled out.

ENDARTERECTOMY

An endarterectomy is a surgical procedure in which the obstructed artery is opened and an atherosclerotic lesion is removed by peeling it away from or cutting it cleanly away from the artery to which it has been adhering. In some cases an ulcerated lesion is also scraped off the arterial wall. This type of operation is usually performed when the obstructive or ulcerated lesion is in the common carotid artery or at the place of origin of the internal carotid artery. Usually the lesions located in these areas occupy only a short portion or piece of the artery, leaving the rest of the artery in a healthy state.

The surgery begins with opening the obstructed artery through a small incision in the neck. Occluding clamps are then placed both above and below the lesion. An incision is then made through the wall of the artery at a point just below the area of obstruction and then on up through that portion of the artery where the obstruction is located to the healthy portion of the artery.

A small plastic tube, which serves as a temporary shunt, is inserted in the opening to allow the blood to flow unimpeded into the brain while the operation continues. The use of shunts is necessary when it appears that there will not be an adequate collateral blood flow.

The obstructing lesion (which is called an atheroma because it consists of atheromatous plaque) is then removed from the arterial wall. If there is an ulcerated lesion, it too is scraped off. The inner lining of the artery may also have to be removed.

The incision that was made in the artery is then closed by suturing, or sewing, the edges of the artery together. The suturing is done with an extremely fine suture, or thread. Sometimes the surgeon sews a small Dacron fabric patch to these edges; this is known as a patch graft.

The plastic tube that has been acting as a shunt is then removed, and the opening is closed up by suturing. Eventually, a new intimal (or inner) coat will grow and cover the entire area, including the inner surface of the patch graft, if one was used.

For those patients in whom the destruction of the tissues of the nervous system has not become irreversible, carotid endarterectomy can prevent a paralytic stroke from developing.

THROMBOENDARTERECTOMY

A thromboendarterectomy is a surgical procedure in which a blood clot that has formed on or is associated with an atherosclerotic lesion is removed from the wall of the artery. The opening that is left in the arterial wall by the removal of the clot is then repaired by suturing together the two edges of the opening and then inserting a patch that will help to widen the arterial lumen (i.e., the space within the wall of the artery) and bring about a return to a normal blood flow through the artery.

CEREBRAL BYPASS

When there are obstructing lesions in any of the major arteries coming from the aortic arch, these obstructions are invariably localized, and the arteries beyond the point of obstruction in the neck are usually healthy and normal. In these instances cerebral bypass surgery is most successful.

In the bypass procedure the ascending aorta is exposed by making a small incision on the right side of the chest between the second and third ribs. A small section of the ascending aorta is closed off by a partial occluding clamp. An incision is then made through this closed-off section into the aortic wall. A tubular-shaped graft made of Dacron is sewn to the edge of the opening that was made in the aorta. Besides being made of Dacron, these grafts can also be made from an autogenous saphenous vein—that is, from a vein taken from the patient's own arm or leg.

The graft is passed through a channel in the tissue at the front of the neck where the neck joins the chest and then on up into the base of the neck. An incision is then made in the neck to expose the healthy artery that lies just beyond the point of obstruction. At this point the other end of the tubular graft is sutured to the opening that was made in the healthy artery, allowing blood to be shunted from the ascending aorta to the healthy artery beyond the point of obstruction and restoring normal blood circulation to the brain. If more than one artery is obstructed, other grafts can then be attached to the principal graft. There is only a 1 to 2 per cent risk attached to cerebral bypass surgery. Instances of complications developing are few, in fact less than 2 per cent.

The operation brings about complete relief from symptoms, and there are very few instances of recurrence of those symptoms. And by improving the blood supply to the brain a cerebral bypass operation can prevent either the first stroke from occurring, or if that has already happened, it can prevent any further strokes from developing.

ARTIFICIAL ARTERIES

Dr. Michael DeBakey, the internationally renowned cardiac surgeon, was the first to make artificial arteries from Dacron. These artificial arteries help to prevent strokes by providing a means for getting sufficient blood to the brain. In the patient who has already had a stroke, an artery that is not capable of carrying its share of blood to the brain can be replaced with an artery made from Dacron. The Dacron artery functions just as the normal artery does in supplying blood, and any further stroke originating from a problem in that area is prevented.

MICROVASCULAR ANASTOMOSIS

Until the advent of the surgical technique known as microvascular anastamosis, cerebral surgery was confined to clots, occlusions, or malformations in the larger arteries, such as the carotid artery in the neck or the artery at the base of the brain, mainly because these areas were the ones to which the surgeon could gain access. The vertebral arteries were considered to be too small for a surgeon to work in.

With the use of the operating microscope, which enables the surgeon to see everything at 20 times its normal size, it is now possible surgically to remove lesions and clots from the very smallest blood vessels and the intracranial arteries. Some of these small blood vessels are only 1 mm in diameter, the equivalent of 0.03937 inch. By using this surgical technique, it is possible to bypass the point of occlusion or blockage in these tiny blood vessels and thus provide some collateral circulation. The procedure is known as cerebral revascularization and was designed for use in both extracranial and intracranial blood vessels. The purpose of the procedure, as with the other surgical procedures, is to restore a normal flow of blood to the brain. When the surgery is done before a stroke has occurred, it can prevent the stroke by actually creating a collateral supply of blood. The procedure is often used in patients who have experienced multiple TIAs, particularly when the lesions causing the TIAs are inaccessible by endarterectomy.

Microvascular anastamosis is also done after a stroke has occurred when the patient is at great risk of having another stroke and the lesion is in one of the small blood vessels. However, no surgery can restore neurological function when large areas of the brain have been irreversibly damaged, nor can it therefore be of help to those patients whose neurological deficits have been present for a long time. The operation itself takes about four hours. The surgical implements or tools that are used are about the size of those in a manicure set. The surgeon works with jeweler's forceps, and the suture he uses is 22 micron wide or 1/10,000 of an inch in diameter.

The end of the superficial temporal artery is located and an incision about the size of a half dollar is made over the area of the recipient artery. This is known as a craniectomy—that is, the opening of the skull. The dura, the outer membrane covering the brain, is lapped over and the surgical microscope is placed over this recipient artery on the surface of the brain. The recipient artery is usually a distant branch of the artery that is occluded and is sufficiently large to be able to retain a graft. The superficial scalp artery is then grafted to the side of the recipient artery, using an ultrafine suture—so fine, in fact, that it is a fifth the diameter of a human hair. All this detailed fine work is made possible only by the use of the surgical microscope.

The blood that then flows from the scalp artery becomes a collateral flow of blood to the nearest point of the middle cerebral artery. It then can provide blood to those areas that have been deprived of blood.

Any surgical complications that might develop usually consist of only scalp discoloration or perhaps some loss of hair due to a neurological deterioration around the area of the surgery.

The operation provides protection against further cerebrovascular incidents in that area of the brain. In fact, the chances of having a stroke on the side of the brain that was not operated on is only 6 per cent whereas on the side of the bypass it is only 1.5 per cent.

ULTRAMICROVASCULAR BYPASS GRAFT

There is yet another procedure known as ultramicrovascular bypass. As its name implies, the procedure is even more delicate and intricate than is microvascular anastomosis. In the ultramicrovascular bypass, a section of the skull about the size of a small coin is temporarily removed, and the scalp artery (with a diameter of only 1.0 mm) is anastamosed, or grafted, to the obstructed cortical artery at a point beyond the area that is obstructed. The suture used is almost invisible to the naked eye.

CHAPTER THIRTEEN
REHABILITATION

THE DEVELOPMENT OF REHABILITATION MEDICINE

Rehabilitation medicine is a relatively new specialty, having been recognized as such by the American Medical Association only in 1951. The pioneer and foremost authority in this field is Dr. Howard A. Rusk, who joined the Army Air Force Medical Corps in World War II. Seeing at first hand the low morale of the convalescing wounded, he recognized the tremendous need for some kind of treatment or therapy that would enable these men to return more quickly to active duty or, if that were not possible, to recover sufficiently to be able to take their place once again in civilian society.

Devastating boredom was undermining the recovery of the convalescents. In an effort to keep both their minds and hands occupied, Dr. Rusk encouraged them to make model airplanes. Along with this went training in the identification of the various types of planes. These efforts were so successful that Dr. Rusk went on to develop a program of study courses that were both service-related and academic, and a physical excerise program tailored to each man's capabilities. The improvement in the morale of the men was immediate. Most of them were able to return to active military duty much faster than would otherwise have been possible. Thus was born the concept of what we know today as rehabilitation medicine.

In recognition of the success of his innovative programs, Dr. Rusk was made Chief of the Army Air Force Convalescent Training Program. In this new position he soon realized that his previously successful program might not be adequate for the severely wounded—the amputees, the blind, the paraplegics, and the quadriplegics who were being sent to the convalescent centers. These were the men who could never be returned to active military duty and who, because of the severity of their injuries, had nothing to look forward to but pensions or custodial care for the rest of their lives. They needed a much different rehabilitation program, one that would prepare them emotionally as well as physically for life as civilians. They needed to be reeducated in the basic facets of daily living in order to make them as self-sufficient as possible.

To describe the scope and breadth of his proposed program, Dr. Rusk introduced the concept of the "whole man." Rusk believed that the natural powers of compensation that every person possesses must be used. The wounded or impaired person must be trained to make use of his remaining resources, and above all efforts must be made to help him to become psychologically adjusted to his disabilities. To get his program underway, Rusk hired many different kinds of therapists, and with no previous studies, programs, or even experience to guide him, he devised a program of rehabilitation that has become the model and the standard that all such programs strive to emulate.

It was just one small step from the world of the military to that of the civilian. The impetus Dr. Rusk needed to found a Rehabilitation Institute was furnished when two of his close friends suffered paralyzing strokes. At that time there was little anyone could do for stroke victims except wait for the second or third stroke to kill them. Realizing that what he had been able to accomplish with the military could and should be made available to the civilian population, Rusk set out to improve his program further and to found the institute that bears his name. Stroke patients constitute the second largest group of patients treated at the Institute of Physical Medicine and Rehabilitation in New York.

In an effort to educate the public to accept and support his ideas, Rusk stressed over and over again that those who had had strokes and other disabling diseases should be retrained so that they could become participants in society, not simply because this was a compassionate goal but because it made good sense economically. The person who has been rehabilitated need no longer be a financial burden to his family or to his community. He can instead become a productive, self-supporting, tax-paying member of society.

THE REHABILITATION PROCESS

Rehabilitation has been called a process of adaptation. Although four out of five persons do survive a first stroke, some are left in what can only be called a vegetable-like condition. Others are left with varying degrees of impairment ranging from paralysis and blindness to speech problems. Some recover completely because other parts of the brain are able to compensate for the damaged areas. Often this recovery takes place only after rehabilitation.

The degree of recovery from neurological deficits varies depending on the cause of the stroke. Persons whose brain lesions are tiny ones, such as are seen in lacunar infarctions, make the most notable recovery, whereas those who experience an extensive hemorrhage in the pons area of the brain make considerably less progress.

Emotional factors play a vital role in recovery. The person must be willing and able to adapt to his disability and be convinced that with therapy he is going to improve. His emotional reaction to the stroke is what determines the success or failure of rehabilitation. Often the person considers himself to have been demolished by the stroke; added to this he both fears and resents his dependence on others. This may make him uncooperative in therapy. Talking over the problems and difficulties he will be trying to overcome at each phase in rehabilitation therapy is important to assure his knowledgeable cooperation. Each step on the road to recovery represents a milestone for which he should be both applauded and encouraged.

Rehabilitation cannot cure residual, fixed neurological deficits, but it can help the person to realize his full potential and to adjust to those problems, be they physical or mental, that cannot be eliminated.

The rehabilitation process should begin as soon as medically possible after the stroke has occurred. The earlier it is started, the more effective it will be. Most persons attain maximum neurological recovery within six to eight weeks after the onset of the stroke. This does not mean, however, that this is the end of learning new ways of coping with disabilities. There is always a challenge to find easier ways of doing things.

Rehabilitation is of value to almost every person who has had a stroke. It focuses attention on each neurological deficit while at the same time maintaining and even improving the function of those areas of the body that have not been affected by the stroke.

The resources that are marshaled to deal with the afteraffects of a stroke are indeed extensive and impressive.

GOALS OF REHABILITATION

The success of rehabilitation depends to a great extent on an early and timely application of therapeutic techniques. These include early ambulation, exercises for retraining the affected parts of the body so that they will function to maximum capacity, training in caring for daily needs, and the use of mechanical aids such as wheelchairs, crutches, walkers, braces, and canes when necessary.

The degree of benefit to be derived from rehabilitation varies with each person so that the results that can be expected must be realistic, taking into account both the extent of the disability and the social and vocational needs of the person.

The main goal in any rehabilitation program is getting the person back to living a life as close to normal as is possible, to restore him to as complete physical, mental, social, and economic well-being of which he is capable, to teach him how to enjoy his life by adapting to his disability.

To accomplish these goals there must be a realization of and the means to cope with all the various aspects that are involved, be they physical, psychological, emotional, social, or vocational. Ideally, rehabilitation aims at enabling the person to live independently at home, or at least to live with the least amount of assistance and supervision possible.

Rehabilitation seeks to prevent or at least to minimize the difficulties that result from an inability to use an arm or a leg in a normal manner. The person is taught how to compensate for his deficits: if he has a sensory loss to teach him to judge distances, to regain his power of speech if that has been lost, to substitute one function for another, and to retrain his muscles when necessary so that he will be able to return to a useful occupation, and finally to teach him how to maintain interpersonal relationships. The rehabilitation program is graded to increase the person's physical and mental activities along with helping him to make the necessary adjustments to his disabilities and to eventually become independent and self-sustaining.

Ninety to 95 per cent of those persons with hemiplegia can be trained to walk again with or without assistance. Forty to 45 per cent of these people can return to the work force.

As soon as the neurological deficits have stabilized, the rehabilitation process actually begins with the proper positioning of the arms and legs, and with passive movements and exercises designed to prevent contractures and to speed up ambulation (See Chapter 12).

After the acute phase of the stroke has passed and the person becomes ambulatory, a more rigorous program of rehabilitation is begun. The average person whose stroke is uncomplicated by medical problems such as diabetes and heart disease may become ambulatory within a week to 10 days after the onset of the stroke. The average length of stay in the hospital does not usually exceed three weeks.

REHABILITATION FACILITIES

Rehabilitation can take place in a large teaching hospital that has the necessary facilities, a rehabilitation center or institute, a skilled nursing facility, on an outpatient basis, or at home. Not all methods of rehabilitation are alike. The therapy provided in nursing homes is markedly different from that in a rehabilitation center.

With the newer and more comprehensive methods of rehabilitation available in the large rehabilitation centers, the average stay is about 27 days, during which time rapid progress is made.

Rehabilitation centers are independent facilities apart from a hospital; they provide treatment facilities as well as counseling and vocational training.

Between 75 and 85 per cent of the people in the United States live within 75 miles of an urban rehabilitation center, making skilled care only a few hours away.

The person who enters a rehabilitation center with a very limited degree of function in those areas of the body that have been affected by a stroke can, within a very few weeks, develop sufficient function in those areas to be able to take care of himself. The extent of the person's disability, his economic situation, and the ability and willingness of his family to provide care determine the place where the rehabilitation process takes place.

The person who has minimal neurological deficits with no loss of memory or sensory function, no visual problems, no speech impairment, and no damage to the intellect can receive rehabilitation therapy on an outpatient basis, either in a general hospital or rehabilitation center or at home where a visiting therapist can come and instruct both the person and the members of his family who are involved in his care on the various aspects of the rehabilitation process.

Because the primary purpose of rehabilitation is to return the person to his family and community as soon as possible, going straight home from the hospital can be a great morale booster. It enables the family to assume a more active role in the person's care, and it enables the person who has had a stroke to become a part of the family setting, with all that this entails.

Wherever rehabilitation is undertaken, there must be provision for periodic evaluation and long-term management.

THE REHABILITATION TEAM

To oversee the rehabilitation process there are a number of highly skilled, trained professionals who constitute the rehabilitation team. A great many persons are involved—from the nurse who teaches the person bowel and bladder control, dressing, and physical hygiene, to the physical therapist who teaches the person to walk again, to the speech therapist who teaches him to speak again. The roles of these therapists overlap, and any one therapist may be involved in several different areas of therapy.

PRIMARY PHYSICIAN

In probably no other illness is a person so dependent on his physician as when he has had a stroke. The family physician is usually the first one to see him. Although the family physian may use the services and expertise of other physician specialists as the need arises, it is the primary physician who continues to oversee the treatment, receive the reports from the consulting physician specialists, and correlate all aspects of the person's care.

This is why it is so important when one is healthy to find a physician with whom you feel comfortable and in whom you have confidence, so that in the event of a catastrophe an interested, concerned, and knowledgeable friend will be there when you need him.

OTHER PHYSICIANS

As other medical problems surface, physicians trained in the necessary specialties are consulted. These may include an urologist to treat diseases of the kidney, an ophthalmologist to treat diseases of the eye, a psychiatrist to treat mental and emotional disorders, and an orthopedist to design splints and braces as needed.

NURSES

The nurses who work with stroke patients are particularly knowledgeable and skilled in rehabilitation medicine, and they are a vital part of the rehabilitation team. The moment-to-moment care of the patient is in their charge. It is the nurses who first involve the patient in the passive range of motion exercises while he is still bedridden, who train the patient in bowel and bladder control, and who aid in the first steps toward ambulation.

SOCIAL WORKER

The social worker is a trained professional with a graduate degree in social work. When the time comes for the patient to leave the hospital, it is he or she who will contact the appropriate agencies for community medical services such as visiting nurses, transportation to rehabilitation sessions, and the like. The social worker also makes the arrangements for nursing home or rehabilitation care, determines the social and psychological needs of the patient, and assesses the economic resources of both patient and family to determine just what outside financial assistance is needed. The social worker is also the one who, when the patient has made sufficient recovery and is ready for the job market, helps him to find suitable work.

Because of the social worker's close involvement with the patient's family, she or he can tell the physician and other medical personnel involved about any family or social problems that might hinder or prolong the patient's recovery.

DIETITIAN

The dietitian is college trained in the scientific use of diet in both health and disease. The role of the dietitian is extremely important when it is considered that diet is one of the many ways to handle such risk factors leading to a stoke as obesity, hyperlipidemia, hypertension, and diabetes. A patient with these diseases must be on a special diet, one that takes into account not only the disease itself but the necessity of maintaining a well-balanced nourishing diet. Additionally, in some cases the patient cannot swallow with ease or cannot chew food. The resources of the dietitian's training come into play in seeing that despite these handicaps that patient remains well nourished by providing him with easily swallowed and nutritious food.

It is the dietitian who also provides dietary counseling for both the patient and the family when the patient returns home. She or he also sees that an appropriate community agency continues a dietary follow-up once the patient has been discharged from the hospital.

THERAPISTS

Therapists practice the art of therapeutics—that branch of medicine concerned with the application of treatment for disabilities designed to bring about specific results. There are many specialists involved in the rehabilitation of the stroke patient, and their functions often overlap. Not all of these various therapists are needed for every patient.

PHYSICAL THERAPIST

The physical therapist uses exercise along with other physical measures both to alleviate pain and to restore function to those parts of the body that have been disabled. These measures include the application of heat with ultrared lamps, diathermy, microwaves and ultrasound, moist pads, steam baths, and massage. Exercise ranks as one of the most important aspects of physical therapy, especially for the person with hemiplegia.

The goal of the physical therapist is to restore the patient to as productive a lifestyle as is possible so that he can become a contributing member of society.

The physical therapist performs various tests to determine the patient's functional motor abilities and his degree of muscle strength and weakness. He or she assesses the degree of incoordination, if such be present, the patient's breathing capacity, the condition of the circulatory, sensory, and respiratory systems, all of which are vital in determining the patient's ability to engage in rehabilitative exercise. The therapist instructs both the patient and the patient's family in the methods to be used in the therapy program so that these procedures can be carried out when the patient is at home.

It is the physical therapist who sets up a program of range-of-motion and strengthening exercises that vary from the simple to the complex and are designed to maintain or increase joint mobility, muscle strength, coordination, and endurance.

Muscle reeducation, which begins as passive exercise with the range-of-motion exercises, encourages the patient to move the affected limbs. When there is a return to voluntary function, muscle activities involving the arms, hands, and legs are begun.

The exercise program also includes activities to enable the patient to perform essential functions of getting out of bed, dressing, and using crutches, canes, and wheelchairs or walkers. The therapist also provides the necessary training in moving about and walking.

The person who has had a stroke needs to relearn how to button a shirt, zip a zipper, tie a shoe. Many of these so-called simple tasks can present formidable stumbling blocks. Self-help is a major step on the road to recovery.

Throughout therapy each person is treated as an individual with all exercises programmed to overcome his or her particular disabilities.

OCCUPATIONAL THERAPIST

It is the occupational therapist who analyzes and endeavors to remove any obstacles that develop and that might become a deterrent to the patient's progress. The techniques used are designed to enable the patient to successfully manage and overcome these difficulties and thus be able to take full advantage of the benefits of the rehabilitation program.

For example, handling clay may be one way of strengthening weakened finger muscles. And working with crafts is an excellent way to relieve boredom when forced idleness must be endured.

The occupational therapist is also involved in assessing the patient's range-of-motion and sensory deficits, the ability to perform motor tasks and to follow simple directions, and the range of his attention span and recall.

Occupational therapy usually begins after the patient has learned to become somewhat independent through physical therapy exercises. In some instances it is the occupational therapist who teaches the techniques of self-care, such as using one hand to perform functions normally done by two, and the use of devices and equipment that assist in self-care. The occupational therapist is involved in determining the advisability of making any environmental changes or changes in the overall rehabilitative program to further assist the patient.

When maximum improvement has been attained through the various methods of therapy and the patient still has only partial function in those areas of the body damaged by the stroke, he is then taught how to use these partially functioning parts of his body to the utmost and to further compensate by using other parts of his body that are unaffected to do some of the necessary tasks.

The occupational therapist provides assistance and advice on recreational methods and facilities. The therapist also provides instruction to the hemiplegic housewife so that she can resume her household activities after leaving the hospital.

SPEECH THERAPIST

The speech therapist deals with problems in communication. It is she who suggests various methods of language stimulation to the family in order that they may continue the work begun by her during speech therapy.

The need for speech therapy is determined by the effect that the aphasia has had on the patient's progress in overcoming his handicaps.

THE FAMILY

The last but by no means least member of the rehabilitation team is the patient's family. In fact, the family is considered to be the most supportive resource the patient has.

The family has the greatest motivation in getting the patient to function once again. As active participants in the rehabilitative process, family members are part of all conferences dealing with the patient's progress and thus are better able to cope with any problem that might arise. They know and understand the patient's limitations and are better able to decide as a family whether they feel capable of taking care of the patient at home or whether for a time he could have better care in a facility designed to give the type of care required.

Each family must conscientiously examine its own feelings to determine just how much anxiety or even resentment there is that a stoke has incapacitated one of its members. The family may find that they are actually facing what to them are intolerable physical and financial burdens. They may have ambivalent hopes about the patient's recovery. Talking these feelings over with a physician is a necessary step toward achieving what is best for the patient and what is best for the family unit.

REHABILITATION METHODS AND TECHNIQUES
IN APHASIA

SPEECH THERAPY

Although the results from speech therapy vary depending on the severity of the aphasia, if therapy is started early enough and continued long enough, the benefits that accrue are well worth the time and effort expended. The more severe the aphasia, the less chance there is of recovering normal speech. Total loss of speech, an inability to identify objects, or an inability to write words that are dictated are symptoms, which if they persist for several weeks do not present a very hopeful outlook for full speech recovery.

In the process of evaluating the degree of aphasia present in the person's language impairment, communication skills still available to him are tested by the therapist, making use of several testing procedures such as the Language Modalistic Test for Aphasia, the Minnesota Test for Differential Diagnosis of Aphasia, the Neurosensory Center Comprehensive Examination for Aphasia, and the Porch Test for Communicative Ability. The results of these tests guide the speech therapist in instituting a program of speech therapy based on specific needs and designed to bring about a return to normal speech function as soon as possible.

Several types of speech therapy are currently in use. In the stimulation approach, the therapist selects material that is both interesting and relevant in an effort to stimulate the patient's motivation to learn to speak again. Both auditory and visual means are used. Words can be spelled out aloud, reading can be done together. The therapist endeavors to get the patient to assemble his thoughts into complete phrases and sentences rather than expressing his thoughts in single words.

Speech therapy is started as soon as the person shows that he has the capacity to understand and to respond to what is said to him. By waiting until this time, a great deal of the anxiety that would be present if the person were unable to fully comprehend what was happening is eliminated. With no feelings of anxiety, there is a better chance of speech recovery. On the other hand, if speech therapy were to be delayed for an extended period, such as a year, the chances of its being successful would be significantly reduced.

The speech therapy program must of necessity be tailored to

the individual's needs and rate of response. Initially the sessions are conducted once or twice a day for a period of from 15 minutes to an hour, but never any longer so as to avoid fatigue.

Family encouragement is an integral part of the speech therapy program. The person who has aphasia needs understanding and encouragement. In the last analysis it is the individual's own motivation and drive to be able to speak again that helps bring about his speech recovery. The rate of speech recovery is faster for those who have had an ischemic stroke than it is for those who have had a cerebral hemorrhage.

The person with aphasia has periods when his energy fluctuates from high to low. His motivation is closely tied to these periods. It is not very profitable to try to work with a person who is fatigued. It is far better to wait for those times when his energy is high, when he will then be more alert and vigorous. The time spent on speech therapy then will have far more satisfactory results.

IN DYSARTHRIA

Because dysarthria is an imperfect articulation of speech that is characterized by weakness and slowness in speech caused by the incoordination of the muscles that produce speech, the treatment consists of teaching the person to make the most efficient use of remaining motor skills, thus compensating for those that have been lost.

The speech therapist endeavors to build on the person's memory of pre-stroke speech patterns. The patient is taught how to adjust his rate of speech so that the paralyzed muscles are able to produce difficult sounds as accurately as possible.

Purposeful articulation is taught by encouraging a slow, deliberate speech with every syllable in a word enunciated. This aids the articulatory muscles to maintain the correct position.

Key words are emphasized to help with the understanding process. By exaggerating the consonants, intelligibility can be improved.

SPEECH APRAXIA

Apraxia is the loss of a previously acquired ability to perform an intricate, skilled act—in this case, speaking. Apraxia is considered by some to be a form of aphasia that can be recognized by a dysarthric type of speech. It occurs when there has been a lesion in the left hemisphere of the brain. Other authorities consider it to be an independent condition that exists in conjunction with aphasia.

With this type of speech disorder, the person is not capable of programming speech movement nor is he able to maintain speech in a proper sequence. He knows what he wants to say but is unable to get his speech muscles into the correct position to say it. Many times the initial sound of the word cannot be pronounced.

In aphasia the difficulty is in processing the words to be spoken, whereas in apraxia the difficulty is in programming what is desired to be spoken.

THERAPY FOR SPEECH APRAXIA

Therapy for speech apraxia is designed to reestablish the lost motor patterns of speech by demonstrating the required phonetic placements of the word, which the person then tries to initiate. Progress can be made much more rapidly by practicing in front of a mirror. Visual, touching, and muscular sensory aids are all used by the therapist and are invaluable tools.

The therapist begins the program with getting the person to utter isolated sounds, then to progress to uttering syllables, then words, and finally groups of words that begin and end with the same sound. The next step is teaching how to shift from one sound to another.

RECOVERY FROM APHASIA

Predictions as to how much improvement can be expected in the person's speech or how long it will take for improvement to take place are not possible to make with any degree of accuracy. The greatest, most obvious progress is made during the first year of therapy. Some patients regain almost completely normal speech, whereas others will have far less satisfactory rates of progress. Even though there appears to be no outstanding improvement, there is always some improvement being made during therapy, however small it may seem.

The active assistance of the members of the person's family is of the utmost importance to the success of speech therapy. It is they who must provide the encouragement and support when the therapist is not there. It is they who have to continue the work the therapist has begun.

The person who has aphasia has a handicap that is almost impossible for those who can speak with ease to fully understand. He feels truly isolated because he has no way of communicating his feelings, of joining in the give and take of life. To become once again a fully functioning member of society he must learn to overcome his language problems. This is why he needs all the support he can possibly receive from everyone with whom he comes in contact.

PHYSICAL THERAPY

Leg weakness accompanied by foot drop and a turning in of the ankle often presents problems for those with hemiplegia. With foot drop there can be difficulty in going up steps and a tendency to trip. When the ankle turns inward, it then becomes unstable and can easily become injured.

Straps can be looped around the toe of the shoe and fastened to the upper part of the calf so as to elevate the toe. A wire foot drop brace can also be used. A short leg brace can be fitted, along with a pair of sturdy shoes. The brace enables the person to avoid touching the floor during the swing phase of walking and will also ensure that he puts his weight on the affected leg when he is standing.

GAIT TRAINING

When there has been some return of strength to the muscles, gait training can commence. Gait training involves learning how to step over thresholds or inclines, to climb stairs, to rise from a chair, to pick up objects from the floor, and finally to get outdoors. Of itself, gait training is an excellent exercise for the legs.

Once a person who has been unable to walk learns to walk again he not only gains more independence but his sense of optimism increases. At first he needs some mechanical aids such as a hemi-walker (a four-legged aluminum walkerette), a quadriped cane (a cane with four tips), a unilateral forearm crutch, and then a regular cane. All these aids should be adjusted for the correct height and should be equipped with rubber tips or suction cups. The person is taught how to get himself up off the floor should he fall and how to use a cane or crutch to get around. Having mastered these techniques, he can safely be left alone and not require constant attention.

WALKING

When the patient first begins to walk, the affected or paralyzed side of the body should be toward a wall. This gives the person a greater sense of security, particularly if he has a visual deficit, such as one-sided vision. Sturdy, broad-heeled shoes (not slippers) should be worn. Rubber soles on the shoes provide a greater sense of security. Learning how to shift the body's weight from one leg to another is an important part of learning balance. By leaning toward the affected side of the body, it is easier for the patient to maintain this sense of balance.

The person who has had only a moderate degree of paralysis and who has regained good-to-moderate recovery of motor function may be able to learn to walk with only a modest amount of assistance and with no special equipment. The person who has had a more severe form of paralysis may first have to be taught to walk between two parallel bars. He is taught how to lean slightly forward by pulling himself forward along the bars with his unaffected hand. He is then taught how to move his legs as he makes his way along between the bars.

Some people have an inclination to bend their knee and also to bend their foot backward during the so-called "swing phase" of walking instead of swinging the leg out with the knee extended and the toes scraping the floor. The proper gait must be observed so that walking can become automatic. It should not take longer than three to four weeks to perfect this technique. When a good gait pattern has been established, the person is then ready to begin walking outside the parallel bars with the use of a cane.

WALKING WITH A CANE

The cane should always be held on the side of the body opposite the affected leg to achieve both balance and weight bearing.

A broad based or quadriped can provides greater stability than a cane with a single, thin base. After the person has learned to walk safely with the specialized cane, he can then switch to a regular cane.

A heavy wooden cane with a good, thick handle is preferable to a lightweight aluminum one, mainly because the aluminum cane does not provide an adequate reception for the nerve impluses that travel from the floor to the hand. The height of the cane from the floor to the person's hand should be such as to allow the elbow to be slightly bent. The cane should always be placed on the floor in front of the stronger, unaffected foot and slightly to the side of the body. The person then steps ahead by putting the weak foot out in front All the weight is then on the weak leg and on the cane as he steps ahead with the unaffected foot.

Another way of walking with a cane entails placing the cane and both feet side by side in a line. Then the person steps ahead with both the cane and the weak foot at the same time. The weight of the body is then on both the weak leg and the cane as the person steps ahead with the strong, unaffected foot. The weak foot must never be permitted to get ahead of the cane. The foot and the cane should always be in line. As these steps are repeated slowly and consciously, the person gains in confidence and gets around with increasing ease.

USING A WIDE-BASED QUADRIPED CANE The wide-based quadriped cane should always be placed a few inches ahead of the strong, unaffected foot. The weak foot is then brought forward and placed opposite the cane. The weight of the body is then shifted to the weak leg, and then the cane is placed a few steps forward and the person steps ahead with his strong, unaffected foot. When using a cane, short steps are much easier to handle than are long ones, and the steps should be kept uniform in length.

GOING UPSTAIRS WITH A CANE The person who has made a good recovery of both strength and balance on the affected side of the body is now ready to learn how to climb a flight of stairs. Climbing stairs is done it by putting first one foot on a step and then bringing the other one up beside it on the same step.

The cane can be hung from a shirt pocket or from an opening above the chest line at the front of the clothing so that it does not impede the climbing. The unaffected hand then grasps the railing or banister and the strong, unaffected foot is placed on the first step. With the strong hand still grasping the railing or banister and using the strong leg that is already on the step for support, the person then leans forward and straightens out his strong knee. The weak foot is then placed beside the strong foot on the same step. It is important to place the feet carefully on each step and to be certain that the affected knee is straight whenever the weight of the body is on it. In climbing stairs, the strong, unaffected foot is always placed on the step first to be followed by the weak foot placed on the same step.

GOING DOWNSTAIRS WITH A CANE When the patient goes downstairs, he grasps the handrailing or banister with the strong, unaffected hand. The toes of the strong foot should overlap the edge of the stair before any attempt is made to start down.

The weak, affected foot always goes first. It is put on the step below, and the knee of the strong, unaffected leg is bent as the weak foot goes down onto the step. The weak foot is then placed firmly on the step. The knee must be straight so that this leg can support the weight of the body. Then the strong, unaffected foot is brought down onto the same step alongside the weak foot.

STEPPING UP ONTO A CURB

The strong unaffected foot is placed on the curb. The weight of the body is then shifted to the strong, unaffected leg. The weak foot is placed on the curb beside the strong foot together with the cane.

STEPPING OFF OF A CURB

The cane should first be placed on the street below and slightly away from the curb. The toes of the strong foot should overlap the curb. The weak foot is then put down from the curb to the street. The strong knee is bent while the weak foot goes down to the street. When the weak leg is stable enough to support the weight of the body, the strong foot can then be brought down from the curb onto the street.

WALKING WITH CRUTCHES

There are several gaits used in walking with crutches. Among them are the following.

When *the four point gait* is used, only one crutch or foot moves at a time. When the left crutch is moved forward, the right foot is then moved forward. The right crutch is moved forward followed by the left foot.

When using the *alternate two-point gait* method, the right

crutch and the left foot move together. Then the left crutch and the right foot move together.

The *weight-bearing three-point gait* puts the least amount of weight possible on the affected leg because both the crutches and the affected leg can be moved forward together. Then by putting the weight of the body on the crutches, the unaffected or good foot can be brought forward.

The *nonweight-bearing three-point gait* keeps the affected foot off of the floor. Both crutches are placed ahead and then leaned on, while both the legs are swung through the crutches.

When the *swing-to gait* is used, the crutches should be placed 8 to 10 inches in front of the body. Then the legs can be swung to a point just behind the crutches.

In the *swing-through gait* maneuver, the crutches should be placed 8 to 10 inches in front of the feet. The muscles of the arm and shoulder are used to swing the body through the crutches. The feet are then brought down 8 to 10 inches in front of the crutches. Then the movement is repeated.

GOING FROM A CHAIR TO STANDING WITH CRUTCHES

The crutches should be hooked onto the back of the chair while the person is sitting. When he goes to rise from the chair, the good, unaffected leg should be slid backward slightly under the seat of the chair. The person then pushes his arms down against the armrests of the chair and bends his body slightly forward as he places weight on his good leg. Holding onto the arm of the chair with the right hand, he pivots the body around until he faces the chair. While he bends over and simulataneously braces himself, he can pick up the crutches with his free hand. Both crutches are then placed under the arm on the affected side of the body. Then one of the crutches can be shifted to the other arm.

GOING UPSTAIRS WITH CRUTCHES

Both crutches should be tucked underneath the stronger arm. The handrail or banister is used to support the weight of the body on the affected side. Leaning slightly forward, the person swings the good leg up one step. He lifts the body weight by straightening the hip and the knee of the unaffected leg just as is done when climbing stairs in the normal manner.

GOING DOWNSTAIRS WITH CRUTCHES

Both of the crutches should be placed on the unaffected side of the body while the hand on the opposite side of the body is placed on the railing or banister.

The person then stands on his good, unaffected leg, leaving the affected leg on the step above. He bends slightly forward and moves the crutches down one step. While the crutches support the weight of the body on the unaffected or good side of the body and the handrail or banister supports the affected side, the unaffected leg can be swung down to the next step. The head and shoulders should be kept back and upright to prevent any pitching forward.

As a precaution against accidents all throw rugs should either be removed or else fastened to the floor. Toys or other small objects that could get in the way of the person with crutches and throw him off balance should be kept in some place other than where he will be walking.

CONTINUING TRAINING IN WALKING

Training in walking can be continued at home using heavy chairs as a substitute for the parallel bars. Training should be done twice a day, even if only for a few minutes each time. Sometimes the use of an aluminum pickup walker is recommended for a time for the person able to use both arms, but dependence on the walker should be discouraged lest it retard the person's independence.

When a good walking pattern has been achieved on level ground, there can be a graduation to climbing and descending stairs, ramps, and curbs. If the person has a good sense of balance and sufficient strength, he can be taught to climb and descend stairs using alternate stairs—the step-over-step routine that is normally used. If he has had a more severe form of paralysis, he should be encouraged to proceed just one step at a time. As a matter of safety, handrails should be placed on both sides of the staircase.

During the course of learning to walk again and until a level of proficiency has been achieved that makes it safe to let the patient try walking alone, a strap or belt can be fastened to the person's waist. Then whoever is assisting, can grasp this belt and help the patient to regain his balance instead of grabbing his arm or encircling his waist and, in effect, half-carrying him along.

HELPING THE FAMILY TO COPE

If the person who as had a stroke is unable to care for himself, it must be decided whether he will be cared for at home or in a nursing facility. The answer largely depends on the family and whether they have the means of providing what may be very demanding care. In some instances, there is no choice because financial resources are such that nursing facilities are beyond the family's means. Home care does necessitate that there be someone in the home who is physically and emotionally able to care for the patient. And home care necessitates that arrangements be made for transporting the patient back to the hospital or rehabilitation center for further therapy and evaluation.

In home care the family must guard against the harm that can come when the well-meaning family becomes overzealous in their concern, which might actually prevent the person from trying to help himself and in so doing cause him to be more incapacitated than he would otherwise be.

NURSING HOMES

Several kinds of nursing homes provide various levels of care. In the majority of cases any rehabilitation therapy that is provided does not help the patient to progress much beyond a low level of functioning.

SKILLED NURSING FACILITIES

A skilled nursing facility provides continuous nursing care and a limited amount of rehabilitation. Some assistance is given in feeding and self-care. Medications are administered and diets are followed as prescribed. When there is little hope of any further recovery of function, but the person can get along with a minimum amount of assistance, this type of facility is excellent.

INTERMEDIATE CARE FACILITIES

Intermediate care facilities generally provide protective care without skilled nursing on an around-the-clock basis. For the person who needs only minimal medical or nursing care, this type of facility is suitable.

HALFWAY HOUSE

Some halfway houses are actually boarding homes whose facilities have been adapted for dealing with the handicapped. This type of facility is often ideal for the elderly person who cannot live alone and for whom a nursing home is not necessary.

CHRONIC CARE INSTITUTIONS

A very small percentage of patients, because of the severity of their neurological deficits, are not able to benefit from rehabilitation and cannot be cared for at home. For them the next step after hospitalization may have to be a chronic care institution. These institutions are generally maintained by state or local governments. They provide medical and protective care. For the person who has no other place to go, these institutions provide a much-needed service.

THE PATIENT AT HOME

Experience in many rehabilitation centers has shown that it is possible for as many as 80 per cent of those persons who have had a stroke to return to their homes and to function adequately. The person should continue to perform range-of-motion exercises daily. The diet furnished by the hospital dietitian should be adhered to faithfully. Once the regularly supervised therapy has been concluded, the family should encourage and assist the person in joining community-sponsored programs designed to aid those who have had a stroke.

In some areas of the country Stroke Clubs have been formed for both the patients and the members of their families. These clubs usually meet once a month, and the members discuss various aspects of rehabilitation. There are often guest lecturers who discuss various forms of therapy, as well as social functions and trips to interesting places. These gatherings help to alleviate the sense of isolation that most stroke patients have.

Having had a stroke does not necessarily mean that sexual capacity has been affected. Many stroke victims believe this to be true, which contributes to the development of deep-seated depression. The rehabilitation centers as well as the family physician can offer practical advice so that this facet of living is not denied to the person who as had a stroke.

CHAPTER FOURTEEN

SOME SELF HELP AIDS

DRESSING

In an endeavor to encourage increasing independence, the people taking care of a person who has had a stroke should encourage him to dress himself. Some patients prefer to dress while sitting on the edge of the bed, while others prefer the greater security of sitting in an armchair.

PUTTING ON A SHIRT OR BLOUSE The shirt or blouse should be laid across the lap with the collar away from the body. The weak hand is placed in the armhole by the strong hand, which is also used to pull the sleeve up over the weak arm. It is always easier if the weak arm is put into the sleeve first. The rest of the shirt or blouse is then thrown back behind the body, and the sleeve on the weak arm is then pulled up all the way by the strong hand. Using the strong hand, the person then reaches behind and places the strong arm in the armhole of the sleeve. The rest of the sleeve can then be worked into place until it covers the arm. Shirts and blouses for stroke victims should have larger-than-normal buttons to make for ease in fastening.

A coat or dress is put on the same way as a shirt or blouse except that the person must stand up with or without support in order to straighten out the skirt part of the dress or coat.

TAKING OFF A SHIRT OR BLOUSE When taking off a shirt or blouse, the person again either sits on the edge of the bed or in a chair and with the strong hand pushes the shirt or blouse off the shoulder on his weak side. With his strong hand, he then grasps the middle of the front edge of the shirt or blouse and pulls it out to the side. He can then pull it off his strong shoulder, and work the strong arm out of the sleeve. Then with his strong hand he can grasp the right cuff of the sleeve and pull it off the arm.

PUTTING ON TROUSERS OR SLACKS It is easier to put on trousers or slacks if the weak leg is put into the pants leg first. While sitting on the edge of the bed or in a chair, the person lifts the weak leg by the strong hand and places it across the strong leg. If this is not possible, the weak leg can be placed on a stool. Using the strong hand, the patient pulls up the pants leg over the weak foot. The weak leg is then taken off the strong leg, and the strong foot is then placed in the pants leg. The pants are then pulled up as far as possible. The person then stands with or without assistance and pulls the pants all the way up with the strong hand.

TAKING OFF TROUSERS OR SLACKS While the patient is standing, he pulls down the pants on both sides using the strong hand. Then while sitting on the edge of the bed or in a chair, he can push the pants leg off the strong leg by the strong hand. He then lifts the weak leg across the strong leg by the strong hand and pulls the pants off the leg.

PUTTING ON SOCKS Using the strong hand, the patient lifts the weak leg and crosses it over the strong leg so that the weak foot is hanging out over the strong leg. In this way it can be more easily reached by the strong hand. Using the strong hand, the person holds the sock over the toes of the weak foot and pulls it up over the foot. The weak leg is then uncrossed and the weak foot placed on the floor. The strong leg is then crossed over the weak leg. Using the strong hand, the person puts the sock on that foot in the same manner as it was put on the weak foot.

PUTTING ON SHOES Oxford-type shoes with elastic strings or with buckles are easy to put on and are much sturdier than are slippers or loafers. The tongue of the shoe should be sewn to the top of the shoe at one side in order to prevent it from doubling under while the shoe is being put on.

Using the strong hand, the person crosses the weak leg over the strong one so that he can more easily reach the weak foot. The shoe is then slipped on the foot as far as possible. Sometimes a shoe horn is helpful in getting the shoe up over the heel. If the shoe does not go all the way up over the heel, the weak foot can be placed on the floor and the person can then push down on his knee to work his foot into the shoe.

The other shoe can then be placed on the floor by the strong hand, and the strong foot can then be slipped into the shoe. Here, too, a shoe horn may be helpful in preventing the heel of the shoe from rolling inward. Long-handled shoe horns are available that are attached to a loop of cord. The strong hand can be put through this loop for a firmer grasp and better leverage.

EATING A number of aids are available to make eating easier for the stroke patient. Among these is a special knife known as a rocker knife, which enables the food to be cut with one hand. A food-guard fastener on the plate helps to keep the food from falling off the plate. Rubber suction cups can be used to keep dishes and glasses steady.

TELEPHONING Telephone companies have a shoulder-rest attachment for the telephone that can be permanently attached. The attachment allows the person both to hear and to talk without having to hold the phone in the hand.

The Speakerphone is another device that has proven to be most helpful. It has a microphone that amplifies the voice of the person talking and a loudspeaker that amplifies the voice of the person at the other end of the telephone. The handset never has to be removed from its place on the phone. All that is necessary is to push the "ON" button to answer the phone and the "OFF" button to end the conversation.

CHAPTER FIFTEEN

FAMOUS PERSONS WHO HAVE HAD STROKES

A stroke is no respecter of a person's station in life. Nor are its effects any different. Many notables have overcome their disabilities and have continued to lead useful and productive lives. Several of this group are discussed in the following paragraphs.

SIR WINSTON CHURCHILL

Churchill's health was always of great concern both to himself and to his physician. And well it should have been, for he had a predilection for attacks of pneumonia. Added to this was his inheritance of the curse of the Marlboroughs—deep, deep depression, which he called the "black dog."

In 1941, just after Pearl Harbor while Churchill was visiting President Franklin Delano Roosevelt in the White House, he experienced a dull pain over his heart while trying to open a window that required considerable force to pry up. His doctor, Lord Charles Moran, believed that Churchill had had a possible coronary, his first heart attack. Because he was at that time 67 years old, atherosclerosis undoubtedly had been a contributing factor.

Yet after this episode Churchill remained as the war-time prime minister and guided England and the Allies to victory. He also produced some notable oil paintings and wrote the first two volumes of his memorable history of World War II, *The Gathering Storm.*

This coronary episode led to Churchill's stroke. The first stroke he experienced occurred in 1949 when he was 74 and out of office as Britain's prime minister. It happened while he was playing cards during a vacation in Monte Carlo. He was quite unsteady when he got up from the card table and complained of a severe cramp-like sensation in his right arm and leg. The next morning he was unable to write. It was determined that a small clot had blocked one of the smaller arteries in his brain. Churchill recovered sufficiently well from this stroke to paint still more landscapes and to write Volume III, *The Grand Alliance.* In 1950 after another moderate disturbance to his cerebral circulation, he wrote Volume IV, *The Hinge of Fate,* and Volume V, *The Closing of the Ring.*

The second stroke occurred in July 1952, followed in June 1953 by a third stroke. At the time of the third stroke Churchill was attending a state dinner and was unable to rise from his chair. This time the stroke left him unable to walk, yet he did retain some use of his arms and legs. His mouth sagged noticeably, and he experienced difficulties with his speech. His physician felt that this time along with a sluggish cerebral circulation Churchill had also experienced a spasm of one of the small arteries in his brain. He became paralyzed for a time.

Several days later he complained that his hands were clumsy—the classic clumsy-hand syndrome. He was unable to put his ever-present cigar in his mouth, which for him was a disaster. There was a developing loss of power in his left hand that had not been present when the stroke had occurred three days before. He also had attacks of giddiness. The diagnosis this time was a cerebral thrombosis whose effects were spreading and affecting other parts of his brain. However, once again he recovered, resumed painting, and wrote the final volume of the series, Volume VI, *Triumph and Tragedy.*

After resigning the office of prime minister in April 1955, Churchill experienced episodes of further loss of memory and became notably fatigued. But, after all, he was at this time 81. In July 1956 he had yet another stroke. His collateral circulation was so extraordinary that after this stroke he actually could do more than had been possible for quite some time.

In April 1959 more wandering clots (emboli) brought on some speech difficulties. At this time a neurologist examined him and determined that a small artery had once again become blocked and had cut off the circulation to the speech control center of Churchill's brain.

Sir Winston's health continued to deteriorate until the end came in January 1965 when a final stroke felled this once-great man in his ninety-first year. Sir Winston fought the effects of his strokes as he fought the war—with everything he had. He never gave up but continued to live a full and active life long after most men have retired.

Not all strokes have such happy endings as these related on the previous pages. Some result in a lifetime of agony for the victim and for his family. Such was the case with those persons discussed in the following paragraphs.

JOSEPH P. KENNEDY, SR.

In 1961 a stroke left Joseph P. Kennedy almost completely incapacitated for the remaining eight years of his life. While playing golf at Palm Beach, he remarked to his niece who was playing with him that he really did not feel too well. He blamed this on having a cold. On the sixteenth tee he sat down on the grass, saying that he now felt really quite ill. His caddy quickly rounded up a golf cart and took the former ambassador to his car. With his niece doing the driving, he arrived home within minutes. He told his daughter-in-law Jacqueline that he would go upstairs to rest and insisted that she not phone for a doctor.

Fortunately, the family seeing how ashen his face was ignored his order and phoned his physician, who immediately ordered him to be taken by ambulance to the hospital. Several times in the preceding months Kennedy had had warnings of an impending stroke, and his physician had prescribed an anticoagulant for him, which he stubbornly refused to take.

At the hospital it was determined that he had had an intracranial thrombosis—that is, a blood clot in an artery within the brain itself. The presence of a clot in the left cerebral hemisphere (i.e., the left side of the brain) was disclosed by X-rays and an angiogram. This was the dominant side for the right-handed Kennedy. The condition was declared to be inoperable because of the location of the clot. His entire right side was paralyzed, and he was unable to speak.

At New York's Institute of Physical Medicine and Rehabilitation, Kennedy received intensive therapy as a patient of Dr. Howard A. Rusk, but he made little progress. From a dominant, domineering, energetic, and vital man he was now and would continue to be until his death a frustrated cripple.

DWIGHT DAVID EISENHOWER

Most people remember that Eisenhower had a heart attack while he was president, but few know that he also had a stroke during his term of office. One cold, windy November day in 1956 he drove to Washington's National Airport to greet Mohammed V, the King of Morocco. Upon returning to the White House, he complained of feeling chilled but nonetheless went on with his usual activities. Then he had lunch and his usual post-lunch nap. It was when he returned to the Oval Office that he experienced a sensation of sudden dizziness. He was unable to hold his pen nor could he pick up a piece of paper that had fallen to the floor. He could not speak a coherent sentence. For a time this man was almost helpless. His basically good constitution helped him to recover fully from what his physician described as a slight stroke or spasm in the brain, probably caused by atherosclerosis.

FRANKLIN DELANO ROOSEVELT

In 1944 Roosevelt was examined by a Navy cardiologist who diagnosed his patient as suffering from hypertension, hypertensive heart disease, cardiac failure in the left ventricle of the heart, and bronchitis. At that time, Roosevelt's activities were curtailed, rest periods were instituted, and a low-fat diet was ordered. Ten hours of sleep a night were also deemed to be necessary, as was the avoidance of irritation and tension. In the office of the presidency the latter was, of course, impossible.

In April 1945, while on his annual spring vacation at Warm Springs, Georgia, Roosevelt's physician noted that his blood pressure tended to fluctuate widely from 170/88 mm Hg to 240/130 mm Hg. While simultaneously signing some state documents and posing for a portrait, the president complained of an excruciating headache and a stiff neck. His left hand, which was pressing against his forehead, dropped limply to his side. He tried to raise his hand again, this time to press the back of his neck. He was pale, his skin was clammy, and he was perspiring profusely. His breathing was stenorous. His blood pressure rose at an alarming rate. His next words were his last, "I have a terrific headache." His arm dropped, his head fell to his chest, and he slumped over in his chair. The cause of death was a massive cerebral hemorrhage.

If the drugs in use today to treat hypertension and to dilate arteries had been available in 1945, the course of history might have been profoundly changed.

DR. PAUL DUDLEY WHITE

Dr. Paul Dudley White, who achieved international status as a pioneer in cardiology and became recognized as the father of modern cardiology, was the most respected and revered of physicians. He treated the great and the humble throughout the world. It was he who once said that no one under 80 years of age should ever experience either a heart attack or a stroke.

His writings were voluminous, contributing so much in the way of information to physician and layman alike. He wrote *Heart Disease* in 1931 which for many years was considered the bible of cardiology, as well as many other books dealing with electrocardiology, rehabilitation, and the diagnosis and treatment of heart disease. His autobiography *My Life and Medicine* was completed two years before his death in 1971. His articles and monographs on cardiac subjects number well over 600.

He was truly a Renaissance man—a man for all seasons. As a young doctor at the Massachusetts General Hospital, he eagerly accepted an invitation to study the electrocardiograph in man and experimental animals (dog and cat) with the renowned Dr. Thomas Lewis at the University College Hospital Medical School in London. It was Dr. White who brought back the first ECG machine into the United States.

Throughout Dr. White's long life, he traveled widely and was at home in any part of the world. Many were the stories he could tell of his experiences. Always closely involved with the American Heart Association, which he and several of his close associates had founded, he was a founder along with Dr. Louis Katz, of the International Cardiology Federation, headquartered in Geneva. To Dr. White, medicine knew no geographical boundaries. His awards and honors received from every country in the world would fill several pages in this book.

Although a fragile-looking man who liked to describe himself as a "bag of bones," he enjoyed remarkably good health throughout his long life. Scarlet fever and diphtheria in childhood, twice yearly bouts with a virus, a leg broken while playing softball, an ankle sprained while skiing, pneumonia while in the nation's capital, an attack of *herpes zoster* (shingles), a minor heart attack at Christmas in 1970, and a slight amount of angina (chest pain) in the last few years of his life comprise his entire medical history up to his eighty-seventh year, when he experienced several strokes. The only medication he ever took was a vitamin mixture for malnutrition.

Dr. White's interest in medicine prompted him to start collecting rare medical books dating back to ancient Greece and Rome. This became recognized as one of the finest collections and upon his death was given to the Countway Medical Library of Harvard Medical School. He traveled widely and took as much to the countries he visited in goodwill and knowledge as he ever received.

Dr. White's first stroke was a minor one, occurring in May 1973. Although hospitalized at the time, he recovered quickly and once again began seeing patients several days a week at his Boston office. The following August he had what his physician thought was another stroke but which Dr. White vehemently insisted was not.

Dr. White was among the first patients to have the benefit of the brain scan, which disclosed the presence of several hematomas (blood clots) on his brain. He believed these resulted from a fall that occurred during one of his daily walks. These clots were removed surgically.

For many years Dr. White was my husband's cardiologist and also had as his patient our beloved little Lhasa Apso dog Mei Ling, whom he treated for congestive heart failure and atrial fibrillation. He always proudly referred to Mei Ling as his only dog patient. Dr. White was convalescing from hematoma surgery at his Belmont home when we all saw him for the last time. We had a lovely visit with both him and his charming and gracious wife on October 12. He talked of their recent trip to China, of how right he had been on his own diagnosis of himself, as confirmed by Dr. Paul D. J. New of the Massachusetts General Hospital, a pioneer in nuclear medicine, and finally on my writing the introductory paragraphs for a collection of his medical articles to be published in book form.

Then he smilingly announced that he had decided it was time for him to write a sequel to *Hearts—Their Long Follow Up,* published by Saunders Company in 1967 in which he had written of the progress of his many patients throughout the years. In this sequel he said he intended at last to tell the story of Mei Ling.

The only noticeable difference in Dr. White's demeanor was his tendency to doze off once in a while. But he was as alert and as outgoing as ever. When it was time to leave, my husband carried Mei Ling out to the car and as I turned from bidding goodbye to Mrs.

White, I saw that Dr. White was holding Mei Ling's face in his hand and looking deeply into her eyes. An awful premonition hit me then and when he bade us goodbye at the car, I walked back with him to the chair where he had been sitting in the sun when we had arrived and once again said goodbye for what turned out to be the last time.

Two days later on October 14, while we were celebrating Mei Ling's thirteenth birthday at a party, Dr. White suffered a massive stoke. Death came two weeks later on All Hallow's Eve in his eighty-seventh year.

Even though this stroke came in his eighties at a time when he felt anyone could reasonably expect to have a stroke, to those of us who knew and loved him, death at any time was too soon. He left us all a legacy in the advice he gave in his books and in his own life, which was spent practicing what he preached.

The people we have been discussing run the gamut from those who survived a stroke to resume normal or near normal lives to those who spent their remaining years as helpless invalids to those who quickly succumbed. If any lesson is to be drawn from their lives, it is that recognition of the risk factors that bring on strokes and knowledge of the steps that can be taken to prevent them should and must become a part of the daily lives of all of us.

INDEX

A

accelerated hypertension, *see* malignant hypertension
acquired hyperlipidemia, *see* secondary hyperlipidemia
acetohexamine (Dymelor), 136
acetone, 125
Achilles' tendon, 126
acquired hyperlipidemia, 107, 108
ACTH, 44
addictive smoker, 157
Addison's disease, 44
adrenal glands, 44, 176, 182, 183
adrenalin, 44, 182
  in Type A persons, 63
adrenal insufficiency, as disorder that mimics stroke, 44
adrenergic blocking agents
  as antihypertensives, 73
  defined, 77–78
agalculia, 212
ages at which strokes occur, 24, 25, 26
agensic aphasia, 211
ageusic aphasia, 211
agglutination, 39
agraphia, 211
airway, 225
alarm reaction, 178
albumen, 102
alcohol, 39, 41, 102
  effect on acidity of urine, 149
alcoholism, detected by test for cholesterol, 102
Aldactone, 75
Aldomet, 77
aldosterone, 53–54
alexia, defined, 211
alkaline phosphatae, 117
alternate two-point gait, 259–260
alveoli, ruptured by smoking, 150
ambulatory training, 235, 236
ambulation, 233–236
American Cancer Society, 145
American Diabetes Association, 126, 134, 138, 139, 140
American Heart Association, 66, 113, 114, 118, 147, 149, 150
American Medical Association, 69, 114, 243
amnesic aphasia, 211
analgesics, during stroke treatment, 228
anastomosis, in treatment of stroke, 237, 241, 242
anastomosis, in treatment for TIA, 41
anemia, as disorder that mimics stroke, 19, 43, 44
  sickle cell, 24
aneroid, 60
aneurysm, 20, 21, 88, 236
  in children, 24
  defined, 18
angina, 117
  from antidiabetic drugs, 137
  as symptom of hypertension, 71
angiography, 40, 92, 96, 191, 192, 238
  for cerebral hemorrhage, 238
  procedure, 201
  risks, 201
angiotension, 78, 79
angiotension adosterone mechanism, 79
angiotensinogen, 170
anniversary syndrome, 184
anosmic aphasia, 211, 212
anticoagulants, 36, 38, 39, 40, 227
antidepressant drugs, as treatment for hypertension, 72
antiedema drugs, 229
antihypertensive drugs, 50, 57, 66
  for elderly, 57
  side effects, 72
antilipemic drugs, 115, 116
antitension, 53
antiplatelet drugs, 36, 38, 39, 40, 41, 96
antismoking pills, 159
antithrombin III, 36
Anturane, 36, 38, 39, 40, 43
anxiety,
  as cause of hypertension, 56, 80
  as result of stroke, 272
aortic arch, 11, 240
aortic arch catheterization technique, 202–203
aphasia, 7, 31 (*see also* loss of speech and difficulty in understanding)
  defined, 33
  detected by ophthalmodynamometry, 195
  anosmic, 211
  motor aphasia, 211
  recovery from, 255–256
  as result of left-brain injury, 205–208
  sensory, 207
  speech therapy, 253–255
  types, 210–212
apoplexy, 3, 18
appetite, 43
apraxia, 254–255
Apresoline, 76
arrhythmia, *see* cardiac arrhythmia
  caused by nicotine intake, 146
  detected by electrocardiography, 200
arterial lumen, 240
arteries
  of the brain, 11–14, 84
  artificial, 241
  basilar, 12, 17
  brachial, 61
  capillaries, 13–14
  carotid, 11, 17, 29, 31, 32, 40, 198, 238
    external, 11, 199
    internal, 11–12, 33, 196, 197, 199
    endarterectomy, 40
  diseased, 18
  eye, 87
  fragile, 18
  middle cerebral, 13, 17, 41
    effects on motor activities, 13
  posterior cerebral, 13, 17
    effects on memory and reading, 13
  superficial temporal, 41, 199, 242
  supraorbital, 199
  vertebral, 12
    basilar artery, 12
    Circle of Willis, 12
    vertebral basilar, 31, 226
arteriograms, 171, 202
arterioles, 76, 84, 147
arteriosclerosis, 15 (*see also* atherosclerosis)
  distinguished from atherosclerosis, 86
artificial arteries, 241
aspirin, 36, 38, 40, 96
asthenia (lack of strength), as symptom of adrenal insufficiency, 44
asthma, from smoking, 144, 150
ataxia, 32
  Broca's aphasia, 210–211, 212
  as result of left-brain injury, 207, 210–211
asymptomatic, in connection with hyperlipidemia, 108
ataxia, 22, 31
atheroma, 239
atheromatous plaque, 239
atherosclerosis, 14, 18, 25, 27, 34, 35, 38, 39, 57, 63, 85, 86–96, 129, 130, 133
  at all ages, 89–90
  causes, 91–92
  in children, 24
  controversy over role of fat, 118–119
  diet and, 109
  as effect of stress, 180
  and environment, 63, 95
  as factor in embolus formation, 38
  incidence in women who smoke, 182
  from taking oral contraceptives, 169–170
  in TIA, 30, 35, 103, 118
  prevention, 93–96
  and race, 89–90, 91, 95
  in relation to diabetes, 129–131
  reversibility, 92–93
  role in strokes, 88–89
  and smoking, 150, 151
  treatment, 96
  in Type A persons, 63
Atromid-S, 96, 116, 117
auditory aphasia, 211
avoidance in reaction to stroke, 223
axon, 7

B

Babinski sign, 21
balance center in cerebellum, 8–9
Banting, Dr. Frederick G., 133, 134, 175
baroceptors, 50, 77
basal ganglion, 238
basilar artery, 12, 17
behavior in left hemiplegic, 217–218
behavior modification, 158
behavior patterns, 62, 63
behavior problems, from aphasia, 210, 215
Benson, Dr. Herbert, 81
Best, Charles H., 11, 133, 134
beta blockers, 77
beta receptors, 77
bicycle ergometer, 71
benzestral (Chemestrogen), 164
Beth Israel Hospital, 81
Biguanide, 136
bile acids, 98
biofeedback
  to combat stress, 185
  for hypertension, 83–84
Biofeedback machine, 83, 84
Biofeedback Research Study, 83
Blacks
  and incidence of atherosclerosis, 89–90
  and incidence of diabetes, 121
  and incidence of hypertension, 65
blindness, as sign of stroke, 8, 13, 31, 34, 39
blindness and diabetes, 131
blood circulation, 10
blood clot, 3, 19, 21, 168, 169
blood gases, 187
blood lipids, *see* lipids
blood pressure
  defined, 47–49
  elevation, 55, 58, 170
  fight-or-flight, 49, 50, 80, 182
  labile, in children, 55
  malignant, 51
  maintaining during stroke treatment, 226–227
  measuring, 59–60
    during biofeedback, 83–84
  methods of reducing, 65–78
  in Type A persons, 63
blood sugar, 126, 128, 130
blood supply to brain, 10
blood tests
  for cholesterol level, 187
  for diabetes, 128–129
  for hemoglobin level, 187
  for hemacrit, 187
  for leukocytes, 187
  for prothrombin time, 187
  for triglycerides, 187
blood types, 169
blood urea nitrogen (BUN), 75
blood vessels, 85
blood viscosity, 36, 41
boils, as symptom of diabetes mellitus, 126
brachial artery, 61, 84
bradycardia, 31
bracing, 235
brain
  cerebellum, 8–9, 19, 29
  cerebrum, 6–8, 29
  left brain injury, 205–216
  right brain injury, 216, 220
  medulla, 9
  membranes, 6
  pons, 9, 238
  regions, 6
  spinal cord, 9, 11
  stem, 9, 19
brain scan, 188–191, 272
  advantages, 190–191
  procedure, 189–190
brain tumors, 23, 43, 122, 198, 236
Broca's aphasia, 210–211 (*see also* ataxia)
Broca, Dr. Paul, 206, 210, 212
bronchitis, from smoking, 150
bruit, 16
  detected by Doppler technique, 198
Buerger's disease, 147
BUN, *see* blood urea nitrogen

C

cadmium, 95
calcium, 75, 95, 117
Canadian Cooperative Study Group, 38
cancer
  in connection with oral contraceptives, 173
  similarity to plaque growth, 88
cane, use of, 257, 258, 259
canned foods, salt content, 65
capillaries, 13, 131
carbohydrates, role in diabetes, 128
carbon dioxide, 42, 43
  decrease in elimination during TM, 82–83
carbon monoxide
  effects-on-smokers, 146, 151, 152, 161
  effects of, in nonsmokers, 161
  increase in intake from filter cigarettes, 156
  role in atherosclerosis, 150–151
  role in heart disease, 145–146
cardiovascular disease, 15
  effect of isometric exercise, 71
  in relation to hypertension, 67
  role in TIA, 35
carbuncles, as symptom of diabetes mellitus, 126
cardiac arrhythmia, 31, 43, 117, 146 (*see also* arrhythmia)
  as disorder that mimics stroke, 41
carotid arteries, 11, 17, 29, 31, 32, 40, 196, 197, 198, 238
carotid endarterectomy, 40
Catapril, 79
Catapres, 77
Castelli, Dr. William P., 102, 106
CAT, *see* computerized axial tomography
cataracts, from diabetes, 131
catheter, urinary, 227
cavernous sinus thrombosis, in women, 173
CBC, *see* complete blood count
Center for Disease Control, 153, 171
central nervous system, 77
cereals, 64, 110
cerebellum, 8, 9, 19, 29, 40
cerebral angiography, 201–203 (*see also* angiography)
  advantages, 203
  risks, 201–202
  technique, 202
cerebral bypass, 238, 240–241
cerebral edema, 22
cerebral embolism, 14, 17–18, 207
cerebral hemorrhage, 14, 18–21, 38, 40, 41, 48, 182, 238, 271
  in atherosclerosis, 89
  as example of hypertensive stroke, 84
  intracerebral, 19–20
  parenchymatous, 20–21
  recovery speed, 254
  subarachnoid, 21
cerebral infarctions, 3, 21, 30, 238
cerebral ischemia, 238
cerebral occlusion, 88
cerebral revascularization, 241
cerebral scintigraphy, 191–192
cerebral thrombosis, 14–17, 19, 207, 226, 268, 269
  arterial, 16
  in atherosclerosis, 88–89
  stenosis, 16
  venous, 166
cerebrospinal fluid, 6, 9, 194
  tests, 188
cerebrovascular accident (CVA), 3
  as result of oral contraceptives, 168–169, 173, 242
cerebrovascular occlusion, 15, 17
cerebrum, 6–8, 19, 29
change in personality and emotions, 34–35
chemical diabetes, 126
  as result of oral contraceptives, 172
chest pain, as sign of stroke, 169
Children's Crusade, 55
chlorpropamine, 136
chlorthiazide, as antihypertensive, 73
chloestyramine (Questran), 116, 117
chlormicrons, 104
cholesterol, 91, 95, 96, 111, 124
  effects of oral contraceptives, 170

  and atherosclerosis, 87, 88, 92, 95
  dangers when elevated, 100
  defined, 98
  elevation
    dangers of, 100
    due to stress, 183
    in women who smoke, 152
  as factor in hyperlipidemia, 113
  functions, 98
  role in hypertension, 66
  in connection with lipoproteins, 104–107
  normal levels, 103
  and smoking, 150
  and stress, 183
  role in strokes, 117–119
  sources, 100–101
  tests for, 102–103, 187
  types, 99–100
Chlormodinone acetate with mestranol, (C-Quens), 165
chronic care instructions, 263
Churchill, Winston, 80, 267–269
chylomicrons, 104
cigarettes, 34, 67, 91, 143–147, 150, 151, 171
Circle of Willis, 12
circulation, 3, 4, 10–11
  in atherosclerosis, 86
  collateral, 10
  in diabetes, 132, 133
claudication, from antidiabetic drugs, 137
clinical diabetes, *see* overt diabetes
Clinitest, 127
clofibrate (Atromid-S)
  for hyperlipidemia, 116
clonic epilepsy, 20
Clonidine, 77
clonic movements, 20
clot (thrombus), 3, 14, 15, 16, 17, 18, 19, 21, 23, 36, 38, 70, 84, 87, 227
  coagulability, affected by oral contraceptives, 167, 168–169
  detection by angiography, 201
  detection by brain scan, 190
  fibroanalysis, affected by oral contraceptives, 169
  from smoking, 148
  removal
    by thromboenarterectomy, 240
    to treat motor aphasia, 207
clumsy hand syndrome, 22, 268
cluster headache, 34
coagulation, 36
Colace, 228
cold pressor test, 94
"cold turkey," 157
collateral circulation, 10, 70, 91, 242
colorimeter, 103
coma, 42, 225
  from juvenile onset diabetes, 125
  treatment for, 225
combination type contraceptive, 165
Committee of the National Institute for Neurological Diseases and Stroke of the National Institutes of Health, 3
communication with stroke victim, 209–220
complete blood count (CBC), 43–44
completed stroke, 204–205
compression, 23
computed tomography (CT), 188, 189
computerized axial tomography (CAT), 188, 189, 192, 202
computerized transaxial tomography (CTT), 188, 189
computerized transverse axial tomography, 189
conduction aphasia, 211–212
confusion, 42
congenital heart disease, 24
congestive heart failure, 46, 130
conjugated estrogens, 164
constipation, 159
  as complication in stroke treatment, 228
  as side effect of adrenergic blocking agent, 78
contractures, 230, 231
contraceptives, *see* oral contraceptives
convulsions, 43
  in aphasia, 210
  as sign of stroke, 5
  after stroke, 228
  as symptom of eclampsia, 59
Corbutamide (BZ 55), 136
coronary, 18, 130
cortex, 7
corticosteroids, to prevent edema, 229
cortisone, 44, 132
Coumadin, *see* coumarin
coumarin, 36, 38
Coxsackie virus, role in diabetes mellitus, 124
C-Quens, 165
craniectomy, 242
crutches, 256, 259–261
crutch smoker, 157
CT, *see* computed tomography
CTT, *see* computerized transaxial tomography
CVA, *see* cerebrovascular accident

D

Dacron, 41
  in artificial arteries, 241
  in cerebral bypass, 240
  in endarterectomy, 239
dairy products, 18, 112
  potassium content, 74
  salt content, 64, 65
DBI, phenformin, 136
DeBakey, Dr. Michael, 88, 241
deafness, 8
Dehydration, as symptom of adrenal insufficiency, 44
Deney-Brown, Dr. Derek E., 29
denial mechanisms, 222–223
Demulen, 165
depression, 222
  due to aphasia, 210, 219
  due to hypertension, 72
  as side effect
    of adrenergic blocking agents, 78
    of The Pill, 16
  as result of smoking, 159
  treatment by MAO inhibitors, 76
Diabenese, 136
diabetes, 120–140
  and aging, 131–132
  and atherosclerosis, 91, 129–131
  as cause of hyperlipidemia, 108
  and diet, 69
  and drugs, 78
  effect of oral contraceptives, 172, 173
  as factor in embolus formation, 38
  and hypertension, 129
  incidence of, 120
  kinds, 122–125
  methods of control, 133–140
  as risk factor, 35
  and smoking, 132–133
  and stress, 132
  symptoms, 125–127
  testing for, 127–129
diabetes insipidus, 122–123
diabetes mellitus, 15, 35, 102, 123–124
  types of, 124–127
diagnostic equipment and procedures, 41, 188–203
diarrhea, as side effect of adrenergic blocking agents, 78
diastolic end point, 195
diastolic pressure, 47–48, 49, 59–60, 68, 73, 82, 170
  in middle age, 57
  on sphygmomanometer, 62
  in young adults, 56
diathermy, 250
diazepan, 228
dicoumarol (Dicumarol), 36
diet
  in atherosclerosis, 89–92
  as factor in hyperlipidemia, 107, 108–110
  as factor in hypertension, 69
  role in stroke treatment, 249–250
  in treatment for diabetes, 138–140
dietition, 249
diethylstilbesterol, 164
difference between heart attack and stroke, 12
difficult breathing, as sign of stroke, 5
Dilantin, 228
diplopia
  defined, 34
  as sign of stroke, 4, 5
  as sign of TIA, 31
dipyridanole, 43
disorders that mimic stroke, 41
displacement, in reaction to stroke, 223
distress, 179, 180
diuretics, 41, 42
  as antihyptensives, 73–74
  effect on blood sugar levels, 132
  types, 74–76
diuril trichlormethiazide, 74
dizziness, 31, 43, 44, 122
  defined, 33
  in elderly, 57–58
DNA, 134, 140
drop attack, 33
Doppler technique, 197, 198–199
  advantages, 199
  procedure, 199
double vision, *see* diplopia
dressing, after stroke, 246–266
driving after TIA, 39
drop attacks, 32, 33
drug
  antidepressant, 72, 76
  antihypertensive, 50, 57, 66, 73
  antihyperlipidemic, 115, 116, 117
  antidiabetic, 135–138
  atherosclerosis, 96
d-thyroxine, 96, 116, 117
Dymelor, 136
dynamic rapid serial scintigraphy, 191
Dyrenium, 75
dysarthria
  from left-brain injury, 208–210
  therapy for, 254

E

eating, after stroke, 266
ECG, *see* electrocardiography
echoencephalography, 197, 198
eclampsia, 59
ECV, *see* extracellular fluid volume
Edecrin, 75
edema
  cerebral, 22, 228–229
  in hyponatremia, 42
  from malignant hypertension, 85
  as symptom of preclampsia, 59
EEG, *see* electroencephalogram
eggs, 115
  salt content, 64
Eisenhower, Dwight D., 80, 270
EKG, *see* electrocardiography
elastic stockings, 227
EMI, 189
electrocardiogram, 58, 71, 74, 148
electrocardiography (ECG or EKG), 199–200
  advantages, 200–201
  procedures, 200
electroencephalogram (EEG), 192–193
  advantages, 193–194
  procedures, 193
electrolytes, 117, 225, 226
electrolytic unbalance, as disorder that mimics stroke, 41
electrophoresis, 104
embolic infarction, as complication in stroke treatment, 227
embolism, 29, 38, 168, 205
  as cause of motor aphasia, 207
  as cause of TIA, 30
  defined, 17
  pulmonary, 22, 168, 227
emotional factors in hypertension, 49
emotional factors in rehabilitation, 245
emotional instability from atherosclerosis, 89
emotional stress, 180
emphysema, from smoking, 144, 150
encephalitis, 15, 24
encephalopathy, 85
Enduron, 74
endarterectomy, 40, 238, 239
endocrinology, 175
enemas, 228
Enovid, 165
environmental influence on cardiovasculare diseases, 94–95
environment and blood pressure, 51
environmental stress, 179, 180
enzymes, 78, 123
epilepsy, 193
  defined, 20
  as disorder that mimics stroke, 41
epinephrine, 73, 77, 146
eruptive xanthoma, 108
essential hyperlipidemia, *see* primary hyperlipidemia
essential hypertension, 51–52, 54, 170
estradial, 165
estrogen, 96, 164
  balance with progesterone, 166
  role in menstruation, 162–163
Eutonyl, 76
evolving (progressing) stroke, 4
exercise, 185
  balancing, 235, 250
  passive, 230
  range of motion, 231, 232, 250
  isometric, 71
  isotonic, 71
  as treatment for hypertension, 67 69–71
  for Type A persons, 63
excessive crying, as result of brain damage, 220
extracellular fluid volume (ECV), 66

F

facial thermography, 196
  advantages, 197
  technique, 197
fainting tendency symptom (*see also* syncope)
  of adrenal insufficiency, 44
  of anemia, 43
familial hyperlipidemia, *see* primary hyperlipidemia
fat
  in blood, 88
  effects of oral contraceptives, 170
  and hypertension, 66
  as normal part of diet, 114
  role in diabetes mellitus, 123–124
  role in juvenile onset diabetes, 125
  types, 99, 100, 101, 113
fatigue
  accompanying hemiplegia, 222
  as side effect of The Pill, 166
  as symptom
    of anemia, 43
    of diabetes, 126
    of hypertension, 72
fatty acids, 116
fear, after stroke, 222
Federal Health Agency in West Berlin, 51
femoral arteries, 92
fibrillation, 31
  from nicotine intake, 146
fibrin, 39
  in plaque, 87
fight-or-flight, 49–50, 80
  in reaction to stress, 178, 182
filter cigarettes, 155, 156
fish
  salt content, 65
  in treatment of hyperlipidemia, 111, 112, 114
flashing lights, as sign of stroke, 169
flatulence, as symptom of hyperventilation, 43
Fleet's solution, 228
fluent aphasia, 212
fluids, 225, 226
fluroscopy, 202
FDA, 136
foods
  rich in potassium, 41, 74
  high in salt, 65
  low in salt, 66
  low in cholesterol, 110
  high in cholesterol, 111
  low in triglycerides, 111, 112
  high in triglycerides, 112
Ford, Gerald R., 70
formalin, 176
four-point gait, 259
Framingham Heart Study Group, 27, 46, 67, 103, 105, 106, 107, 118, 120, 130, 148, 149
frontal-lobes, 6
frozen shoulder, 231
fruits, 64, 110, 112
  potassium content, 42, 74
  salt content, 66
furosemide, 75
functional position, 229

G

gait training, 256–257
gall bladder disease, 69
ganglionic blockers, 77
GAS, *see* General Adaptative Syndrome
gastrointestinal disorders, as side effect of diet, 116
gelatin, in treatment of hyperlipidemia, 110
General Adaptative Syndrome, 178, 184
generalization, 214
Georgia Heart Association, 55
gerontologists, 179
glaucoma, 126
global aphasia, 212
Globin, insulin, 134
glucose, 10, 24, 102, 123–125, 128, 187
  in diabetics' blood, 127–128
  effect of diuretics on, 74
  regulated by insulin, 123–124
glucose tolerance level
  abnormal results for women on oral contraceptives, 172
  as test for diabetes mellitus, 126, 128
glycerine suppositories, 228
glycerol, 102
glycogen, 124, 146
glycosuria, 127
gout, 75
grafts, 140, 239
  in cerebral bypass, 240
  as treatment for TIA, 40–41

grand mal, 20, 194
guanethedine, 77

H

habitual smoker, 157
halfway house, 263
handling smoke, 157
hard water, 95
HDL, *see* high density lipids
headaches, 20, 34, 47, 75, 76, 122, 195
as anemia symptom, 43, 210
as disorder that mimics stroke, 41
cluster, 34
migraine, 33, 42
as side effect
of The Pill, 166, 173
of vasodilating agents, 76
as sign of impending stroke, 5, 169, 173
as symptom of TIA, 31
after stroke, 228
"The Health Consequences of Smoking," 161
Heart attack, *see* myocardial infarction
heart disease, 24, 117
hematoma, 23, 34, 43, 238
defined, 23
hematocrit, 43
hemianopia, 230
hemiparesis, 10, 19, 32
hemiplagia, 20, 21, 22, 229
catastrophic, 205
detected by ophthalmodynanometer, 195
left, 216–221
right, 18, 19, 20, 21, 24, 48, 84, 85, 153, 168, 182, 190, 194, 205–215, 238, 271
hemaglobin, 43, 44, 187
heparin, 36
heredity, as factor in hyperlipidemia, 107
as a factor in stress, 178
high blood calcium, *see* hypercalcemia
high density lipids (HDL), 103, 105–107, 117
effects of oral contraceptives, 170
lowering level by smoking, 150
role in diabetes, 131
high density lipoproteins (HDL), *see* high density lipids
high uric acid level, *see* hyperuricemia
Hippocrates, 3, 67, 121, 206
hormones, 44, 163–164, 166, 172, 175–176, 182–184
Hounsfield, Godfrey N., 189
Hydergine, 229
Hydralazine, 76
hydrogenation, 99
Hydromax, 74
hydrometer, 122
Hygrotin, 74
hypercalcemia, 75
hypercholesterolemia, 107, 112
as TIA risk factor, 35
hyperlipidemia, 15, 102, 103, 140, 227
causes, 107
defined, 107
diet as treatment, 107, 108–115, 118
and HDL, 105
incidence among diabetics, 140
kinds of, 107–108
as risk factor, 35
symptoms of, 108
treatment by drugs, 115–117
Types I through IV, 108
hyperlipoproteinemia, 107
as factor in embolus formation, 38
Hyperstat, 76
hypertension, 15, 18, 20, 22, 27, 45–87
and atherosclerosis, 91
characteristic personality, 62–63
caused by nicotine intake, 146, 149
juvenile, 24, 54–56
elderly, 49, 57
middle age, 57
brain, 46, 84–86
heart, 46
kidneys, 46
effects of oral contraceptives, 58, 149, 169, 170, 173
effects of stress, 180
as factor in hyperlipidemia, 110
incidences of, 45
kinds of, 51–54,85
labile, 45
malignant, 51
methods of treatment, 64–87
in middle age, 57
personality characteristics, 62, 63
renovascular, 53, 54
in relation to diabetes, 129
as risk factor, 35
role of environment, 51
role of stress, 49–50
in women, 58–59, 68, 169
in women who smoke, 152
in young adults, 25, 56–57
hypertensive stroke, 84
hypertriglycemia, 107, 112, 116
hyperventilation,
as disorder that mimics stroke, 42–43
in electroencephalogram, 193
hyperuricemia, 30, 75, 227
hypnosis, to quit smoking, 160
hypnotic drugs, used in electroencephalogram, 193
hypoglycemia, 10, 78
as cause of stroke, 24
and diet, 69
as disorder that mimics stroke, 41
detected by glucose tolerance test, 129
from too much insulin, 135
as symptom of hyperventilation, 43
hypokalemia, 41, 75
hypolipidemia, 102
hyponatremia, as disorder that mimics stroke, 42
hypotension, 31, 42, 44, 76, 84, 95
in elderly, 58
postural, as disorder that mimics stroke, 41
from alcohol consumption, 39
as symptom of adrenal insufficiency, 44
hypothalmus, 122
hypothyroidism, 91, 102, 108
in connection with atherosclerosis, 91
hypoxic, 225
hysteria, 20

I

impairment of memory, 89
incoordination, as sign of dysarthria, 268
Inderal, 77, 78
IND, *see* Investigative New Drug
Infarction, 3, 15, 21, 22, 130, 190, 238
defined, 15–16, 21
lacunar, 21
myocardial, 22 (*see also* myocardial infarction)
pulmonary, 22, 227
inner ear, 9
Institute of Physical Medicine and Rehabilitation in New York, 245, 269
insular (Island of Reil), 7
insulin, 133–135, 138, 139
role in diabetes mellitus, 123, 124, 126, 131
role in juvenile onset diabetes, 125
intermediate care facilities, 262
International Atherosclerosis Project, 150
International Atomic Energy Agency, 95
International Cardiology Foundation, 271
International Institute of Stress, 174
Intoxication, as disorder that mimics stroke, 41
intracerebral hemorrhage, 3, 19, 20, 190
intracranial hemorrhage, 3, 24
intracranial pressure, 85
intraocular pressure, measured by ODM, 195
Investigative New Drug, 137
irritability
as earmark of stress, 151
as symptom of hypertension, 72
ischemia, 3, 16, 29, 236
detection by electrocardiography 199
as result of vasospasm, 85
speed of recovery, 254
islets of Langerhans, role in diabetes mellitus, 123, 124, 134, 135, 139
Ismelin, 77
isometric exercise, 71
isotonic exercise, 71
itching, as symptom of diabetes mellitus, 126

J

jaundice, as side effect of Corbutamide, 136
juices
potassium content, 74
salt content, 66
in treatment of hyperlipidemia, 110, 112
junk foods, 112
sale content, 65
juvenile onset diabetes, 124–125, 134

K

K-Ciel, 41
Kempner rice diet, 72
Kennedy, John F., 44, 80
Kennedy, Joseph P., Sr., 269–270
kidney function, 44
kidney, role in stress, 176
kidney disease, *see* renal disease
K-Lyte, 41
Kopel, Dr. Steven, 158, 159

L

labile hypertension, 45, 55
Laboutatieres, 135
laboratory tests for stroke, 41, 187–188
lactic acid, 136
lactic acidosis, as side effect of Biguanide, 136
lactose, 127
lacunas, 22
Laënner, René, 61
language, distinguished from speech, 32, 208
language center in brain, 7
Language Modalistic Test for Aphasia, 253
Laragh, Dr. John, 170
Lasix, 75
latent diabetes, *see* chemical diabetes
LDL, *see* low density lipoproteins
lecithin, 97
left brain injury, *see* right hemiplegia
left hemiplegia, 216–221
leg pains, as sign of stroke, 169
Lente, 134
lesions, 23, 89
access by microsurgery, 237
as cause of change in behavior, 218
as cause of dysarthria, 208
as cause of fluent aphasia, 212
brain, 21, 22, 40
detection
by angiography, 201
by brain scan, 190
by cerebral scintigraphy, 191
by skull X-ray, 192
formed by carbon monoxide, 151
removed by microvascular anastomosis, 241
removed by endarterectomy, 239
surgery for, 238
treatment by cerebral bypass, 240
tuberous, 108
ulcerated, 238
xanthoma, 131
lethargy, 42
leukemia, 19
leukocytes, 43–44, 187
Librium, 78
"Licit & Illicit Drugs," 158
light headedness, 33
Link and Campbell, 36–37
lipids, 76, 87, 97, 118
elevation due to stress, 105–107, 180, 182
chloromicrons, 104
high density lipids, 103
low density lipids, 104, 105
very low density lipids, 104
role in atherosclerosis, 92
plasma lipids, 109
lipoproteins, 98
broken down by clofibrate, 116
types, 104–107
"little stroke," *see* transient ischemic attack
liver
affected by oral contraceptives, 172, 173
and bile acids, 98
and cholesterol, 100
disease, 102
metabolizer of estrogen, 164
role in chemical diabetes, 172
role in stress, 176
and triglycerides, 101
lobelin, 159
lobes of brain, 6–8
loop diuretics, 74, 75
loop of Henle, 75
Lopressor, 78
loss of appetite, as stress symptom, 175
loss of speech and difficulty in understanding, 33–34
as sign of stroke, 5
loss or dimness of vision, 34
as sign of stroke, 169
low blood pressure, *see* hypotension
low blood sugar, *see* hypoglycemia
low density lipoproteins (LDL), 104, 107, 116, 117
role in diabetes, 131
low-fat diet
as factor in hyperlipidemia, 109
role in reversing atherosclerosis, 92
low potassium, *see* hypokalemia
LP, *see* lumbar puncture
lumbar puncture,
after effects, 195
procedure, 194
lymph nodes, role in stress reaction, 176

M

MacLeod, Professor J. J. R., 133, 134
Macronar, 167
Maharishi Mahesh Yogi, 81
mainstream smoke, 161
major stroke, 4
malignant hypertension, 51, 52, 170
as result of vasospasm, 85
Mallenkrodt, Inc., test kit for triglycerides, 103
magnesium, 95
manganese, role in vascular disease, 95
Mannitol, 229
manometer, 60
MAO, *see* monoamine oxidase inhibitors
massage, 250
maturity onset diabetes, 124, 134
maximal stroke, 4
Mayer, Dr. Jean, 114
Mayo Clinic, 147
Meat
salt content, 64, 65
in treatment of hyperlipidemia, 110, 111, 112, 115
medical treatment for stroke, 224–236
meditation, to fight stress, 185
meditative response, 80–83, 185
medulla, 9
membranes of brain, 6
meningitis, 15, 194
menopause, 166
and hypertension, 58, 59
menstruation, 162, 163, 165
mental activities in the cerebrum, 8
mental confusion, as sign of stroke, 5
Meprobamate, 9
Meprone, 164
Metaprolol (Lopressor), 78
methyeldopa, 77
Metropol, 79
microsurgery, 237, 238
microvascular anastomosis, 237, 241–242
microvascular bypass, 238
midbrain (mesencephalon), 9
middle cerebral artery, 13, 41
migraine, 33, 41, 173
milk, *see* dairy products
minipill, 167
Minipress, 76
Minnesota Test for Differential Diagnosis of Aphasia, 253
minor stroke, 4
Minoxidel, 76
monoamine oxidase (MAO) inhibitors, 76–77
mononucleosis, in connection with oral contraceptives, 173
monounsaturated fats, 99–100
motor activities in cerebrum, 8
motor aphasia, *see* ataxia, Broca's aphasia
Multiple Risk Factor Intervention Trial Program for the Prevention of Heart Disease, 158
multiple sclerosis, 22–24
muscle coordination, 8–9
muscle weakness, 44
myocardial infarction, 14, 22, 47, 53, 78
from antidiabetic drugs, 137
compared to stroke, 14
detection
by brain scan, 190
by ECG, 200–201
from diabetes, 125, 129, 130
effects of oral contraceptives, 153, 166, 171, 173
from juvenile onset diabetes, 125
in Type A persons, 63
from withdrawal from adrenergic blocking agents, 78

N

National Commission on Diabetes, 120
National Heart, Lung and Blood Institute, 55, 66, 102
National Institutes of Health (NIH), 137
natural estrogen, 164
Natural Protamine Hagedon Insulin, (NPH), 124

85%

nausea
as side effect
of adrenergic blocking agent, 78
of thiazide diuretics, 75
as sign of stroke, 5
as stress symptom, 175
negative effect smoker, 157
nervousness, as symptom
of adrenal insufficiency, 44
of hypertension, 46
of stress, 151
neurological deficit, 15, 20, 30
Neurosurgery Center Communicative Ability, 253
Neurosurgery Center Comprehensive Examination for Aphasia, 253
neutral fats, *see* triglycerides
new learning, 213–214
New, Dr. Paul F. J., 272
niacin, *see* nicotenic acid
nickel, role in vascular disease, 95
nicotiana, *see* tobacco
nicotine, role in heart disease, 145–149, 152
nicotinic acid (niacin), 96, 116–117
Nitroprusside-D, 76
nominal aphasia, *see* anosmic aphasia
noncatheter, retrograde arterial technique, 203
noncholesterol sterols, 114
nonfluent aphasia, 212
nonketatic maturity onset diabetes, 137
nonweight-bearing three-point gait, 260
norepinephrine, 76, 77
normotensive person, 66, 68
NPH, 134
nuclear medicine, 188
numbness,
as sign of stroke, 5, 8
as sign of TIA, 31, 32, 33, 43
nursing facilities, 262
nursing homes, 262
nurses, 249
nuts
potassium content, 74
in treatment of hyperlipidemia, 111, 112

O

obesity
and atherosclerosis, 91
and hypertension, 67–69, 115
role in diabetes, 132
occipital lobes, 7
occlusion, 15, 18, 196
in atherosclerosis, 88–89
detection by Doppler technique, 199
need for surgery, 40
of verterbrobasilar artery in women, 166
occupational therapist, 251–252
ODM, *see* ophthalmodynamometry
old learning vs new learning, 213
one-sided neglect, 215
ophthalmodynamometry (ODM), 195
advantages, 196
procedure, 195–196
ophthalmologist, 18
ophthalmoscope, 87
Oracon, 165
oral antidiabetic drugs, 135–138
oral contraceptives, 25, 35, 38, 162–173
and atherosclerosis, 169–170
considerations for use, 173
and diabetics, 172
effects on parts of body, 167–168, 172–173
and hypertension, 58, 59, 170, 171
and myocardial infarction, 171
and smoking, 152–153, 171–172
types, 165–168
use of pills, 167
and venous thrombosis, 168–169
oral pharyngeal tube, 225
Orinase, *see* Tolbutamide
Ortho-Novum SQ, 165
orthostatic hypotension, 41, 58
Osler, 109
ovaries
affected by oral contraceptives, 172
in stress experiments, 176
overt diabetes, 127
Ovral, 165
oxygen, 10
in blood, 14
in brain, 14, 43, 89, 148, 226
decrease during TM, 81, 82
to eyes, 131

P

pain, as stress symptom, 44, 175, 228
palpitation, as side effect of vasodilating agent, 76
pancreas, 123–125, 131, 135, 140
pancreatitis, 102
Papaverine, 76
papilledema, a symptom of hypertension, 52
parallel bars, 236, 257
paralysis
as a sign of stroke, 5, 20, 22
left-sided, 216–222
right-sided, 205–216
as result of clogged artery, 89
paraphasia, 212
parenchymal hematoma, 238
parenchymatous hemorrhage, 20–21
pargyline, 76
parietal-lobes, 7
Parkinson's disease, 22
role in diabetes, 122
paroxysmal, 34
partial thromboplastin time (PTT) test, 37
patch graph, 239
pectin, 113
pentaquine, 72
perceptual deficits, 216
periarteritis nodosa, 10, 19
PeriColace, 228
peripheral dilators, as antihypertensives, 73
peripheral vascular disease, 126
Persantine, 39
personality of stroke victims, 25
PET, *see* positron emission tomography
petit mal, 20, 194
pH (acidity), 42–43
phenobarbitol, 228
Phenformin (DBI), 136
pheochromocytoma,
as cause of renovascular hypertension, 54
test for, 188
phlebography, 202
phonation, 208
phospholipid, 97, 105
physical stress, 180
physical therapist, 250–251
physical therapy, 256–261
The Pill, *see* oral contraceptives
pitressin tannate, use against diabetes insipidus, 122–123
pituitary, 122, 132, 172
pituitary gland, effects of oral contraceptives, 172
pituitary extract, 122–123
plasma cholesterol, 100, 104
plaque, 17, 21, 30, 38, 40, 46, 85, 88, 89, 91, 98, 102, 130, 151, 183
detection by Doppler technique, 199
platelets, 40
contribution to thrombosis, 96
effect of oral contraceptive, 169
pneumonia, as complication in treatment for stroke, 227
polycythemia, 15, 19, 31
polydipsia, 122, 126
polyphagia, as symptom of diabetes mellitus, 126
polyunsaturated fats
factor in hyperlipidemia, 113
role in diabetes treatment, 138
polyuria, as symptom of diabetes mellitus, 122, 126
pons, 9, 238
poor appetite, as symptom of anemia, 43
positron emission tomography (PET), 191
posterior cerebral artery, 12
post ganglionic blockers, 177
positive effect smoker, 157
postural hypotension, *see* orthostatic hypotension
postural (orthostatic) hypotension
in elderly, 57–58
as disorder that mimics stroke, 41
potassium, 41
eliminated by diuretics, 73–74
hypokalemia, 75
potassium-sparing diuretics, 74, 75
potassium determination test, 75
Practolol, 78
pre-diabetes, 126
preeclampsia, as symptom of hypertension, 59
pregnancy
and diabetes, 132
and hypertension, 59
and smoking, 152
and stress, 166
pressure, 177
pressure sores, 230
prevention of strokes, 26, 27
primary hyperlipidemia, 107
primary hypertension, *see* essential hypertension
primary physician, 248
PRIND, *see* prolonged reversible ischemic neurological deficit
Profile, 12, 102, 114
progesterone
balance with estrogen, 166
role in birth control, 162–163
role in menstruation, 162
progressing stroke, 4
projection, as reaction to stroke, 223
prolonged reversible ischemic neurological deficit (PRIND), 29
promesthestral (Meprone), 164
propranalol hydrochloride, 78
prosody, 208
protein, 105
Protein Zinc Insulin, (PZI), 134
proteinuria, as symptom of preeclampsia, 59
prothrombin time tests, 37, 187
in treatment of hyperlipidemia, 117
"pro time" tests, *see* prothrombin time test
pseudo bulbar palsy, 22
P/S ratio, 113
psychological reaction to stroke, 221
psychometrics, 207
psychomotor seizures, 194
psychotherapeutic drugs, as treatment of hypertension, 72
psychotherapy, for hypertension, 72
pseudo bulbar palsy, 22
PTT test, *see* partial thromboplastin time test
Puerto Rican Family Planning Center, 162
pulmonary embolism, 22, 168, 227
pure motor hemiplegia, 4, 22
pure sensory stroke, 4
putamen, 19
PZI insulin, 134

Q

QRS complex, 199–200
quadriped cane, 256, 258
quantitative urine determination test, 127
Questran, 116, 117
quitting smoking, 156–160

R

radioactive isotopes
in cerebral scintigraphy, 191, 192
in positron emission tomography, 191–192
rash, as side effect,
of adrenergic blocking agent, 78
of Corbutamide, 136
rationalization, in reaction to stroke, 223
rauwolfia serpetina, *see* reserpine
rectal temperature, decrease during TM, 83
red blood cells, 19, 43, 44, 146
redness of skin, after stroke, 229
regions of brain, 6
regression, reaction to stroke, 223
regular insulin (RI), 134
rehabilitation, 204, 243–263
with cane, 256–259
with crutches, 259–260
dietitian, 249
emotional factors, 245
facilities, 247–248
goals, 246–247
in-home care, 263
methods and techniques, 253–261
nurses, 249
physical therapy, 256–261
primary physician, 248
role of family, 252, 255, 262–263
self-help, 264–265
social worker, 249
therapists, 250–252
relaxation response, to fight stress, 81, 185
renal disease, 52, 53, 91, 125
in children, 54
in elderly, 58
in women, 58
renal glycosuria, 127
renin, 53, 170
renovascular hypertension, 53–54
reserpine
asadrenergic blocking agent, 77
as antihypertensive, 73
rest and relaxation, as treatment for hypertension, 80
to relieve stress, 185
retinopathy
diabetic, 131, 168
as symptom of malignant hypertension, 52
revascularization, 241
reversible ischemic neurological deficit (RIND), 29
RI, *see* regular insulin
right-brain injury, *see* left hemiplegia
RIND, *see* reversible ischemic neurological deficit
risk factors, 26, 119
need for control, 227
Rock, Dr. John, 162, 167
Rogers, Jacquelyn and Dr. Jan, 159–160
Roosevelt, Franklin Delano, 270, 271
Royal Victorian Hospital (Belfast), 130–131
Rusk, Dr. Howard A., 2, 243, 244, 269
rutin, as antihypertensive, 72

S

saturated fats, 99
as factor in hyperlipidemia, 113
salt, effect on blood pressure, 42, 63–66, 74
scintigraphy, 191
seasonings, salt content, 65
secondary (acquired) hyperlipidemia, 107, 108
secondary hypertension, *see* malignant hypertension
seizures, 20
from aphasia, 210
detected by electroencephalogram, 192–194
after stroke, 228
Selacryn, 75
self help aids, 264–266
Selye, Dr. Hans, 174–178, 179
senescence, 131
senility, 89
sensory activities, 8
septicemia, 24
Sequential Multiphasic Analysis (SMA), 187
sequential type contraceptive, 165
serial angiography, 92, 96
serum cholesterol, *see* plasma cholesterol
shortness of breath, as sign of stroke, 169
shoulder and forearm exercises, 231–232
side stream smoke, 161
slowness, as sign of dysarthria, 208
slow healing, as symptom of diabetes, 126
SMA, *see* Sequential Multiphasic Analysis
Smithwick, Dr. Reginald, 50, 66
SmokeEnders, 159–160
smoking, 34, 35, 67, 141–161
advantages of not smoking, 154–156
and atherosclerosis, 91
background, 141–144
cause of hypertension in women, 59
diabetes, 132–133
effects
on body, 144–145
on cholesterol, 150
on circulation, 147
on heart, 145–147
on kidneys, 149
on lungs, 150
on nonsmoker, 161
of oral contraceptives, 171–172, 173
as factor in embolus formation, 38
and life expectancy, 153–154
in New World, 141–142
and oral contraceptives, 152–153
quitting, 159–160
in relation to stress, 151–152
types, 157
and women, 152
Smoking and Health: A Report of the Surgeon General, 155, 157–158
snack foods, *see* junk foods
Social Readjustment Scale, 184
social worker, 249
sodium, retention due to sodium chloride, 170
sodium chloride, *see* salt
soft water, 95
spasticity, after stroke, 230
spatial deficits, 216
SPE, *see* sucrose polyester
specific gravity test, 122
speech, distinguished from language, 208
speech apraxia, 254–255
therapy for, 255
speech difficulties in stroke, 4, 206, 208
speech center in cerebrum, 8
speech therapist, 252, 254, 255
sphygmotonometer, 60, 62
spinal cord, 6, 9, 11
spinal tap, *see* lumbar puncture

spironolactone, 75
spleen, role in stress, 176
stable stroke, 4
stage of exhaustion, 178
stage of resistance and adaptation, 178
stenosis, 16, 40, 196
"stepped care" approach to therapy, 73, 77
stethoscopes, 61
Stillman diet, 118
stress, 71, 94, 174–186
affected by smoking, 151–152
body's reaction to, 182–183
and death, 183–184
and diabetes, 132
and hypertension, 49, 50
distinguished from pressure, 177
General Adaptative Syndrome (GAS), 178, 179, 180, 184
coping with, 185
response of men versus women, 181
as risk factor, 181–182
theory, 175–178
types, 179–180
value of recreation, 184–185
stress tests, 71
Stress of Life, The, 174
stroke
ages when occurring, 24–26
from antidiabetic drugs, 137
classifications, 4
causes, 23–24
completed, 204–205
coping with, 221–223
defined, 3
early warning signs, 28
effects
on brain, 3–4
on emotions, 219–220, 245
on generalization capability, 214–215
on judgment, 216–217
on memory, 212–213
on personality, 218–219
on retention span, 213
on speech and language, 205–208
on thinking and perception, 212
on vision, 215
hypertensive, 84
from juvenile onset diabetes, 125
occurrence in elderly, 25–26, 30
personality characteristics of victims, 26
during pregnancy, 166
prevention, 26, 27
preventing recurrence, 236
probable ages, 24–26
psychological reaction, 221
recognition, 5, 28–44
risk factors, 27, 227
in TIA, 35
as side effect of The Pill, 166, 173
and stress, 181, 182
survival, 1–2, 4
treatment of, 224–242
thrombotic stroke, 168
stroke clubs, 263
understanding, 2–3
stroke in evolution, 237–238
stuttering (stammering), 8
subarachnoidal hemorrhage, 21, 194
risk in women who take The Pill and smoke, 153
rupture of aneurysm, 228
subclinical diabetes, *see* suspected diabetes
subdural hematomas, 24
as cause of TIA, 23
as disorder that mimics stroke, 43
submaximal stroke, 4
sucrose polyester, 117
sugar diabetes, *see* diabetes mellitus
Sulfenpyrazone, 38 (*see* Anturane)
sulfonylurea, 135, 136
suppression, in reaction to stroke, 223
Surgeon General's Report on Smoking, 155, 157, 161
surgery
for cerebral hemorrhage, 238
to examine arteries for atherosclerosis, 94
as a last resort, 236–237
for perenchymal hematomas, 238
for subdural or cerebral hematomas, 238
as treatment for TIA, 40
as treatment for stroke, 236–242
types, 238–239
suspected diabetes, 126
swing-through gait, 260
sympathectomy, 50, 66
syncope (sudden fainting), as sign of stroke, 31
systolic end point, 195
systolic pressure, 47, 48, 49, 59–60, [illegible]8, 73, 82, 84, 94, 170
[illegible]dle age, 57
and obesity, 68
on sphygmomanometer, 62
in young adults, 56

T

tachycardia, 31, 71, 76
telephoning, after stroke, 266
temporal-lobes, 7
Testape, 127
thalamus, 19, 21
thermography, 196, 197
therapists, 250–252
thiazide diuretics, 74–76
thromboendarterectomy, 238, 240
thrombophlebitis, 167, 168, 173
thrombosis, 84, 205, 207, 226, 268, 269
deep vein, 168
defined, 14
retinal, 167, 173
thrombotic stroke, 168, 173
thrombus, *see* clot
thymus, role in stress, 176
thyroid, 132
TIA, *see* transient ischemic attack
ticrynofen, 75
tissue cholesterol, *see* cholesterol
TM, *see* transcendental meditation
tobacco, 141, 142
redrying, 144–145
Tolazamide (Tolinase), 136, 137
Tolbutamide (Orinase), 136, 137
toxemia, in connection with hypertension, 59
tracheotomy, 225
tranquilizers, for hypertension, 56, 73, 78, 228
transcendental meditation techniques, 81–83
transient ischemic attack (TIA) (*see also* prolonged reversible ischemic neurological deficit, reversible ischemic neurological deficit)
cause, 31, 46, 85, 96, 195, 196
defined, 16, 28, 29
detection by ophthalmodynamometry, 195
and driving, 39–40
frequency, 29
incidence, 30
significance, 29
symptoms, 31–35
treatment, 35–41
by microvascular anastomosis, 241
treatment of stroke
ambulation, 233–236
ankle exercises, 232
bracing, 235
fingers and thumb exercises, 232
getting into bed, 234
learning to stand, 234–235
leg and knee, 232
lessening disability and deformity, 229–230
limiting brain damage, 226–229
medical problems, 227–228
need for fluids, 225–226
objectives, 224
passive exercises, 230–231
preventing pressure sores and contractures, 230, 233
range-of-motion exercises, 231, 233
surgical methods, 238–242
toes exercise, 232
treadmill testing, 71
triad of effects, 176–177
triamterine, 75
triglycerides, 87, 91, 96, 98, 101–103
effects of oral contraceptives, 170
elevation due to stress, 183
normal level, 103
role in strokes, 117–119
tests for, 102–103, 187
types of, 104–107
tuberous lesion, 108
tumor, *see* hematoma
detection
by angiography, 201
by encephalography, 198
by scan, 191
removal to treat motor aphasia, 207
turbidity, 104
twitching, as symptom of adrenal insufficiency, 44
Type A personality, 62, 215
and atherosclerosis, 91
loss of traits due to right hemiplegia, 215–216
reaction to stress, 181
Type B personality, 63
types of hyperlipidemia, 108

U

ulcers, 42
from smoking, 144, 152
treated by diet, 69
ultramicrovascular bypass, 238, 242
ultrasonography, 197–199
unconsciousness, 43
United States Air Force study on blood pressure, 62–63
on stress, 183
United States Food and Drug Administration, 137, 167
United States Health Service, 81
United States Public Health Service Clearing House for Smoking, 156
University Group Diabetic Program (UGDP), 137
unsaturated fats, 99
urinary tract infections
as complication in treatment of stroke, 227–228
as side effect of The Pill, 166
urates, 75–76
uremia, 227
uric acid, 38, 75
uricosuric diuretics, 75–76
urinary tract infections, 227
urine test, for diabetes, 127–128
urinometer, 122
uterus, role in mentruation, 162

V

vaginal bleeding, as side effect of The Pill, 166, 173
vaginal discharge, as side effect of The Pill, 166, 173
Valium, 78, 228
vanilmandelic acid (VMA) test, 188
vascular disease, 129, 130, 151
vasodilators, 36, 39, 76
vasospasm, 85
vegetables, 64
potassium content, 74
salt content, 66
venography, 202
vertigo, 31–32
defined, 33
as disorder that mimics stroke, 41
very low density lipoproteins (VLDL), 104, 116, 140
increase in diabetic, 140
viscosity, 36, 41
effects of aspirin, 38
vision, 31, 32, 43, 125, 126, 159, 215, 230
Vitamin B, as source of nicotinic acid, 116
Vitamin C, 113
effect on acidity of urine, 149
Vitamin D, 98
Vitamin E, 113
Vitamin K, 36
VLDL, *see very* low density lipoproteins
VMA, *see* vanilmandelic acid test
vomiting, 20, 75
as side effect of adrenergic blocking agent, 78
as sign of stroke, 5

W

walker, 256
walking, 70, 71, 257, 261–262
warfarin, 36
water
hard, 95
soft, 95
intoxication, 42
weakness and numbness, 75
defined, 32–33
as sign of dysarthria, 208
weight-bearing three-point gait, 260
weight gain, as side effect of The Pill, 166
weight loss
as symptom
of adrenal insufficiency, 44
of diabetes insipidus, 122
of diabetes mellitus, 126
of stress, 175
in stroke treatment, 226
weight reduction, as treatment,
for diabetes, 138–140
for hyperlipidemia, 113
for hypertriglyceremia, 115
for hypertension, 67–69
Wernicke, 206
Wernicke's aphasia, 211, 212
White, Dr. Paul Dudley, 55, 70, 86, 93, 154, 271–272
white blood cells, 19, 40, 43, 44, 187
Willis, Thomas, 121, 133
word deafness, *see* auditory aphasia
World Health Organization, 56, 95, 181
wrist exercises, 231

X

xanthomas, 108, 131
X-rays, 42
in aortic arch catheterization, 202
in CAT scanning, 189–190
in cerebral angiography, 201
of skull, 192